T010052b

THE
OPEN
HEART
CLUB

———

ALSO BY GABRIEL BROWNSTEIN

The Curious Case of Benjamin Button, Apt. 3W
The Man from Beyond
The Secret Mind of Bertha Pappenheim: The Woman Who
Invented Freud's Talking Cure

THE
OPEN
HEART
CLUB

---

*A Story About
Birth and Death
and Cardiac Surgery*

GABRIEL
BROWNSTEIN

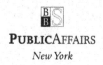

PUBLICAFFAIRS
New York

Copyright © 2019 by Gabriel Brownstein
Cover design by Pete Garceau
Cover images copyright © iStock/Getty Images
Cover copyright © 2024 Hachette Book Group, Inc.

Hachette Book Group supports the right to free expression and the value of copyright. The purpose of copyright is to encourage writers and artists to produce the creative works that enrich our culture.

The scanning, uploading, and distribution of this book without permission is a theft of the author's intellectual property. If you would like permission to use material from the book (other than for review purposes), please contact permissions@hbgusa.com. Thank you for your support of the author's rights.

PublicAffairs
Hachette Book Group
1290 Avenue of the Americas, New York, NY 10104
www.publicaffairsbooks.com
@Public_Affairs

Printed in the United States of America
Originally published in hardcover and ebook by PublicAffairs in October 2019
First trade paperback edition: April 2024

Published by PublicAffairs, an imprint of Hachette Book Group, Inc. The PublicAffairs name and logo is a trademark of the Hachette Book Group.

The Hachette Speakers Bureau provides a wide range of authors for speaking events. To find out more, go to hachettespeakersbureau.com or email HachetteSpeakers@hbgusa.com.

PublicAffairs books may be purchased in bulk for business, educational, or promotional use. For more information, please contact your local bookseller or the Hachette Book Group Special Markets Department at special.markets@hbgusa.com.

The publisher is not responsible for websites (or their content) that are not owned by the publisher.

Print book interior design by Jeff Williams.

Library of Congress Control Number: 2019026725

ISBNs: 9781610399494 (hardcover), 9781610399470 (ebook), 9781610399487 (paperback)

LSC-C

10 9 8 7 6 5 4 3 2 1

For Marcia, Lucy, and Eliza,
and in memory of my father, Shale Brownstein

CONTENTS

PART ONE

——

Near Encounters with the Real

1.

B Y THE TIME his son Danny was born, Ludwig Spandau had lived three lives. He was fifty-three years old, with a young new wife, Sali, and a year-old daughter named Ruthie. He rented a walk-up apartment in Flatbush, Brooklyn, and worked on Long Island as a pharmaceutical chemist. He was a refugee, once divorced and once widowed. He spoke English with a thick German accent. Most of the people he had known had been murdered. On his forearm he had frightening scars where—so his son later suspected—Ludwig had removed his concentration camp tattoo.

Ludwig had been born to well-to-do Berlin Jews. His family had owned a paper business. He had served as a radioman in World War I, in a U-boat. After the war he had attended Humboldt University in Berlin, when Albert Einstein was on the faculty. Ludwig liked to dance. He met a girl named Friedel at a dance hall in Berlin in 1922 and got her pregnant. Their daughter, Inge, was born in 1923, and not long after her birth, the couple came to terms on a divorce. Soon after the divorce from Friedel, Ludwig married again, and his second wife, Lani, converted to Judaism.

They were assimilated, cosmopolitan people, raising two boys. The Nazis came to power, and Lani was murdered by the SS, and Ludwig's father was killed at the concentration camp at Sachsenhausen. Ludwig, strong and able, was kept in Berlin, a slave on a work crew, repairing the city's roads when they were bombed. After the war, he and his two boys—who had been in hiding in

Bavaria—were reunited by the Jewish Agency in London, and all three came to the United States together in 1948.

Ludwig started a business formulating chemicals and trying to sell them. His English was poor. His business failed. He traveled across the country, looking for work. He returned to New York, and at a dance sponsored by a resettlement program, he met Sali. She was in her mid-twenties, almost half Ludwig's age, the child of a refugee family from Hamburg; after years in Palestine, Sali had recently been reunited with her father in New Jersey.

War and calamity had erased whatever traces of religion Ludwig might once have had, but Sali was observant. In their Flatbush apartment, they kept a kosher home. Their building was busy with Yiddish-speaking immigrants, many with concentration camp tattoos. The crowded hallways smelled of onion and roasted garlic.

The Spandau's second child, Daniel, was born in 1954. He would have been the final piece to cement their new American lives, but something was wrong with the baby. Little Danny was sickly and weak. He struggled for breath. He was prone to fainting spells. The more he was able to move around, the more frequently his lips and fingers turned blue.

At the local hospital, little Danny was X-rayed and given an electrocardiogram. Nurses fed the toddler vanilla pudding mixed with crushed radium pills and put him in a fluoroscopy machine: a kind of moving-image X-ray projected onto a screen. Their boy's heart was deformed, the doctors told the parents, a cluster of four specific defects: (1) a hole in the center between the ventricles, the two largest chambers of the heart, (2) a narrowing in the pulmonary valve, the passage between the heart and the lungs, (3) a displacement of the aorta, the big artery that took the blood from the heart to the body, and (4) an enlarged right ventricle, the bottom right chamber. This complex of heart defects was called a tetralogy of Fallot, "tetralogy" for its four elements and "Fallot" for a nineteenth-century French physician, Étienne-Louis Arthur Fallot. Danny's heart was shaped like a boot, and it was incapable of pumping sufficient oxygen to his body. In 1955 in Brooklyn, there was no cure for this condition, no such thing as open-heart surgery.

There was, however, a new kind of procedure that might alleviate his symptoms, one that had been invented a decade earlier. It was an operation not on the heart itself—an operation on the heart was impossible—but on the great arteries right above the heart. The newspapers called it a "blue baby operation." The doctors called it a "Blalock shunt." It had been invented by a remarkable team at Johns Hopkins University in Baltimore. Dr. Helen Taussig, a deaf, dyslexic pediatrician, had conceived of the procedure; Taussig, a rare woman in medicine in the 1940s, had been put in charge of these children doomed to die and figured out how to make their lives better. Vivien Thomas, an African American technician, had designed the tools and developed the surgical technique; Thomas, the only black man to wear a white coat at Hopkins in the Jim Crow South of the 1940s, could not use the main entrance to the building where he worked and was supposed to use only the water fountains and restrooms marked "colored." Dr. Alfred Blalock, for whom the shunt was named, was the white southern surgeon who led the team and performed the first operations under Thomas's careful guidance.

A Blalock shunt, the Brooklyn doctors explained to the Spandaus, would not cure their child. After the operation, Daniel's boot-shaped heart would still have a hole in its center, a blocked passage, and a misplaced aorta, but the shunt would reroute the blood so that more of it went to the lungs. If everything worked out, the blood that fed his body would have a higher oxygen content. The surgery was risky. There was a chance of infection, pneumonia, brain damage, or death. The long-term prospects were uncertain. The first procedures had been done in the mid-1940s, and the oldest surviving patients were mostly in their late teens.

The surgery took place in 1956, when Danny was two years old. The incision began at Danny's left nipple and cut across his side, under his left arm, all the way to his back. The doctors entered the chest cavity between the third and fourth ribs, deflating the lung and sectioning membranes until they had a clear view of the beating heart.

A Blalock shunt (sometimes called a Blalock-Thomas-Taussig shunt) is not an implant but a suture, in medical terms an anastomosis, between the two of the largest blood vessels that run right above the heart. The doctors dug into Danny's chest and located the pulmonary artery, the artery that brings blood to the lungs. They clamped the artery. They had to move fast. The operation had to be done quickly to reduce the chances of damage to the child's brain. A second incision was made in the left subclavian artery, the big artery that fed blood to Danny's left arm. The surgeons sewed the two arteries together so as to divert more blood from the subclavian artery to the lungs. Too large an anastomosis, and too much blood would flow through, overwhelming the lungs and the heart. Too small, and not enough blood would flow through, and the procedure's effect would be negligible. The racing doctors completed their sutures. Quick as they could, they released the clamps. The blood from the subclavian artery joined the blood from Danny's starved pulmonary artery. More blood than ever flowed to the boy's lungs.

When a Blalock procedure is effective, the oxygen-rich blood feeds the body, and the results are visible right away. On the table, the child's skin turns from blue to pink. But that didn't happen to Danny Spandau. He lingered listlessly in the hospital. He came home small and weak and blue. He was two years old and could barely walk.

Back home in Brooklyn, the bloodless, blue-skinned little boy, skinny as a skeleton, cast a shadow across the building of traumatized refugees. Ludwig carried little Danny everywhere. The boy rode on his father's shoulders up to the apartment, and if anyone asked what was wrong, why the father would not let the boy climb the stairs on his own, Ludwig would bark at them in his German-accent English, "None of your business!"

Danny's sister, Ruthie, remembers those years after the first surgery as frightening and sad. The apartment was dark, and the mood was bleak. She thought—as everyone must have thought—that Danny was going to die. Danny thought more about his father.

"I never thought about me," Danny remembers. "I thought about him, and how it made him feel when other people commented. I don't think I ever thought of myself as sick." But he was always terrified of going to the doctor. "I remember the blood drawings. I was all skin and bones and it hurt. They were always doing blood tests and X-rays. All sorts of crowds came to look at me."

He was a curiosity, a learning tool for the doctors and medical students, who could not cure his condition but were nonetheless fascinated by its progression. Every time he was supposed to go to the hospital, little Danny hid. His mother would plead for him to come out. His parents had to hunt for him and drag him from under the couch.

2.

THE SPANDAUS WERE referred to Dr. Aaron Himmelstein, an amiable-looking, bald, round-faced man with glasses, who was beginning to perform experimental open-heart surgery at Babies Hospital, part of the Columbia Presbyterian Hospital in upper Manhattan, about a mile south of the George Washington Bridge and across the street from Harlem's Audubon Ballroom. Dr. Himmelstein accepted Danny as a candidate for open-heart surgery. The boy must have been a desperate case. He was scheduled to be Himmelstein's twelfth tetralogy of Fallot patient. Seven of the previous eleven had died.

Danny was tiny at four years old, fragile and skeletal. His sister Ruthie was his babysitter. Danny remembers the courtyard of the apartment building, where there were concrete walkways separated from grass lawns by low-slung chain barriers. He described for me his immobility: one day, he went for a walk, his sister on one side of him, her friend on the other. Two boys on bicycles came speeding toward them. The girls darted to either side of the path. Both called to little Danny, but he was too slow to join either of them. The bicycles knocked him down.

The odds were not good for his survival. In the late 1950s, birth defects of the heart ranked as one of the top ten causes of death in the United States. In March 25, 1957, *Time* magazine's cover story was "Surgery's New Frontier." It was all about hopeful new break-throughs in heart surgery: "rib-spreaders," "rib-shears," and a heart "red and purple with a greyish cast, glistening under the lights, squirming and rippling." Alarming photographs showed patients plunged into ice water in preparation for surgery. One patient, according to the article, was put into a six-foot-long kitchen freezer until her body temperature dropped to seventy-five degrees. The article mentioned but misspelled Danny's deformity, "the most famed of all congenital defects, Pallet's tetralogy," in which "the blue baby has an amazingly consistent pattern of four anomalies combined." The magazine noted grimly that "the death rate inevitably is high in heroic operations on patients already in poor condition."

The cover illustration showed Dr. Charles Bailey of Hahnemann Hospital in Philadelphia, one of "the most daring innovators in heart surgery," pushing against "the limits set by nature" far beyond anything that had previously been thought possible. In the front-cover portrait, Bailey's comb-over was concealed by his white surgical cap; his shoulders were drawn as broad as Superman's, and even his glasses looked like futuristic armor—a vision of the doctor as warrior, scientist, spaceman, and explorer of the unknown, "mummified," as the article put it, "in sterile gear."

The magazine issue, with its neo-Frankensteinian cover, hung on every newsstand in every train and subway station in New York City. It piled up on tables in doctors' waiting rooms. In breathless prose, it recounted the history of heart surgery. Since 1944, Blalock and Taussig in Baltimore had put over 1,000 shunts into the great arteries above the hearts of blue babies, with an 85 percent long-term survival rate—a rate that could have given no cheer to Ludwig Spandau, as the procedure had not helped his son. In 1948, according to the article, Charles Bailey had performed the first-ever cardiac surgery on a human being by punching through the wall of a beating heart and clearing a clogged valve with his gloved finger. That remarkable feat was only prelude to the era of bypass surgery, when the heart was disconnected from the patient's body and repaired.

Open-heart surgery was a postwar American invention, as miraculous as space travel and as bloody as the Battle of the Bulge. It began with children. The first series of successful surgeries happened in the mid-1950s in Minnesota, and the patients were all kids, blue babies like Danny who had been born with defective hearts. The advances in pediatric cardiac surgery led to operations on adults. In 1954 at the University of Minnesota in Minneapolis, Dr. C. Walt Lillehei had begun performing bypass procedures by laying out two operating tables: one for the patient and one for the patient's parent. Lillehei connected the parent's and child's bloodstreams to each other. The parent's heart filled the child's body with oxygenated blood, while Lillehei cut into his patient's little heart and repaired its deformities, sewing shut holes in the walls between the chambers. The parents risked their lives for their kids. A mother had gone brain-dead. Once, when Lillehei could not get a parent to participate, he had used the lung of a dog to oxygenate his patient's blood.

By 1957, Lillehei's two-patient bypass procedure had given way to use of the heart-lung machine. Three hundred miles south of Minneapolis at the Mayo Clinic, Dr. John Kirklin's heart-lung machine procedures had progressed to the point where the majority of his patients with simple defects survived. In 1957, complex conditions like tetralogy of Fallot were just beyond medicine's reach, but operations with these new machines were now being performed around the country. *Time* magazine described Charles Bailey's heart-lung machine as "an odd-looking device":

On the front edge of its table was an electric motor flanked by pumps. Behind was the oxygenator—an arrangement of plastic cylinders and tubing. "Ready?" asked Bailey. The moment had come to bypass the heart and lungs to give the surgeon a dry field and to let the machine take over. As the first pump was switched on, the surgeons tightened the tourniquets around the great veins so that the blood, shut off from the heart, was forced out of the body along tubes leading to the machine. In the artificial lung, the blood picked up fresh oxygen. As the tourniquet on the subclavian was tightened, the machine forced the blood back into the patient: the major inflow went to the aorta to supply blood to the head, arms, and lower body; a small additional pump sent blood through the small tube into the coronary sinus, from which it nourished the heart muscle by reverse flow into the veins. . . . The patient's lungs went limp; the oxygenator was doing their work, as the pumps were doing that of the heart.

Not long after the magazine came out, the date for Danny Spandau's surgery drew near. In preparation for the operation, Danny had a cardiac catheterization. The inventors of the cardiac catheter were two Columbia doctors, Andre Cournand and Dickinson Richards, and they had won the Nobel Prize for their invention just two years before. Danny was strapped down on the operating table, while the doctors cut a hole in his thigh and guided a wire up inside him. Through the catheter, the doctors released dye into his bloodstream. Neither Danny nor I remember our early catheterizations, but I have spoken to other patients who do, and they recall feeling the dye as it released and how that was painful and terrifying. The masked doctors gathered around Danny's gurney, put on lead vests, and with giant X-ray guns shot images of his chest from two different angles, one from above and one from the side, a dozen X-rays per second, to get a sense of the flows and dynamics of his heart.

Not long after the catheter exam, the hospital called the Spandaus with bad news. Dr. Himmelstein had taken sick. He had brain cancer. He would not be able to operate. The surgery would have to be postponed. The family had to wait another year, with their fainting blue baby at death's door. Columbia was not able to find a replacement heart surgeon. Danny's case was taken over by Himmelstein's young chief resident, Dr. James Malm.

In 1960, six-year-old Danny Spandau was listless and weighed just twenty-seven pounds. When he rested, he tended to draw his legs up against his chest, a squat typical of children with tetralogy of Fallot; it relieves some of the pressure on their chest. The Spandaus met Dr. Malm up in Babies Hospital. He was tall and graceful, precise in his speech, elegant, and well-mannered. His hair was parted neatly. He had high cheekbones. His features were small, feminine, almost Asiatic, and his skin strangely flawless. In blue and red pens, Malm drew careful pictures of Danny's heart and described to the Spandaus the surgery he would perform. He showed the four chambers of the heart, the big ventricles below and the small atria above.

In a normal heart, the blood flowed in through the vena cava, down into the small chamber on the right side, the right atrium. From the right atrium, it descended into the right ventricle, the big powerful pumping chamber that sent the blood up through the pulmonary artery into the lungs. From the lungs, the blood came back into the left atrium, then down into the big left ventricle, which shot the blood out through the aorta to fill the body with life. Danny's heart, Malm explained, had four defects, but Malm focused on two of them. There was a big hole in the ventricular septum, the wall between the two big beating chambers of the heart, so the oxygenated and unoxygenated blood comingled and went out the aorta together. There was also a narrowing, a stenosis, in the valve between the right ventricle and the pulmonary artery—that stenosis limited the amount of blood that could get to Danny's lungs. Malm was going to patch the hole in the middle of the heart, and he was going to widen the gap between the pulmonary artery and the right ventricle.

He called this operation a "complete repair." What the Spandaus did not know in that first meeting was that Jim Malm had never in his life performed open-heart surgery.

3.

HEART DEFECTS ARE the most common of all life-threatening birth defects, affecting 1 in every 110 babies. Roughly one in every three kids born with a heart defect requires surgery, which means (more or less) that there's now a kid with a surgically repaired heart at every school in the affluent world. Pediatric cardiologists and pediatric heart surgeons are good at what they do: these days, in the United States, over 85 percent of kids with deformed hearts survive surgery into adulthood. Still, congenital heart defects remain, of all birth defects, the number one cause of infant death.

Congenital heart disease is among the most common chronic diseases in the United States. People with repaired hearts are living long lives—healthy, give or take, but in need of constant monitoring and attention. You probably have a neighbor, a relative, a friend, or a coworker with a repaired heart defect. Most of us look entirely ordinary, even when we're in deep trouble. We are invisible. Approximately nine in ten Americans with moderate to severe heart defects do not get the lifelong care and monitoring that they need.

Tetralogy of Fallot is the most common complex congenital heart defect. Fifteen years before Jim Malm, all the kids with tetralogy died—most died in infancy, but the healthiest lived crippled lives into their teens. Fifteen years after his breakthrough surgeries, almost all the tetralogy kids in the United States survived surgery, and many of us have thrived—snowboarder Shaun White, a three-time Olympic gold medalist, was born in 1986 with a tetralogy of Fallot.

In 1960, when Danny was rolled into surgery, a good portion of tetralogy patients didn't make it through the operation. Mortality rates varied from hospital to hospital, but they were so bad that Helen Taussig—the most prominent pediatric cardiologist of all—argued that corrective surgery on "tet" patients wasn't worth attempting. At Columbia under Himmelstein, more than half of the patients died.

In 1960, blood could not be stored safely long term. The donors had to be on hand for surgery, so Danny was accompanied by his older brother Stevie, one of the two sons from Ludwig's first marriage—as a child during World War II, Stevie had hidden from Nazis. Now he was a US marine. He came to the hospital with twelve of his Marine Corps buddies, all of them ready to donate blood.

In those days at Columbia Presbyterian, there were no operating rooms specifically designated for cardiac cases. "Every operating room was occupied every day," Malm remembered. "Gall bladders, colon cancer, breast surgery, thyroids." He had to fight for operating room space. "There was no room at the inn. If I increased my volume, then one of the other surgeons couldn't do his thyroid, couldn't do his breast."

Danny was rolled in. The anesthesiologist put a mask over the boy's face and told him to count down from ten. Something extraordinary happened as he passed out. "I'm a scientific guy," Danny told me. "I'm an analytic chemist by training. So I've explained it not as an out-of-body experience, but maybe it was. Who knows? It may have been the reflection in an overhead lamp. All of a sudden I wake up and see the reflections of all the doctors around the table. I see the top of the doctors and me lying on the table. It was so clear. It was literally like being with my back on the ceiling of the OR looking down at the operation. I saw the doctors in all

their scrubs. And I saw myself lying on the table, being worked on."
He felt completely removed from his body, a spirit looking down
at the surgery. "And that's a memory I've had essentially all my life."

Carefully, Malm sectioned the little boy's chest. The heart-lung
machine was of the new disc oxygenator type, a device about
the size of a big fat salami, stored in something the shape of an
industrial-sized sewing machine. It sat on a rolling cabinet, and
from it extended long clear tubes. The machine was primed with
a mixture of blood and blood thinners. One tube's canula was inserted into Danny's aorta, the other into his vena cava above his
right atrium. Danny's blood came into the machine and coursed
over a series of discs. Each bloody disc was perfused with oxygen,
and the oxygen-rich blood was sent back into Danny's circulatory
system. The heart-lung machine regulated the speed of blood flow,
and by slowing down the blood, Malm lowered Danny's body temperature to eighty-two degrees. The induced hypothermia slowed
Danny's metabolism and gave him some protection from damage
that might come from oxygen deprivation during surgery. The
heart was drained entirely.

Malm cut right through the pericardium, the rough sack of
protective tissue that contains the heart. Now he had to attack
the heart muscle itself. Other surgeons had favored a "median," or
horizontal, slice across the right ventricle, but instead of going side
to side, Malm made a "vertical right ventriculotomy incision." He
had devoted himself to study of the heart's electrophysiology—
the system of electrical currents that control the heartbeat—and
this seemed less likely to interfere with the circuitry of the heartbeat. It also gave Malm a better view of the hole in the septum.

The interior of the right ventricle wall is not smooth but, in
doctors' terms, trabeculated, which means it's made of a criss-
cross web of muscle fibers. Even with today's powerful imaging
technology, it can be difficult to locate the boundaries of each
ventricular septal defect. Malm found Danny's by feel. He took
a Teflon patch and stopped the gap in the middle of the heart,
between the muscular wall at the bottom of the ventricles and

the soft tissue at the top. He used mattress sutures to attach the patch, the kind of big, railroad-track loops that are inelegant but extremely secure. Once Malm was sure there was no leak at all, he attacked the stenosis of the pulmonary valve, the blockage on the right side of Danny's heart.

He made a generous hole between the right ventricle and the pulmonary artery, slicing any tissue that was in the way and putting in an outflow patch to smooth the passage of blood toward the lungs. He wanted to get as much blood moving as he could, and he wanted the space wide open. Where a normal heart would have a pulmonary valve, impeding blood flow backward from the lungs, Danny would have an open passageway.

Malm shut the hole in the ventricular septum. He relieved the pulmonary stenosis. He sewed Danny's heart shut, doing as little damage to the muscle as he could, and he stitched up the pericardium. The boy was taken off the heart-lung machine. Blood filled his heart and the chambers began to beat. The boy's temperature returned to normal, and his blood pressure did too. The whole operation had taken about an hour and a half. The crucial thing, according to Malm, was to get the blood flow as near normal as possible. "No leaks!" he barked at me over the phone when I asked him his secret to keeping a child alive.

There was no special recovery room for cardiac patients in 1960. Danny recalls a big room with lots of other kids. He woke up under a clear plastic oxygen tent. For the first two days after surgery, he lived in a high-humidity bubble. His parents hovered close by but could not touch the top of his body. IV tubes replaced his lost blood and body fluids and gave him the necessary sugars and electrolytes. Nurses came by with shots of penicillin and streptomycin and delivered the shots to the muscle of Danny's legs.

"I pinked up right after surgery," Danny told me.

For a time, after the oxygen tent was removed, Danny was confined to a wheelchair. "I remember my hands were so dirty from wheel-chairing, and it was so disgusting that I never sucked my thumb again." After six days, he was allowed to walk. When Danny came home from the hospital, everything had changed. He could climb the stairs to his apartment. He began to put on weight and to grow. The darkness was lifted from the Spandaus' lives. When Danny was strong enough, his brother Stevie took him to a marine ball to celebrate his resuscitation, and Danny was shown off in front of all the young men who'd given their blood to him.

In the late 1950s, a new era had begun, the era of open-heart surgery, and in the early 1960s a new kind of person was invented, a person like Danny Spandau, a person like me, who would live a whole lifetime with a surgically repaired heart.

4.

I WAS BORN WITH tetralogy of Fallot, the same defect as Danny Spandau, but I had the good fortune to be born a decade later, in 1966. My birth defect went unnoticed in the obstetrics ward. My parents thought I was perfectly healthy when they brought me home. My pediatrician, too, missed the squishy sound in my heart on my first visit. In 1966, there weren't the same protocols for checking for heart defects that there are today—no sonograms, no fetal echocardiograms, just diagnosis with a stethoscope. The doctor caught it on my second visit, when I was already a month old, and he sent my parents to a pediatric cardiologist, Dr. Lucy Swift, at St. Luke's Hospital on Manhattan's Upper West Side.

Women doctors were uncommon in 1966, but not in pediatric cardiology. In the study of deformed babies' hearts, women doctors were the rule. Helen Taussig, the Johns Hopkins doctor who had conceived of the Blalock shunt procedure in 1944, had founded the discipline of pediatric cardiology. She was still alive and at work in 1966, and her students, the so-called Knights of Taussig, dominated the field. Women, most of them Taussig's heirs, ran most of the pediatric cardiology programs in the New York region: at Yale, Ruth Whittemore; at New York University, Janet Baldwin; at Columbia, Sylvia P. Griffiths; and at Cornell, Mary Allen Engle.

My mother remembers Dr. Swift as a small, strange, other-worldly, birdlike creature, but also as a woman of considerable will and professional devotion. Dr. Swift examined my fingers and toes. She listened to my heart with a stethoscope and then pressed her fingers to my abdomen and shut her eyes. Because she had been deaf, Helen Taussig had developed techniques for listening to infant hearts with her fingertips, and those techniques had been passed down to some of her heirs. After palpating my abdomen, Dr. Swift had me sent for X-rays.

My parents received the diagnosis, a heart defect, a tetralogy of Fallot, something neither of them had ever heard of. Untreated, I would probably not live past the age of fourteen. But yes, Dr. Swift explained, it could be cured. She gave my parents the name of Dr. James Malm at Babies Hospital up at Columbia Presbyterian, where Dr. Swift had done her residency. Jim Malm was the one man in the world most qualified to cure me.

I recently met a woman who was born in Chicago the same year I was, with the same condition I have, and when her parents first took her to see a doctor, the doctor advised them to give up. The baby would not live. But Lucy Swift knew exactly where to send us. My parents traveled up to 168th Street, just five subway stops from their apartment. This has been the story of my life: an expert clinician, right there every single time I have needed it.

My parents sat in a large, stuffy New York City waiting room, baby me fussing on my mother's lap. Malm met them in his office. In my recent meetings with Malm, I've found him both reserved and very funny. Even in his nineties, he's quick and intimidating and capable of dominating a room. I've interviewed his colleagues and his patients. Everyone I spoke to seemed to view Malm with affectionate awe. Everyone loved him—except my mother. Jim Malm scared her half to death.

"Something about his eyes," she told me.

They were blue, extraordinarily, clearly, high-sky blue. My mom started seeing a therapist. She told the therapist how the surgeon spooked her.

The therapist nodded. "They give up something to be able to do that."

Malm wanted to take a scalpel to the perfect skin of her baby's chest. With a saw, he wanted to cut through her little boy's breastbone. He'd take a stainless steel spreader and pry open her son's ribcage. Wearing sterile rubber gloves, he'd press his fingers against the muscle of his heart, even as it was beating. He would slice the big vessels around the heart and shove plastic tubes into the holes. With those tubes, he would drain the heart of blood and then connect the child to a newfangled machine with a humming motor and a plug that went into the electrical outlet in the operating room wall, and while the lungs deflated, this weird invention of metal discs and rubber tubes and plastic casing would do the work of the heart, while Malm took his scalpel and cut open the heart's chambers. He'd take a piece of Teflon and shove it in there. He would sew Teflon into the heart with a needle and thread. He would dig into the heart, into the pulmonary valve, and he'd cut a piece right out, her baby's heart sectioned with a knife and a piece of it thrown into the garbage.

Malm was a superb clinician. Colleagues have noted that when things got catastrophic in the operating room, he got more focused and calm. He loved his work—that's what he told me when I talked to him, loved every day in the operating room. There was no place he would rather be than masked and scrubbed, putting his clamp and scalpel into the hearts of young children. "I miss it still," he told me. "The old dog wants to be in the operating room." My mom must have recognized this in him—his uncanny cool, his fascination and eagerness—and these qualities unnerved her. She was required to do something out of folktale: to offer up her child to this handsome stranger, who was going to stick a knife into her son's heart.

Everyone reading this book knows someone who's had heart surgery, who's gone under the knife and come out fine. But in 1966, heart surgery was new. When Jim Malm did his residency, there was no such thing as open-heart surgery. In the late 1950s heart bypass surgery, which is to say surgery where the patient's heart is taken out of the circulatory system, was performed only at a few highly specialized hospitals, and all the patients were children. In 1966, my parents had never met anyone who'd had heart surgery or whose baby's heart had been repaired. This was a thing outside the experience of everyone they knew.

My father was a doctor, a psychiatrist, but where he had been in medical school in Buffalo, New York, there had been no open-heart surgery. Someone tried to monkey with it, he told me, but the results had been terrible. He had grown up in a lower-middle-class Jewish enclave in Buffalo, the second child of an insurance salesman, the brightest boy in his school. My mother was the daughter of two Jews from Mielecz, Poland, who spoke Yiddish in their one-bedroom apartment in Queens. She was a Yale PhD in nineteenth-century British literature and an English professor at City College. Her dissertation had been on Lord Byron.

My parents were brilliant, educated people who through diligence and education had broken out of the cloistered worlds of their beginnings. They were scientific, assimilated, secular Jews who saw their parents' lives as rife with primitive mumbo jumbo. On an early date, my dad won my mom over by taking her out on Yom Kippur, the Jewish day of fasting and atonement, and ordering bacon and eggs. Their friends were Upper West Side artists and intellectuals. These were people who could talk about anything: Keats, Vietnam, orgasms, Robert Rauschenberg, Thelonious Monk, marijuana, or Freud. But this, tetralogy of Fallot, was beyond meaning. Even for an English professor, even for an MD, it verged on gibberish. "Tetralogy" is an English word, but the kind that no one ever speaks or writes, and if used at all, it's for artworks and not medical conditions. (William Safire wrote the "On Language" column in the *New York Times* when I was growing up, and I remember when he discovered the word in 2002: "Now I know," he wrote in a column when he was eighty-three years old, "three volumes is a trilogy, four is a tetralogy.") But "Fallot"? "Who was Fallot?" my mother asked me last summer. This was like "Rumpelstiltskin," a heap of syllables indicating nothing. And there was Malm sitting at his desk, with his neatly combed hair, his fine features, and his carefully clipped speech.

The story he was telling was not to be believed. Malm cast himself as the hero, but wasn't that just what a devil would do: appear so supercompetent, urbane, and helpful when what he really wanted was the blood of her child? My parents were frightened, and in their fear, victims of an obscure, atavistic guilt.

My father, the MD, believed it was a curse. One night before the diagnosis, I had been crying in my crib, and he hadn't come to get me—that was why it had happened, he decided. He didn't get out of bed to respond to the crying baby. So the finger of God had come and punched a hole in his son's heart. My grandma, Rose, my mother's mother, rode the subway from Queens to visit the baby. She lifted me from my crib and said to my mom, "The baby is blue."

My mother snatched me from my grandma. "No, he's not," my mother said, blue baby in hand.

The good news was that Malm could fix my heart. The less good news was that the surgery could not take place until I was five years old and big enough to be attached to a heart-lung machine. In the interim, my doctors could do nothing. As my dad remembers it, he was told that the doctors would monitor the pressures in the chambers of my heart and hope that things kept working until 1971. For all that time, my life would hang in the balance of those pressures.

As I began to crawl, to toddle, and to walk, things became more obvious. The more I exerted myself, the more often my lips and fingertips turned blue. I got tired. I rested in that same squat that Danny Spandau had, relieving some of the pressure on my heart and lungs. (It's a squat I can still do. I can do it as flexibly as anyone in any yoga class.) When I was two, I had my first cardiac catheter exam.

For the exam I was sedated and laid out on an operating room table. An incision was made in my groin—the first time a scalpel ever cut into my flesh—and the doctors loaded a thin guide wire into my femoral artery. Then the catheter tube followed the wire and traveled all the way up my little torso, through the abdominal aorta, over the aortic arch, and into the chambers of my heart. With the catheter, doctors measured the heart chambers' pressures in millimeters of mercury. They squirted dye through the catheter, and with X-rays and fluoroscopes, they photographed the blood flow through the deformed chambers. They saw the hole in the wall between my ventricles, the ventricular septal defect, and they measured its size. They watched how the oxygenated and deoxygenated blood mingled in my heart, and they measured the function of my stenotic pulmonary valve—the point at which in a normal heart blood would flow from the right ventricle to the lungs. They looked at my aorta, how it hovered right above the hole in the middle of my heart. A mixture of arterial and venous blood flowed out into the body. The doctors tried to quantify all this. How much oxygen was in my blood? How compromised was my cardiopulmonary system?

If necessary, Malm and his team would sew a shunt into my great arteries and see if that would increase my blood oxygen levels—the same sort of shunt sewn into Danny's great arteries when he was two years old, the sort of shunts developed by Helen Taussig and Vivien Thomas and Alfred Blalock at Johns Hopkins in the 1940s. But I was fortunate. My tetralogy was, as the doctors put it, "well balanced." The stenosis wasn't terrible. Enough blood was going to my lungs. It looked like I would live until I was five. For now, the doctors were not going to intervene. Three uncertain years spanned out before my parents. And after the surgery? No one knew. The number of surgically corrected hearts was tiny. By 1970, the oldest repaired tet kids had lived ten years past their corrective surgeries. So far, things looked good. They were doing well.

My parents were of a generation raised not to talk about their kids' mysterious diseases. They lived those five years between diagnosis and surgery stoically. From 1966 to 1971, they mentioned the problem to no one. My father, the psychiatrist, was concerned about my emotional development. He didn't want me to be singled out, ever. He didn't want anyone to fuss over me or worry. He didn't want me to think of myself as sick.

My grandma came in from Queens every Monday. She knew my favorite foods, my favorite games, and my friends. She knew which of my friends liked chicken soup and which didn't like lima beans. She must have known—my blue lips, my blue fingers, my energy and stamina decreasing year after year—but some strange unspoken pact grew between her and my mother. They didn't talk about my illness; they just pretended it wasn't there. My parents didn't even tell my preschool teachers about my heart.

My mother is a warm, social woman, a champion conversationalist. She makes friends everywhere she goes and keeps them forever. While I played in the sandbox, she sat on a park bench. The other mothers on those park benches became her lifelong friends. They had gone to college together, some of them, and their husbands scored each other dope. In the late 1960s, they threw each other dinner parties. They traded recipes and manuscripts. They protested the war. To this day, my mom lunches with those same women who sat on those park benches. But all through the late 1960s, through that period of intense, diaper-changing intimacy, she never mentioned my crisis to her friends, that her baby needed heart surgery.

I said to her once, "That must have driven you crazy."

"I think it did," my mother said.

I laughed.

She grew serious. "I think it drove me crazy," she insisted. "I think it was the craziest thing in my whole life."

My condition wasn't subtle.

"I remember your blue lips," my best friend's mother said to me years later—and how could she not? There I was in her apartment, playing with her children after school, every day.

In *Illness as Metaphor*, Susan Sontag discusses the unmentionable nature of incurable disease, or as she puts it, "a disease not understood." Sontag writes, "The very names of such diseases are felt to have magic power." Even in medical circles, the dread words were taboo. She quotes the eminent psychiatrist Karl Menninger, from his 1963 book *The Vital Impulse*: "The very word 'cancer' is said to kill some patients who would not have succumbed (so quickly) to the malignancy from which they suffer." My father's colleagues at the William Alanson White Institute of Psychiatry, Psychoanalysis, and Psychology would have likely agreed with Menninger that the best thing to do with a condition like mine—a bizarre, unheard-of condition—was never to say a word about it. In Menninger's formulation, to say its name would be to make me sicker, the syllables themselves taking on esoteric power. Furthermore, people might not want their children to play with me if they knew I was dying.

Sontag writes, "Contact with someone afflicted with a disease regarded as a mysterious malevolency inevitably feels like trespass; worse, like the violation of a taboo." Secrecy was the course of wisdom and propriety, best for my health and social development.

The Orthodox Jews in my grandparents' synagogue in Queens would have agreed. In Judaism there is a concept called *lashon hora*: a Jew shall not speak ill of another Jew. You cannot gossip idly about your own child, about the evil things that have befallen him. For my grandparents it would have been sinful to tell anyone that their little grandson had a mysterious heart condition. All the social forces around my parents, all authorities, familial and professional, rabbinical and secular, agreed: they had to hide my heart condition like Anne Frank in the attics of their minds. My father confessed it one time, in confidence, to his buddy Leo.

"Oh, Gabriel?" Leo brushed him off. "He'll be fine."

As in Lorrie Moore's story "People Like That Are the Only People Here," about a child with a dread illness, my parents were plunged into a linguistic vacuum: "What words can be uttered? You turn just slightly and there it is: the death of your child. It is part symbol, part devil, and in your blind spot all along, until, if you are unlucky, it is completely upon you. Then it is a fierce little country abducting you; it holds you squarely inside itself like a cellar room—the best boundaries of you are the boundaries of it. Are there windows? Sometimes, aren't there windows?"

I certainly don't remember thinking of myself as ill or crippled. I knew, but I didn't acknowledge. I was limited, but I didn't ever believe I was sick. I developed strategies to hide my weakness, to live with it, and to cope with it. I never tried to climb the monkey bars in the playground. I never ran races. When they were playing tag, I sat on my tricycle, playing games of my own. I was never stigmatized. I was happy. I had great friends.

"You got slick," said my dad. I learned to pretend to be healthy.

Outside school, I spent a lot of time on his shoulders. I can still imagine it, my hands on his forehead, his head as big as my whole torso. I was a spoiled, doted-on child. I don't remember feeling much self-pity, though my dad remembers that I turned on him once, when he asked me to close the refrigerator door. "I have a whisper in my heart," I said. When my father tells that story, he grabs his own chest.

When he tells the story of the heart surgery, he always mentions that it came during the Attica prison riots. I picture my dad, a big, sleepless, bearded guy in a sweaty Oxford shirt, standing outside the hospital in September, across from the Audubon Ballroom, where Malcolm X had been assassinated the year before I was born. His whole world was turning upside down.

Mine was only disrupted slightly. Heart surgery when it came didn't feel like a relief or a cure. It felt like an intrusion. I was Gaby Baby. I was so adorable. People were always nice to me. Then suddenly, they were sticking needles in me and knives, and no one cared if I was comfortable, and I was not allowed to play or get out of bed or go home for eleven days.

5.

I REMEMBER MALM'S OFFICE as a dark place, and I only remember visiting there once, right before surgery. I don't remember his face, probably because I wasn't looking at him. Probably I was hiding in my mother's lap.

They didn't describe it to me as heart surgery. They said it was an operation to make me run faster. After the meeting, I left Dr. Malm's office in slow motion, with big strides and elbows pumping, imagining my future speed. After the operation, I'd move like Batman, like the Flash.

My parents tell me I spent the night before surgery in the hospital chattering on the phone with my friends. I imagine my little skinny self with my 1970s poof of dark hair, buck-toothed and smiling on the hospital bed, big phone pressed against my ear. The next morning I was wheeled into the operating room. The gas mask was put over my face, a triangular mask, attached to an accordion-stretch plastic hose of the same pale transparent blue.

I woke up screaming, outraged to find myself immobilized and full of needles and tubes and wires. The post-op room was busy with nurses in white uniforms, all at work with tools and trays. One hissed at me, "Will you be quiet?" In my mind she is blond and pretty enough to be on television (maybe I confuse her with a television nurse), and she says to me, "Look at that little baby," pointing to one in a crib beside my bed. "That baby's not crying."

They rolled me down the hallway, past the Winnie-the-Pooh stickers on the tiled walls. There was Muzak playing through the loudspeakers, "Never on Sunday." I hate that dippy melody still. My memories of the hospital stay are thin and fragmented and vague: curtains around the bed, other beds across the room, a television set playing in a corner, and my mother beside me devotedly, religiously.

My mom needed a ginger ale. Never in her life before or since has she *needed* a ginger ale. She said, "I'll be back before you can say Jack Robinson," another thing my mom has never done before or since. I went, "Jack Robinson Jack Robinson Jack Robinson Jack Robinson," and when she came back, I complained that I had said it seventy-two times.

I was a thumb sucker, and that's what pissed me off most about the hospital, that my left hand was encased in tubes and tape. They kept that hand tied up above me so that (they explained) I wouldn't pull the IV out when I was asleep.

"Suck your right thumb," said the doctor, like he knew anything about it. The left was the only thumb to suck.

From the bed I was moved to a wheelchair and started wheeling around the hospital. I got good at it. Someone suggested that I could race my parents' paraplegic friend, Richard Brickner. I imagined the finish line and breaking the tape and me pumping my hands over my head in victory.

In 1971, recovery from open-heart surgery called for penicillin shots each day. Penicillin is very thick going in, and the shots were painful in my five-year-old groin. I remember the sound of the rolling tray just beyond the curtain, outside the area of my vision, the nurse coming in to administer the shot. I remember pleading for them not to do it.

The last time they tried to give me the shot, I threw a fit, and they had to hold me down, a nurse or orderly for every limb, and as my dad held my head, he laughed. I remember being outraged by the enormous smile spreading out under his beard. Wasn't he on my side? Now I understand: this must have been the happiest sight in the world for him, all he had wanted for five years, his baby boy alive, repaired, and fighting.

One night at home, not too long after the hospital, I woke up to notice a sore in my scar, a little red swelling like a bug bite. My mother wanted to call the hospital, but my father took me to the bathroom and made me stand on the toilet seat, and with a pair of tweezers he took the black suture out from under the skin. For thirty years, until my second open-heart surgery, I had a little hole there, a cavity in the scar, a little burrow where the thread had been.

I got presents. One was an adding toy, not a calculator or an abacus but a little plastic man on a board like a square clock face, and when you moved his legs to the numbers below, his big pencil would move across the top of the board and show the sum. I also got a special pillow—I believe it's called a husband pillow—the kind with armrests and a back like a chair, and I sat against that pillow and watched television. Every night, in the bathroom before bed, my mother ran cocoa butter on the scar to smooth it. The cocoa butter came in a stick, and she pressed it up from the bottom through an aluminum tube. I loved that cocoa butter smell.

The ordeal was over, and I was back home, back to normal. One of the doctors had said something ominous to my mother—"They all get off the operating table"—but my family was insistent. The hospital stay was done, and I was well. We called it "the operation," which is slightly more euphemistic than "the surgery," and as far as I could tell, the operation, and not the heart disease, was the bad thing that had happened to me. The good thing for me as a five-year-old boy was not that I had been cured of a potentially fatal condition—I never allowed myself to think in those terms, that without the operation I would have been crippled and then dead—the good thing was that I was home and safe. My normal life, I believed, was comfort and not illness. After the first corrective heart surgery in 1971, I had to see the doctor regularly, but I lived in a dream world of good health.

I had a scar on my chest, but that was it. By the time I was nine, it seemed the operation had happened in a different historical epoch. I barely remembered first grade, just vague images of guinea pig cages and hooks in a closet to hang up coats. Second grade, that's when my life began.

———

The triumph over congenital heart disease is one of the great victories of modern medicine. Because pediatric open-heart surgery led to adult heart surgery, its effects are widespread. Maybe you have an uncle with a new heart valve, a grandmother with a pacemaker. Maybe the woman at your deli counter had a bypass. This all started with kids like me.

Pediatric cardiology changed the world. It was invented by two women, Helen Taussig and her predecessor, Maude Abbott, both of whom were initially denied admission to medical school on account of their sex, both of whom were prevented by the male medical establishment from practicing the kind of medicine they wanted to practice, both of whom were forced to look at children with defective hearts because no male doctors deemed those hearts significant enough to look at. Kids born with bad hearts were dead-end patients, for whom nothing could be done, until Abbott and Taussig, with genius, patience, and discipline, learned to diagnose and to treat those conditions. Vivien Thomas, who invented most of the original equipment for pediatric heart surgery, who designed and oversaw some of the great groundbreaking procedures on children with deformed hearts, and who trained many of the most important doctors in the first generation of heart surgeons, never got to medical school himself because he was black and because he was poor. The early pioneers of heart surgery operated on the margins of convention and respectability, risking their medical licenses and their patients' lives and sometimes skirting the law.

Those of us who have survived childhood heart surgery have been repaired but not exactly cured and have lived our lives on the border between sickness and health. I have been absurdly lucky. I am past fifty, not much younger than heart surgery itself. And my luck has held: every time my life has been in danger, doctors have come along and invented something to save me. I have surfed wave after wave of advances in heart surgery and in medical technology. The history of cardiac surgery is inscribed in the muscle of my heart, and in this book I will try to give that carved-up muscle a voice, to tell the history of heart surgery through the story of my heart.

The first half of my life, from my first open-heart surgery when I was five to my second when I was in my mid-thirties, was spent mostly in denial that I had any kind of heart problem. The second half has been punctuated by regular visits to the operating table. What's all this been like?

Scary at times, but on the whole, great. Lucky. Privileged. Like your life, dear reader, only more so, lived (like yours) with the support of medicine and in the shadow of death. I have a job, two kids, and a happy marriage. I climb mountains up above the tree line. I ride my bike around New York City. In yoga classes, I stand on my head. I take five pills a day, and my torso is scarred, and I need to go into an ambulance every so often, and more often into an operating room, and medical devices lodge under my skin, but you can't see any of that when I have a shirt on.

You get used to it. The miracle of modern medicine is a little like the miracle of modern flight. Time in hospitals can seem a lot like time in airports. You sit in waiting rooms. You get antsy in your seat. There's a lot of taking off shoes and going into scanning machines. You remove all the change in your pocket before you get weighed. People poke at you and ask the same questions every time: Swelling in your feet? Shortness of breath? Trouble climbing stairs? The ceremony becomes a recitation you half attend to, like the flight attendants' ritual performed with the safety belts and oxygen masks and floatation devices under your seat, until all of a sudden—CATASTROPHE!!! The engines are dying! Cabin pressure fails! We're going to plummet 39,000 feet! Then the plane rights itself. The crisis passes. You're above the clouds again, cruising at five hundred miles per hour, with your legs uncomfortable, all the way from New York to Los Angeles.

6.

IN THE FALL of 1973, when I was seven years old, my dad and I took the subway from our apartment on 108th Street up to Columbia Presbyterian Hospital in Washington Heights, where just two years before I had had open-heart surgery.

This was before the trains were covered in spectacular graffiti. If my memory is right, there were still gum-vending machines on the platforms. Most of them were broken, the coin slots clogged, but I'd stick my finger in anyway and hope for one of those shiny little brightly colored Chiclets.

My dad and I were a mismatched pair. Brown Beatles bangs covered my forehead. His style was more Allen Ginsberg/Fidel Castro, with his dark hair combed back and a black beard covering his chin. The similarity in the shapes of our faces was obscured. I was tiny, all skin and bones, and he was six feet tall with a hefty gut, strong shoulders, and big hands. His anxiety filled his body with a watchful tension. Mine left me dreamy, not quite present in the physical world. My brother, Daniel, was there too—three years older than me, skinny, with a handsome, serious face and an enormous poof of curly Jewish hair. Daniel recalls the events of that day better than I do, but the truth is I have somehow excised him from my memories.

When the subway came above ground after 116th Street, I spun around on my knees and pressed my face against the window, fogging it with my breath and leaving the print of my nose. On one side were the buildings where I went to school; on the other was the Hudson River. I had been going to the hospital at least once a year, every year since I was an infant, but this time we didn't go to the doctor's office. We went to the auditorium. The place was packed with kids who'd had open-heart surgery. They all seemed very happy to be in the hospital—blond kids, black kids, boys and girls. Everyone seemed to be smiling and making friends. This was very confusing to me. Daniel remembers that lots of sick kids were there, kids not doing as well as me, and it freaked him out a little to see them.

I was shy. I wasn't ashamed of my surgery. I didn't try to hide the big scar on my chest, not at sleepovers or when I went swimming. But I thought the surgery was something private, mine alone, not to be talked about. I also thought the surgery was over, past and done, very unpleasant and nothing to be celebrated.

"Where are the grown-ups who had the operation?" I asked my dad.

"There aren't any," he said, looking around the lobby in undisguised wonder. "There's no one here ten years older than you."

The summer after the surgery was the summer I had begun to read C. S. Lewis. I had stumbled through the back of a wardrobe in an old castle in northern England, and the fur coats had become fir trees, and the mothballs had become snow, and I had entered the kingdom of Narnia, which was the place for me. My favorite of all the books was *The Voyage of the Dawn Treader*. Prince Caspian and the Pevensies sailed toward the end of the world. This idea fascinated me: the earth as a flat disc with a lip over which the oceans fell. When my dad said that there were no kids ten years older than me in the hospital lobby, no grown-ups who had had the same surgery I had, I felt the intimation of something similar, the end of the world, the oceans cascading into oblivion. In the hospital with all those happy, smiling, dying kids, I understood for the first time in my life that my little ship was sailing toward the edge of the world. I don't know what everyone else does with their first childhood intimation of death, but I tried to swallow mine and push it way down deep inside me.

As I recall it, they called us the Open Heart Club—I remember confusing it with the Beatles and *Sgt. Pepper's Lonely Hearts Club Band*. We filed into the auditorium and took our seats. There on the stage were the most famous players from the New York Mets, Tom Seaver and Willie Mays. Willie Mays in 1973 was confusing to me. He had once been the greatest ballplayer ever, but now he was a forty-three-year-old man way past his prime, who couldn't hit or run or throw or field, and it was incomprehensible that someone my dad's age got called "the Say Hey Kid." Tom Seaver, on the other hand, was dominant. My friends and I pretended to be him and Tug McGraw and Cleon Jones and Felix Millan. Seaver was on stage in a suit, smiling and waving at us.

He made a speech. He said something like, "You kids are the real heroes," and I had no idea what he meant. I dreamed of becoming a hero, a baseball player like him (though, as I explained to my friends, I'd work as a veterinarian in the off-season). I didn't want to grow up to be a heart patient.

When Tom Seaver's Mets had won the World Series in 1969, they had been called the Miracle Mets, and this was a name Seaver had objected to. It was no *miracle* he said; they had worked like hell to win that championship. When he looked around the room, did Seaver call us miracles? I didn't feel much like a miracle. I did not want to know how lucky I was to be sitting there in that auditorium with my dad and big brother and all those kids just like me, feeling so confused and alone and alienated.

Sitting up on stage with Tom Seaver and Willie Mays was Dr. Malm. This also confused me. He'd seen me as an infant and right before surgery, and probably he had come by my hospital bed to visit me at least one time after the operation, one of a hundred doctors and nurses poking at me, but I had no memory of Malm's face. His name had been invoked over and over again in our home, and I had thought his name was spelled "Dr. Mom" and not "Dr. Malm," and some of the magic of that misspelling had rubbed off on my conception of the man—the doctor named Mom who had fixed my heart. On stage, he seemed small and ordinary next to the ballplayers. There were speeches. There was clapping. The boy next

to me seemed very excited. That was weird to me. Did he *want* to
be part of the Open Heart Club?

We filed up on stage to get our programs and autograph books
signed by the baseball players. When I interviewed him for this
book, Malm told me a story: he saw a boy at the end of the line,
an old patient of his waiting impatiently, and when Malm said,
"Johnnie, I'll sign your book for you," the kid had refused. No.
He wanted Tom Seaver's autograph. Malm laughed when he told
me the story, and I guess it's a measure of his success. Kids like
us didn't think much about our hearts. We could dream about
baseball. The more we took Jim Malm for granted, the greater his
achievement.

My brother and I were the kind of kids who got everyone
to sign. Daniel has kept his childhood autograph book, and he
showed me Malm's signature. Malm made a little heart under his
name, with two *x*'s in it, like stitches or eyes. It's hard to tell if the
heart is dead or if it's mended. A lot of the kids in the auditorium
had their Mets hats on. A lot of them had brought baseball mitts.
Danny Spandau wasn't there.

In 1961, his family had moved out of Brooklyn to Plainview,
Long Island. He had been followed by Malm in the years immediately after his procedure. Five years after surgery, Malm had
pronounced Danny cured, and Danny came back to the hospital
only once more, in 1971, for a ten-year checkup. He had a good
relationship with his surgeon. "He exuded confidence. He exuded
it," Danny told me. "He had a great smile, and he had this clean-
cut presence. He was a super professional, but also warm and he
had a great bedside manner, and he was genuine. Very, very, very
well groomed, very tight skinned, almost waxy face with perfect
hair. And he had this beautiful smile. He always smiled. And his
hands were always warm and gentle. He was never the one who
stuck me. He was never the one who gave me the shots or drew
the blood or whatever. And he was always writing in his journal. I
remember that because I was always inquisitive. I remember asking
why are you writing that, now you're drawing a picture. What are
you doing?" Malm kept an enormous folder on Danny's case, in

which he kept all the detailed plans and pictures that he drew of Danny's heart.

In their last meeting, teenaged Danny asked a favor of Malm. Could he see an open-heart surgery in process? Malm consented. He didn't let Danny see a child being operated on, and he didn't let him see the actual sectioning apart of the chest, but in the middle of an operation on a grown man, Danny was allowed to walk onto the balcony of the operating theater and look down on Malm in his scrubs, and at the open cavity of the patient's chest, and at the humming heart-lung machine. Danny did not visit a cardiologist again until he was fifty years old, and by that time his heart was in trouble, and Danny was told that he was highly susceptible to sudden cardiac death.

In the auditorium with me that day in 1973 were children with many different kinds of heart defects. We are all lumped together, sometimes, as patients with congenital heart disease, but that is an oversimplification. There is not one single congenital heart disease; rather there are many different kinds of defects, some arising from chromosomal disorders, some from accidents of development in the womb, and some of unknown etiology. There are correlations between certain congenital heart defects and certain genetic conditions: for example, there is a relatively high incidence of tetralogy of Fallot among children with Down syndrome. Because a fetus doesn't breathe in the womb, because the mother supplies the blood with oxygen, an infant can develop and be born with even the most extreme heart defect.

The most common defects are the simplest: a single hole in the central wall between the chambers of the heart. A tetralogy like mine is the most common complex congenital malformation of the heart, and it is usually described as a collection of four distinct defects. In fact it's the result of a single problem in fetal development. The ventricular septum, the wall between the two large chambers at the bottom of the heart, emerges in the developing fetus in two parts, strong and muscular at the bottom and thin and membranous at the top. In a normally developing heart, these two pieces connect and merge, but in my mother's womb, the two parts failed to do so. The top part of my septum, the membranous part called the conal septum, drifted off to the side, blocking my pulmonary valve.

"Tetralogy," as one cardiologist explained to me, "is the anterior displacement of the conal septum."

So I had the same defect as Danny Spandau. If, after failing to knit with the muscular bottom part, the membranous part had moved in the other direction, then a different kind of heart defect would have ensued. My aorta and not my pulmonary valve would have been blocked. The doctors would have called this "subaortic stenosis," and the defect might have caused a narrowing, or coarctation, of my aorta. Jim Malm repaired those too, and kids with subaortic stenosis and coarctation of the aorta were sitting in the stands with me.

So many things can go wrong in a developing heart. Heart valves are made of tiny leaflets, little flaps of flesh that come together and move apart as the heart contracts and expands. The pulmonary valve has two leaflets, and the tricuspid valve has three, and the leaflets open and shut with each heartbeat, allowing the blood to circulate when they open and preventing it from flowing backward when they close. If the leaflets of the pulmonary valves don't develop separately in the fetus, if they fuse together and form a blockage, this is known as pulmonary atresia. If the tricuspid's leaflets fuse, it's tricuspid atresia. A fused valve can affect the fetus like a heart attack. The blood stops running through one chamber of the heart. That chamber fails to develop.

Some authorities claim there are at least eighteen different kinds of congenital heart defects; others will say at least thirty-five. The distinctions between anomalies can be subtle. "Pulmonary atresia with VSD" refers to a defect a lot like mine, a hole in the ventricle (a ventricular septal defect), but with a total blockage in the pulmonary valve. In some cases, the whole right side of the heart can fail to develop, and then the baby comes out with something called hypoplastic right heart syndrome, or HRHS. The kid only has one ventricle. There is no chamber to push the blood to the lungs. In 1973, cardiac surgeons couldn't save kids with just one ventricle.

There are genetic and environmental factors in the etiology of congenital heart disease. People who have heart defects represent about 1 percent of the population, but in their children the incidence of congenital heart defects rises to 3 percent. Exposure to certain kinds of environmental factors may correspond to higher rates of congenital heart defects. If you look around a movie theater or subway car and try to approximate the number of people there with congenital heart defects (something you've probably never done, but something I do frequently), 1 percent can seem a large number, but if you think in terms of the complexity of the human heart and the number of things that can possibly go wrong in the womb, 1 percent seems tiny. It's amazing that babies' hearts develop perfectly more than 99 percent of the time.

There were kids in the Open Heart Club who had been born with startlingly dangerous defects—for instance, transposition of the great arteries, a condition in which the pulmonary artery and the aorta are switched, so that the heart is essentially set backward in the circulatory system, with blood from the veins routed out to the body, and blood from the arteries routed to the lungs. No baby born with transposition of the great arteries can survive long without surgery. Without intervention, these babies will die within the first months, weeks, days, or hours after birth.

Through the 1950s, the great Canadian surgeon Dr. William Mustard devoted himself to the cure of children with transposition of the great arteries. His colleagues called him "Wild Bill" Mustard, and I heard one old doctor say of Mustard that his surgical technique was so powerful that he could sew together two farts. In the 1950s, Mustard experimented with new techniques in experimental heart bypass surgery. He invented an organic heart-lung machine (it didn't work): he cleaned the lungs of freshly killed monkeys so they were translucent and put them in jars, then directed his patients' blood through the cleaned and suspended monkey lungs so as to perfuse it with oxygen. In 1957, he published the results of twenty-one such surgeries; three of his patients were alive at the time of publication, but they all died soon after.

Beginning in 1952, Mustard attempted surgical repairs of babies with transposition of the great arteries. For roughly a decade, he had a 100 percent mortality rate in these operations. Baby after baby died on the table as he struggled to find a way to reroute their blood. On May 16, 1963, after eleven consecutive years of failure, Mustard performed an operation called an "atrial switch" on an eighteen-month-old girl who had been born with transposition. On this girl, Mustard finally succeeded in redirecting the blood flow at the top of the heart, putting a baffle between her left and right atria so that the venous blood would go to her lungs and the arterial blood would go to her body. This procedure, called the Mustard procedure, was the standard treatment for transposition of the great arteries for the next decade.

Malm performed Mustard surgeries in the mid- and late 1960s, so there must have been kids in the audience with baffles in their hearts, and they must have clapped for the ballplayers, too, and lined up for autographs, but no one knew how long the baffles in the tops of their hearts would last. No one knew how long any of our hearts would last, really.

We were the first large cohort of heart-repair patients. After 1973, the technology advanced, and Malm was able to perform surgery on infants. No tetralogy patient younger than me really remembers being operated on as a small child: their defects were repaired when they were babies.

Patients like me and Danny Spandau seemed to do great after surgery, but our hearts were jerry-rigged. None of us had valves between our right ventricles and our pulmonary arteries. In a normal heart, a pulmonary valve opens and closes with each heartbeat. We had an open passageway in that place. Our blood flowed up from the heart to the lungs, and then leaked back into our big, overdeveloped right ventricles. In 1963, Malm had used the term "complete repair" for his tetralogy surgeries, but that terminology was soon dropped and altered to "total correction." We didn't have the right number of heart valves.

Hang a big bookshelf from your wall using just three anchors when you ought to use four, and it's likely that in the first decade the bookshelf will hold up just fine. But after a while it might begin to wobble. And it's a good idea to check on the bookshelf to make sure it's secure. The installation might require some revisions.

We all looked great when we got to Shea Stadium to continue our celebration, but no one knew when our baffles might deteriorate, or how well our hypertrophied right ventricles would do in the long term, or who would go into a sudden fatal cardiac arrhythmia. Danny Spandau lived for decades without worrying. He told me (smiling) that as a teenager he had lived an "experimental life." When he finally saw a heart doctor, thirty-five years after his last visit with Malm, Danny was aware of no symptoms—he'd gone to the cardiologist as part of an insurance application—but the backward leak in his heart had enlarged his right ventricle severely. Not too long after that visit, he was told that he was in need of heart surgery. This scared the crap out of him. The great trauma of his life, long repressed, had returned. My heart repair didn't last as long as Danny's. By my mid-twenties, my heart was pretty wobbly, and no one was quite sure what to do about me.

At the baseball game, the Mets gave us our own section in the upper deck. We sat together happily and were announced to the crowd. They put up on the scoreboard the name of our hospital, and maybe Dr. Malm's name too, and maybe "THE OPEN HEART CLUB." The whole stadium stood and cheered.

Did I worry about how long my heart would survive? Did I think of myself as a medical miracle? No. I asked my dad for a hotdog. I filled out my scorecard. I hoped that the Mets would win.

7.

THE OLDEST SURGEONS and cardiologists I interviewed for this book are now in their eighties and nineties, people who started their careers before Danny Spandau's heart was repaired by Jim Malm at Babies Hospital. These doctors remembered the awful moral calculus they faced at the dawn of the age of open-heart surgery. Dr. Welton M. Gersony, who would later direct the program in pediatric cardiology at Columbia, was completing his medical residency at Boston Children's Hospital in the late 1950s.

"The early patients," he told me, "paid a terrible price."

Tetralogy of Fallot patients in particular presented doctors with a difficult puzzle. The vascular surgical techniques that had been devised by Helen Taussig, Vivien Thomas, and Alfred Blalock in Baltimore in 1944 alleviated a great deal of the tetralogy kids' suffering. By sewing a shunt between the pulmonary and subclavian arteries, doctors could extend children's lives. Some of those kids, like Danny Spandau, saw little improvement, but the vast majority responded well to the treatment and were still going after surgery, living limited but productive lives.

By the late 1950s, surgery to implant a Blalock shunt was a reasonably safe procedure, one that could grant an eight-year-old tetralogy kid another ten or twenty years of life, or more. Meanwhile, in 1958, if you put the same kid on the operating table and tried to fix her heart more permanently, the odds weren't great that the child would make it through the week.

The surgeons, confident in their technical expertise, usually wanted to operate. But for a doctor like Gersony, deciding when to prescribe a risky surgery and on which child was an awful decision.

"It was a tremendous dilemma," Gersony told me. In his mid-eighties, thin and vigorous when I met him, Dr. Gersony still sympathized with the patients and parents he'd seen all those years ago. "When you're ten years old, adding decades to your life means living until you're thirty. And that sounds great when you're ten. The problem is, how much extra mortality do you accept at five or ten years old, or even in a newborn or neonate, to then get potentially another fifty years of life? Would you accept that even 5 percent die there—kids who could have lived another twenty years with the Blalock? How many of those kids would you be willing to sacrifice to do the operation so the next generation would live?"

The early experimental surgeries being done in Minnesota were often performed in lieu of the Blalock. C. Walt Lillehei's first bypass operations risked the life of the parent as well as the child, the two of them hooked up in a complex blood transfusion, the parent's heart feeding the child's body. In some cases, Lillehei performed these procedures when the Blalock shunt was still possible—when the child's life could have been extended for a decade with a safe and simple operation. At Babies Hospital at Columbia Presbyterian, most of Aaron Himmelstein's tetralogy patients died—seven of eleven. Some of these were no doubt desperate cases, but if Himmelstein was like the other heart surgeons in the country, some likely might have lived another decade or two with a safely implanted Blalock shunt. Mortality rates for early open-heart surgery were 25 percent, 50 percent, or more, depending on the defect and the hospital.

But the doctors had to consider not just the patient in their hands but also the next generation of children. This is what made the calculus so awful. If they were too cautious, if they never tried bypass surgery on the blue babies, if they just stuck with the shunts in the great arteries, they'd only be extending sick lives. They'd never cure anyone. With the heart-lung machine, the Holy Grail stood before them. They could grant long, happy, healthy lives to the sick children of the future, but in their present state of expertise, the first open-heart surgeries were almost murderous.

In the late 1950s Welton Gersony was working with one of the most eminent heart surgeons in the world, Dr. Robert Gross, the chief heart surgeon at Boston Children's. For decades Gross had been among the top chest surgeons in the nation, a natty, pompous, strutting genius, the best surgeon at the best pediatric surgery program in the world. But he was having a terrible time with open-heart surgery—connecting children to heart-lung machines and cutting into their hearts while they were on bypass. Gross liked to invent his own equipment and his own procedures, and his results with kids with heart defects were not good. Children were dying. It was too much for Welton Gersony. Despite his junior status, he went to Alexander Nadas, the chief of pediatric cardiology at Boston Children's. Full of trepidation, Gersony emplored Nadas to tell Gross to stop.

"I thought he'd throw me out the window," Gersony told me. "But he did listen." They did stop the program, for a while at least.

My own pediatric cardiologist, Dr. Sylvia P. Griffiths, came to Columbia Presbyterian in 1955. Dr. Griffiths was trained at Yale by Ruth Whittemore, who had been Helen Taussig's assistant during the very first blue baby operation at Hopkins in 1944. Griffiths, along with Whittemore, attended some of the summer gatherings of the so-called Knights of Taussig at Taussig's family summer home in Cotuit, Cape Cod. Griffiths was also a coauthor of Malm's breakthrough 1963 paper on the treatment of tetralogy of Fallot, describing his unprecedented string of effective corrections.

She was at Columbia for Himmelstein's early ventures into open-heart surgery, watching patients before and after the operations, and she too struggled with the high mortality rates. The chief of her pediatrics program summoned her to his office and sent her on a mission to Minnesota, the cradle of open-heart surgery, to see what was happening there. Why were their results so much better than Columbia's?

If, in the 1950s, Minnesota was the fertile crescent of the heart bypass, the University of Minnesota at Minneapolis and the Mayo

Clinic were heart surgery's Tigris and Euphrates, the two great wellsprings. Dr. John Kirklin at Mayo was technically minded and reserved. Walt Lillehei at the University of Minnesota was a wild man, a flamboyant daredevil and risk taker in medicine and in life. Lillehei would stay out all night drinking and dancing and show up in the OR hungover to perform impeccable surgeries. It was Lillehei who had the first successful series of bypasses with his two-patient surgeries—using an adult in place of a heart-lung machine and using transfusion to oxygenate his patients' blood— but by 1958 Kirklin's procedures with a heart-lung machine had surpassed Lillehei's, and Sylvia Griffiths was sent to Mayo to watch Kirklin at work.

I visited Dr. Griffiths in her apartment on Manhattan's Upper East Side, where classical music was playing and the windows looked out over the East River. In her nineties, Dr. Griffiths was tall, fit, and elegant, in a white shirt with a bow and a long, dark pleated skirt. We met on a Thursday. She had done rounds at Columbia's pediatric cardiology wards that Wednesday. She still did rounds every week. Her feral cat curled at my feet. "That one's not for petting," she said. Her hair was neatly cut in a white Prince Valliant bob, and she asked after my health with the same concern and hopefulness that she had when I was a child and she was my doctor. Then she told me about her visit to Rochester, Minnesota.

"It was my first time in an airplane," she told me. "I was given a hundred dollars from each department. I don't know how much that is in present dollars, but right then and there, you could make a telephone call for a nickel. That trip was the most significant experience of my medical life. The operating room was an almost intimate setting. Beside a central bed on which the patient lay and the surrounding equipment, a balcony was in the OR. You were masked, but you were not behind glass. It was like another century. It seemed so advanced to anything I had seen or really understood, but there was remarkable teamwork between Kirklin and the anesthesiologist who ran the heart-lung machine.

"In one week, three children were operated on, each with a ventricular septal defect." That is, a hole in the wall between the two main pumping chambers of the heart. "These were approximately six to ten years in age. The most significant part of the visit was my observation and seeing the children. There were only three—but of course in those days three was a lot to leave the OR and go to the recovery room. Of course, I was familiar with the recovery room, in terms of intravenous and support fluids. In terms of the constant monitoring of the EKG and blood pressure. It was all very orderly, there were no disasters, and all three were discharged from the recovery room and sent back to the ward.

"I went back to New York and said, 'The problem is not one of management in the recovery room. The problem is in the operating room and what the surgeon'—Himmelstein—'was doing.'"

This was a remarkable thing, to have a part-time junior physician criticize the work of the senior surgical staff. But at Columbia at that time, with a whole new world of surgery being invented, they listened to Sylvia Griffiths. A significant part of her critique had to do with the Columbia surgeons' understanding of congenital heart defects.

"The people who started at Columbia weren't schooled in anatomy of the heart," she told me. "In Mayo, Kirklin and whoever was working with him was trained in pathology of the heart. One of the big liabilities of the early surgeries, say for ventricular septal defect, was creating heart block"—that is, destroying the heart's electrical conduction system and thus its ability to beat. "At the Mayo Clinic, when I was there, none of the patients developed heart block. But our people weren't schooled in the proximate location of the conduction system."

In other words, Himmelstein had trained as a chest surgeon. He hadn't studied the complex workings of a child's heart—the complicated interrelations of its muscular and electrical systems—and the hearts of his patients were consequently damaged in surgery. When Himmelstein died and Malm was preparing to take over the heart surgery program, he worked closely with Griffiths, studying congenital heart disease—women's work, the field that Sylvia P. Griffiths was expert in and that Helen Taussig had pioneered.

8.

WHEN I CALLED Jim Malm in 2017 and said that I wanted to thank him for saving my life, the first thing he said was, "What took you so long?"

I stammered. I said I wanted to interview him for a book I was writing. He gave me the phone number for the Babies Heart Fund and asked me to contribute. "Price of the phone call," he said.

I met him the next month at a gathering of Columbia heart surgeons, the fiftieth anniversary of cardiac surgery at Columbia Presbyterian. A number of eminent doctors were in the room—inventors of groundbreaking procedures like Dr. Jan Quaegebeur, who developed the current technique for repair of transposition of the great arteries, and Dr. Craig Smith, who had fixed Bill Clinton's heart. These were men (the heart surgeons were all men, and the old ones were all white) of excessive self-confidence and achievement. Imagine a convention of retired, highly educated, highly decorated fighter pilots who have all made good money together. They were all conservatively turned out, and they all had a gentlemanly air that required no swagger. They had proven themselves. They had played with life and death, and they had won and won and won and won.

In that crowd, the name I heard over and over again was Jim Malm's. "Jim Malm is here!" "Is that Jim Malm?" At ninety-two, though his face was a little rounder than in the old photographs, he stood as tall as me, with a firm grip and a clever eye. His skin was strangely smooth for a man his age, and delicate, with very fine wrinkles.

"Where's that book you're writing?" he said and smiled. "You're going to have to finish it soon if I'm going to read it."

In 1959, when little blue Danny Spandau was awaiting surgery, Malm was a junior member of the Columbia team. His work was kept to closed-heart procedures—operations on the great arteries, like the Blalock shunt. Aaron Himmelstein still ran the program, and Malm didn't have the opportunity to undertake the open-heart cases he yearned for.

"In 1959, our program was floundering, not doing well, a high mortality rate, lots of complications," Malm told me. "I spent much of the whole year waiting for my first patient."

Like Sylvia Griffiths, he traveled the country and looked at other programs.

"I had the opportunity to visit and spend time in centers all over the US, to study techniques in open-heart surgery," he told me. "I had the experience of seeing bad heart surgery, and I had the experience of seeing good heart surgery."

I asked him what the difference was.

"You can't have people shouting in the operating room. It can't be hyperactive. You've got to have peace, quiet, concentration. I saw it. Demeanor in the operating room. It's got to be a quiet environment. Orderly. Someone's in charge. Like any business, you've got to have someone at the helm." For Malm, it came down to the affect of the surgeon. "Not cocky. But confident. But you don't achieve that without a good background and training and discipline."

So Malm educated himself in the anatomy of congenital heart defects. That way he would know what he was going to encounter when he opened his first little blue chest.

The pathology lab at Columbia was run by Dr. Dorothy Hansine Andersen. Andersen had been trained as a surgeon at a time when there were no female surgeons, and the medical establishment had shoved her off into the less prestigious field of pathology. From her lab at Columbia, Andersen changed the medical world. She is best known as the discoverer of cystic fibrosis, but her interests were wide, and she maintained a collection of defective children's hearts in her lab. Every week, Malm, Sylvia Griffiths, and another pediatric cardiologist, Sidney Blumenthal, attended seminars in Dorothy Andersen's lab.

"The focus," Sylvia Griffiths told me, "was to learn anatomy, in mapping the cardiac conduction system, not simply in normal hearts, but looking at the conduction system, say, in the presence of a ventricular septal defect."

Dorothy Andersen was a large woman with a broad, strong-featured face. In photographs, she looks imposing and unsmiling, and she dresses in man-tailored clothes. She was an amateur carpenter and roofer. She did all the repairs on her own house. She was a hard drinker, and her hair and her lab were famously a mess. She seems to have been as much of an out lesbian as it was possible to be in 1959.

It's interesting to me that Malm, alone of the heart surgeons, attended these seminars. He emerged from a very traditional, white, Protestant, male-dominated environment, but he was perfectly happy working each week with a Jew, Sidney Blumenthal, and two women, Griffiths and Andersen, with the gay one, Andersen, running the show. I doubt this had anything to do with a commitment to liberal politics. Unlike the generation of chest surgeons who had come before him, Malm wanted to learn everything about a child's heart's workings. He was interested in only one thing: surgery on the human heart.

James Malm was born in 1925 in Cleveland, Ohio, and grew up in Evanston, Illinois. His father, Royal, was the son of Swedish immigrants, and James was his parents' first child. He suffered from childhood asthma and frequent lung infections, and he admired the local doctors who treated him. By the time he had recovered from those troubles, he knew what he wanted to do with his life.

"It never occurred to me to be anything but a doctor," he told me. "Somehow, I never wanted to be anything else."

By second grade, he had met Constance Martha Brooks, the girl he was going to marry. His purpose was absolutely clear. Young

Jim had about as much uncertainty as a scalpel does. He set up a lab in his basement, with a microscope and slides, and prepared himself for his future profession. He did well in school. He was good with his hands. When the family went off to northern Michigan in the summers, he hired himself out to scale and clean the catch of summer fishermen. He finished Princeton in two years, and in 1949 he graduated with honors from Columbia Medical School. "I excelled in clinical courses, particularly in surgery, so I elected to pursue a career in surgery," he told me. With other interview subjects, I have had to edit their spoken grammar, to make it intelligible on the page. Not so with Jim Malm. Even his syntax was crisp and cutting.

He interned at Pennsylvania Hospital in Philadelphia. "A wonderful clinical experience," he told me. "Every possible wound, gunshot, abortion, alcoholism, drugs, poverty, which you really did not see at Columbia Presbyterian." He was called to active duty in the Korean War. He served as the junior medical officer and the only surgeon on the aircraft carrier *Philippine Sea*. The planes took off and bombed Korean cities. The three hundred seamen were mostly healthy. The most common operations that Malm performed were circumcisions on sailors in whom venereal disease had resulted in infected foreskins. Once, he had to perform an appendectomy during a typhoon.

"It was a big ship, and it was rocking and rolling. We had a whole flotilla, so forty boats had to slow down. That was my only moment of power in my two years at sea," he remembered. "The entire 7th Fleet had to slow down to stabilize the operating table until I finished."

He returned to New York for his medical residency. One winter day, a terrible snowstorm blanketed Manhattan. The regular surgical resident on call for chest surgery could not make it in to work. Malm was technically on vacation, but he had stayed home for his break. His apartment was near the hospital, and he volunteered to help out in the OR, where he assisted on a lung operation.

"I was introduced to chest surgery, and I became enchanted," he said. "That was when I got a bee. I thought this was the greatest thing I'd ever seen. Then and there I decided to become a heart surgeon. It meant a couple of additional years of training, but my wife didn't mind."

During the years that he trained as a thoracic surgeon, the whole discipline of chest surgery changed. The heart-lung machine was introduced. When I asked him about his initial interest in pediatrics, Malm cut me off. "You must understand the original cardiac surgery, the first open-heart surgery, was for congenital heart disease." He wasn't so much interested in kids; he was interested in hearts.

In the late 1950s, Griffiths, Blumenthal, and Malm were all around thirty years old, just beginning their careers in medicine, and heart surgery was medicine's furthest frontier. Then Himmelstein got sick, and Malm—who not long before had been floating in the Korean Sea circumcising priapic sailors—was put in charge. The opportunity he dreamed of was suddenly thrust upon him.

Was he intimidated? I asked.

"Never occurred to me."

What was the hardest thing in learning to repair a child's heart?

"Nothing," he said. "Piece of cake, as they say."

As Sylvia Griffiths described it to me, the first cases that were fed to Malm were simple ones: atrial septal defects (holes between the heart's top two chambers) and ventricular septal defects (holes between the heart's bottom two chambers). Gradually they built up toward more complicated cases, like Danny Spandau's tetralogy of Fallot.

Malm was young, he was strong, he was smart, and he was well trained and observant. One of his students, John Norman, writing about stress that affects heart surgeons, described Malm's preternatural calm. "Cardiac surgery, for cardiac surgeons, was thought of as an emerging specialty aptly characterized by periods of prolonged boredom interspersed with anticipated, or, worse, unanticipated episodes of sheer terror. Even then, we of the lower echelons had noted and remarked (in his absence) that during such moments, [Malm's] affect appeared to become somewhat blunted, while his cognitive processes and technical performances simultaneously became more incisive and effective—admirable and enviable capabilities in coping with sudden intraoperative stress."

As we discussed his breakthrough surgeries, Malm tried to push attention away from his success. "I was in the top echelon of surgeons at the time, but there were other programs doing almost as well." This was not true; he was the best. "Everything just fell into place. I learned the anatomy for congenital heart disease. A lot of people didn't quite understand the anatomy. It wasn't experimental surgery, it wasn't pioneering surgery, it was something carefully planned out and carried out. I found my niche somehow. Everything was easy, fun, exciting, and rewarding. It was all the training in the right time in the history of cardiac surgery, so I felt very lucky to be at the right place and the right time. I came into the program in the 1960s, quite confident that I knew as much as anyone in the field. It was just magic."

Which were his most exciting moments? I asked.

"Every morning. Getting to that OR. You betcha. I miss it today."

There was no apparent learning curve. He was successful right away. Patient after patient survived, their defects corrected and their little hearts beating. Or as he put it, "No one was allowed to die."

Malm's system of repair for tetralogy of Fallot, the algorithm he published with Sylvia Griffiths in 1963, seems almost obvious in retrospect: (1) close the ventricular septal defect so there's no leak; (2) open up the obstruction so blood can flow to the lungs; (3) use an outflow patch in place of the pulmonary valve to let the blood flow freely; and (4) leave the heart muscle intact. The first two are plumber's observations, which holes are to be closed and which opened, but in the early 1960s, closing these holes required extraordinary skill. Even now with 3-D imaging of hearts and echocardiography at the surgical bedside, it can be difficult to identify each hole inside the webby, messy musculature of a deformed heart. Malm had to do it with finger and eye. The third is a risk calculation learned collectively by cardiologists over time: a child could live for decades without a pulmonary valve, with decent function in the right ventricle. The fourth has something to do with Malm's training with Dorothy Andersen and his study of the pathology of the deformed infant heart, but it also has to do with surgical genius, with the hands of the man with the scalpel. No one else was able to do it as well—to get into the heart and reroute the blood flow, to cut and patch and sew, and to do it all so gingerly, so gracefully, that the muscle itself was left undamaged. Those first forty-one straight successful tetralogy cases were an astonishment.

—

Welton Gersony hardly smiled in the first half hour of my interview with him. He was serious in his purpose and careful in his explanations. He was generous with me. There were suitcases half packed on the sofa; he and his wife were heading off to Florida later that day. He had no time to play the jovial host.

Still, when he described reading Malm's article in *Circulation*, he acted it out for me. He turned comedian. His jaw dropped. He looked up from the imaginary journal in his hands and bugged his eyes.

"I couldn't believe it." He grinned.

9.

THESE DAYS I deal with my heart in two ways, mostly the same ways that many people cope with mortality: there's panic, and there's denial. When my heart is healthy, I worry that it's sick. When it's sick, I pretend everything's fine. I have no idea what's happening inside my chest, and I'm not alone. The history of human misunderstanding of the heart is thick with worship, mystification, and denial.

When the Egyptians mummified their dead, they drew out all the organs (the brain was pulled out through the nose so as not to break the head and face) except the heart, which was preserved alone inside the corpse in the sarcophagus. Against the wishes of the popes, crusaders boiled the flesh off their dead but kept the hearts and sent them home along with the skeletons. The heart was the seat of intelligence for Aristotle, of human feeling for Shakespeare, and according to Deuteronomy and Proverbs, the part of the body on which to inscribe the words of God. No one in the West knew how the heart functioned—and if that news ever hit Europe, the Europeans shut their ears in denial. In the thirteenth century in what is now Syria, the great physician Ala al-Din ibn Al Nafis correctly described the pulmonary transit of the blood, but for hundreds of years his discoveries were lost or willfully ignored by the Christian world.

In Shakespeare's *Henry VI, Part 3*, Richard Plantagenet becomes enraged and describes his heart as follows:

I cannot weep, for all my body's moisture
Scarce serves to quench my furnace-burning heart;
Nor can my tongue unload my heart's great burden
For the self-same wind, that I should speak withal
Is kindling coals that fire all my breast
And burns me up with flames, that tears would quench.

As Richard sees it, his heart is a furnace, and his feelings of anger make it burn at high temperatures, causing the hot blood to rush up to his head and evaporate all the water there, so that no tears can come from his eyes. The fire sucks the wind down his throat, too, so he cannot speak. In Stratford-on-Avon in 1591, this was not just high-flown poetry; it was up-to-date physiology. Richard's heart works the way the leading medical men of the time said it would.

For Shakespeare and his contemporaries, knowledge about the heart was drawn from a combination of Christianity and classical learning, from the Bible and from the writings of Galen of Pergamon, the great Roman physician, who in the Renaissance came to dominate European anatomical thought. Galen offered a holistic understanding of the body, a comprehensible system that replaced scattered views of diseases as caused by imps, curses, witches, and sins.

Galen began his career as a gladiator's doctor and rose to become physician to the emperor Marcus Aurelius. He liked to demonstrate his superiority to other doctors through competitive vivisections. Once he sliced open a live ape and eviscerated it, challenging other doctors to put the organs back in their proper places. When they could not, Galen reassembled the animal himself. He showed off his understanding of the nervous system by taking a squealing pig and cutting the nerves of its throat one by one, until finally he severed the laryngeal nerve—cutting the one nerve that would make the pig mute.

According to Galen, the key to good health was balance. Bodies should never get too hot or too cold, too moist or too dry. The body was governed by four humors—phlegm, which came from the lungs; choler, which came from the gall bladder; black bile or melancholy, which came from the spleen; and blood, which came from the liver—and these humors had to stay in equilibrium. Fever and inflammation came from a plethora, or excess, of blood, and so most diseases and infections could be cured by bloodletting.

Because Roman physicians did not cut into human bodies, Galen based his studies on dissections of animals, and this led to some crucial errors in his anatomy. Galen believed, for instance, that the human liver had five lobes, like a dog's, and that these five lobes gripped the stomach. He saw the mass of arteries at the base of the skulls of cattle and believed these existed in human beings. He called them the *rete mirabile*.

According to Galen, digested food traveled from the stomach to the liver in a substance called chyle. The liver turned the chyle into natural spirits, which nourished the body. Blood moved like the tides, back and forth, the organs gathering natural spirits toward them as was necessary. Some of the blood went to the right ventricle of the heart, and some of it went to the lungs. According to Galen, the septum of the heart had tiny, invisible pores within its trabeculated mass of muscle. The blood ran through these pores into the left ventricle, where it mixed with the air from the lungs. Air contained pneuma, the life force. Through a process known as concoction, the natural spirits in the blood mixed with the pneuma from the air. It was heated in the furnace of the heart, and when the heart expanded, the concocted blood shot upward toward the brain. In the *rete mirabile*, the natural spirits and pneuma were converted into animal spirits, which ran from the brain down through the nerves, enlivening the body.

This was what Shakespeare believed, and Leonardo Da Vinci, too. Leonardo, as observant a man as ever lived, drew a five-lobed human liver like a dog's and a heart with tiny passages in the septum, following Galen's descriptions over what he might otherwise have independently perceived with his own hand and eye. Galen's theories were enforced not just through culture but by laws and violence. A doctor in England or France could lose his license for contradicting Galen. In 1553, Michael Servetus published his claim that there were no pores in the center of the heart and that blood and air met and mingled in the lungs. For this, he was declared a heretic and had to flee the Catholic Inquisition in France. He went to Geneva, where the Protestants hated him too. John Calvin ordered Servetus burned at the stake, along with every copy of his book. But even as Servetus was burning to death, three hundred miles to the east in Padua, researchers were beginning to agree that Galen's description of the heart was inaccurate.

My struggle is everyone's struggle: it's so hard to know your own heart.

10.

IN MY LAST visit with Sylvia Griffiths, she tried to indicate something that might be of concern—that my heart might not have been completely repaired in surgery. She put an X-ray of my teenaged chest on the light panel in her office and described the enlargement of my heart.

"Is that a bad thing?" my mother asked.

"From a poetic point of view, no," said Dr. Griffiths.

An X-ray is an imprecise tool. It offers only a shadow, an outline. It indicates the heart's enlargement, but it doesn't say which part is getting bigger. An echocardiogram, too, is imperfect. Especially in the 1980s, when echocardiography was young, it was difficult to say year to year exactly how or whether my heart continued to get bigger. I graduated from Dr. Griffiths's pediatric practice with an unspoken, unexamined conviction that nothing was wrong with me. It was a conviction I had cultivated all my life.

I remember one time when I was little, my friends and I were playing pirates, and we tried to imagine what we would have been like if we had *really* been born in the time of the pirates. I said, "Well, I guess I'd be dead," and that stopped our game for a minute. But then we got right back to it, crossing swords and hopping across furniture and waving the pretend Jolly Roger.

Walking to school with some other boys, I speculated cheerfully that by the time I was fifty, I'd probably be dead—a kind of lunatic, childish boasting. Being fifty seemed as unreal as being dead. A passerby stopped me and said, "Hey, kid, don't talk that way." I was brought up short, and it was embarrassing. Mostly, I tried not to think about my heart and surgery. I was a skinny kid, no great athlete, but in elementary school I could participate— never picked first for a team but never left out. Occasionally, my condition was acknowledged, but this always surprised me. One time at summer camp, the other kids were going to throw me into the lake, but then another camper said, "Careful, careful—he had heart surgery!" It was a bummer. All the cool kids in my cabin were getting thrown in the lake.

A friend of my parents, Zale Bernstein, a big, bearded hippy, sat on the couch in our living room and said, "So he's fine? He just goes on with his life? Jesus—a medical miracle!" I was startled. I didn't think of myself that way—I didn't want to know what those words meant.

Sickness is, historically, a shameful thing. Susan Sontag writes persuasively about the way the healthy tend to blame the sick for their illnesses and also how the sick tend to blame themselves. Again, she quotes Karl Menninger: "Illness is in part what the world has done to the victim, but in a larger part it is what the victim has done with his world, and with himself." For Menninger, illness is the result of a diseased psyche, a willed action on the part of the sick person.

As a kid, as a teenager, as a young adult, I was determined never to be the victim. I had learned from an early age to disguise and deny my symptoms, to act healthy even when unwell. Menninger's belief, as Sontag demonstrates, has a long medical, literary, and philosophical history. She quotes Arthur Schopenhauer: "The will exhibits itself as an organized body... and the presence of disease signifies that the will itself is sick." Patients frequently absorb this idea and come to see their diseases as expressions of the failure of their personalities. Sontag quotes Franz Kafka: "Secretly I don't believe this illness to be tuberculosis, at least not primarily tuber- culosis, but rather a sign of my general bankruptcy." My will was all about overcompensation and a desire to be strong.

If, in my waking hours, I did my best not to think about my heart, in the night it came to me, but not in specific worries about

ventricles or valves. I imagined death, absence, nothingness. I remember crawling out of bed, unable to sleep, and going to my
parents' room and trying to explain my fears. My mother held me
close. Her atheism is real. She was never going to offer me things
she did not believe in. We come from nothing, she said; we go to
nothing.

I remember seventh-grade biology and the diagrams of the
zygote splitting in the womb, a map of oblivion at the cellular level.
I sat there in my little plastic molded chair. I gripped the attached
plywood laminate desk. The floor opened beneath the chair legs.

"Oh, God, oh, God," I'd whisper.

Terry Pratchett says pleading with God for help makes as much
sense as trying to argue with a thunderstorm. I don't disagree, but
prayer is something I do, something I did as a kid every time I
thought of oblivion, and something I still do as an adult every time
I get rolled into an operating room on a gurney. I pray when I'm
frightened the same way I laugh when I'm amused. Intellectually,
I'm agnostic and irreligious. God as bearded, law-giving father
seems no more or less likely to exist than God as elephant-headed
boy who beats a tambourine. Still, I pray. I distrust people who say
they never pray. I distrust them the same way I distrust people who
say they never masturbate. If they're telling the truth, the more
reason to pity them—they've never learned to touch themselves in
a place that feels so comforting.

Every year, I went to the hospital, and walked in my underpants
into the cold, white-tiled X-ray room, and pressed my chest to an
icy pane of glass, left side, right side, front, and back. The technicians in their goggles and lead smocks focused the giant gun, told
me to stand still, then left the room, and the light flashed. Later,
as the technology developed, I got echocardiograms. I lay shirtless
in the dark room on the table, my chest covered with stickers and
electrical leads. A single technician—usually a resident, or an intern,
or a fellow in pediatric cardiology, more often than not a young
woman—applied clear jelly to a transducer wand and rubbed that
wand and jelly across my chest. I was a small, virginal fifteen-year-
old boy, and the pretty young doctor sat close to me on the medical

bed, her hip against my naked side and her hair hanging down. She'd say, "Closer," and nudge me. She'd lean across me, and she'd run the shockingly cold, slimy transducer wand across my chest. On a video screen behind her appeared the sonogram image of my beating heart, of each chamber and of each valve, these images appearing in gray scale in a conical field like a radar screen, with the blood flow plumes illustrated in red and blue, and I would pretend not to be afraid or aroused. I would pretend everything was just normal.

When I was a teenager, when I was in my twenties, I wore what's called a Holter monitor for one twenty-four-hour period annually. In those days the device was about the size of an old Sony Walkman, attached to the hip with a harness and to the chest with stickers and electrical leads, recording each heartbeat over the course of a day. It was so embarrassing to wear that to high school. I wore a big plaid shirt and kept it untucked. I kept my coat on. I kept my distance from everyone in the lunchroom and the subway. I went jogging with it, just to prove to my doctors that all was well. I never had much endurance. It was hard for me to run a mile, but I would push myself in those jogs with the Holter monitor, and at the end of the little jog, I would sprint—determined to prove to my doctors that I was strong. All those tests felt like interrogations, like my doctors were trying to ferret something out of me. The Hungarian writer Frigyes Karinthy, in his 1939 memoir about brain cancer, *Journey Around My Skull*, writes,

> The medical examination and confinement in the hospital of a patient before he is treated exactly corresponds to the detention of an accused man before trial. The accused has only one idea in his head—namely, is he going to be declared guilty and if so, what will the sentence be? Whichever way the verdict runs, he is bound to suffer a certain punishment from the fact that he has publicly come under suspicion.

When I wore those Holter monitors, I never let myself consider the obvious question: What were the doctors looking for? I clung to my innocence, in both senses of the word. I conceived of my good health as a kind of personal virtue. I could not believe that I might be sick. Now I know that if in the 1980s the monitor had turned up what the doctors feared—evidence of the kinds of cardiac arrhythmias that killed other tet kids, the kinds of arrhythmias from which I now suffer—there was really no way they could have cured me. The treatments I get now for my arrhythmias have been invented within the past twenty-five years. Did I know anyone else who had to wear a Holter monitor, who had to submit to echocardiograms? Was this all really just to satisfy doctors' curiosity? My only thought was that I would prove to them that I was normal.

With girls, I was shy and physically restrained. As a little kid before surgery, I always had to restrain myself from any impulse to action—not to run, not to jump, not to dance or get too excited—and I wonder if this reinforced my tendencies to withdraw, to watch, and to stand apart. The more interested I got in girls, the more I thought the scar on my chest would turn them off. Even into my late twenties, I was embarrassed by the scar.

The truth is, no one has ever found it repulsive. Every woman I've ever slept with has touched and run her finger down my scar. My first college girlfriend wrote a poem about it after we broke up, how despite the Teflon in my heart, she was still stuck on me. Friends have used it metaphorically, when they're drunk and expansive, telling me what a good guy I am—despite the surgeries and the scars, wow, Gabe, what a big heart.

The truth is, it's nothing to hide. Most people tend to be sympathetic. If they care at all, women tend to be impressed. Some even find it attractive. Not too long ago, I saw a young barista in Brooklyn dressed to show off his chest and its scar from childhood heart surgery, like it was a cool tattoo, like he was doing a St. Sebastian look. Me, I always kept the second button of my shirt carefully buttoned.

I once heard a cardiologist say that an average repaired tetralogy case functions at about 75 percent the level of an average healthy heart, but that's by nature a fuzzy number, the intersection of two bell curves. As a kid, as a teenager, I wasn't fast. I wasn't strong. I couldn't jump high. My endurance was poor. I was skinny. But all I did every day after school from when I was seven years old to when I was about seventeen was sports. The neighborhood kids and I went to the park, and we played four-on-four games of touch football or soccer. There are narrow strips of dirt on the fields from 107th Street to 109th Street where we beat the ground so regularly that grass could never grow.

The sweet gum trees dropped their burr balls, the muggers stole our calculator watches, the graffiti artists festooned the walls with outrageous letters and faces and raucous colored art, and we played ultimate Frisbee, every day, three-on-three, four-on-four, five-on-five. My friends were good. I was less good. But I was still part of the little club team we formed, and we competed against and beat some of the best high school teams in the city. I was devoted to it, every day, pushing myself to keep up with kids who were faster and stronger and had better endurance than I did, good athletes with normal hearts. I had fun. Heart surgery was something in the past. That's how I thought about it.

Dr. Griffiths was a particularly kind and encouraging soul. In those days her Prince Valiant hair cut was gray, not white, but the East Coast aristocratic drawl was just the same. I never guessed at her eminent status—that she had been there at the founding of the pediatric cardiology program at Columbia, that she had coauthored the major paper on my birth defect. She was a nice older woman with somewhat formal manners, someone else's grandmother substituting for my own. Dr. Griffiths didn't want me to think of myself as a sick person. Other doctors at other hospitals sent kids like me for regular cardiac catheter exams, overnight studies in the hospital to see how their hearts were holding up. Dr. Griffiths didn't want me lying on the operating room table or waking up in recovery. I remember her telling me about one of her patients who had just joined the Marine Corps. She liked me to think there would be no limit to what I could do.

When I was eighteen, I transitioned out of her care, and my case was taken over by Dr. Marlon Rosenbaum. In the early 1980s, there was no such medical field as adult congenital cardiology—the medical discipline that focuses on people like me. In 1975, in England, Dr. Jane Somerville had hypothesized the field, foreseeing that there would be a need for it, that children like me would survive and would need specialized doctors to treat them in their adulthood. In 1980 at the University of California at Los Angeles, Dr. Joseph Perloff founded the first adult congenital heart disease (ACHD) center in the United States, but the number of ACHD patients was relatively small. Very few pediatric heart patients had survived into adulthood.

As I write, there are roughly 2.4 million patients in the United States with congenitally defective hearts. A little more than half of them are adults, and this is new—according to the Adult Congenital Heart Association, enough congenital heart patients have survived into adulthood that we now, for the first time ever, outnumber the kids. More and more of us are surviving longer and longer, living into middle age and beyond. I heard a doctor say that in the next couple of decades, we will begin to need geriatric congenital cardiologists. Our numbers will continue to grow. But the field of adult congenital cardiology is barely out of its infancy. It's only in the past decade that the American College of Cardiology has recognized adult congenital heart disease as a subdiscipline. The first board-certifying exam for adult congenital cardiology was given in 2015. Criteria are just now being established to certify hospitals as being accredited ACHD care centers. To this day, most adult congenital heart disease patients don't see the appropriate specialist. The Adult Congenital Heart Association—the largest US nonprofit association studying the field—approximates that somewhere in the neighborhood of 90 percent of adults living with moderate to severe heart defects are not being treated by the appropriate, qualified physician.

I had no idea how lucky I was. Marlon Rosenbaum had never trained to be an adult congenital cardiologist—that training didn't exist when he was younger—but in the 1990s, in collaboration with Welton Gersony, he was writing one of the early textbooks on congenital heart disease in adults, and he was beginning to train the first generation of residents and fellows in the field. I was as fortunate to fall into his hands as I had been to fall into the hands of Dr. Malm—Dr. Rosenbaum was the only doctor in New York City whose practice focused on people like me—but as a high school senior in 1984, I didn't see it that way. I didn't think of myself as sick, and I didn't like going to doctors.

I have come to admire Marlon tremendously. I trust him about my heart as much as I'm capable of trusting a human being about anything. I have developed a real affection for the man. I love him in all his brilliance and awkwardness. But at first I didn't. Dr. Rosenbaum came to adult congenital cardiology from electrophysiology, a highly intellectualized field studying electrical patterns of the heart. He did not coddle me the way Dr. Griffiths had. He wasn't fatherly or avuncular, and in his early days on the job, he didn't have a great bedside manner. He was a rumpled, distracted guy, young enough to be my cousin, hair uncombed, cheeks sometimes unshaven. Once, when I was on his examination table, he took his stethoscope from my chest and said, "You know, Gabriel, they're not that far from building an artificial heart." I suppose he meant this as comforting and maybe as the sort of thing that might interest an intelligent patient. But I was insulted. He scared the crap out of me. Why the fuck would I ever need an artificial heart? I was healthy! Didn't he know that? My life depended on shutting my eyes to the state of my heart. I quote here from William James:

> Happiness, like every other emotional state, has blindness and insensibility to opposing facts given it as its instinctive weapon against disturbance. . . . To the man actively happy, from whatever cause, evil simply cannot then and there be believed in. He must ignore it; and to the bystander he may then seem perversely to shut his eyes to it and to hush it up.

Dr. Griffiths had seen me as a success story. For her I was part of the march of progress and a break from the sick kids she saw every day, struggling before or after heart surgery. She allowed me to continue in my happiness, in my blindness, and I loved her for it.

Dr. Rosenbaum saw my case more critically. He had to view my life with a longer field of vision. It was in his character to be much more clinical and reserved. What would I be like in the next ten, or twenty, or fifty years, if I lived that long? He was thinking about what might make my heart fall apart, and he was trying to forestall catastrophe.

The difference in the two doctors' views was most evident in the way they saw my right ventricle. For pediatric cardiologists after Malm, it was dogma. Surgeons put an outflow patch in the place of the obstructed pulmonary valve, and the kids did well. Everyone believed that tetralogy patients after surgery tolerated the leakage very well and did not need a pulmonary valve. Through the first decades of pediatric cardiology, doctors had been focused on infants, getting them to adulthood, not on adults, getting them to middle age. So mine was a new kind of problem. People with normal hearts don't typically develop problems with their pulmonary valves. Marlon saw people like me coming into his office— people whose blood was running backward in their hearts—and he wondered if he should take action.

He was in a tricky position, going against the orthodoxy of the 1980s and 1990s. His situation in some ways wasn't that different from Malm's and Griffiths's in 1960, going ahead with open-heart surgery on tetralogy patients when their lives could easily be extended with a Blalock shunt. There was no data on people like me, no sense of what would happen to an enlarged heart like mine as it aged. There weren't enough patients yet. There were no protocols to follow with congenital heart patients my age. The dangers of valve replacement surgery on someone like me were not negligible. Each time a patient is subjected to open-heart surgery, the risks of damage to the muscle and the conduction system increase exponentially. Rosenbaum in 1990 was working in a medical discipline that did not yet exist, but he suspected against the consensus of US pediatric cardiologists that I should be given a new valve before my right ventricle collapsed and I went into right-sided heart failure. For him, the risks of inaction likely outweighed the risks of surgery.

As for me, I had no sense that there was anything remarkable about my heart (except that it had been fixed) and no sense of my doctor's strange place in the world of US cardiology. I felt fine in my early twenties. It was nearly impossible for me to believe that I was in danger. I had no limits on my activities. I had no symptoms, no palpitations. I drank a little too much alcohol and never went to the gym, and the one time I decided to reform myself and go jogging in the park, I pulled up after a quarter of a mile. I remember my roommate saying, "Gabe, what are you going to do about that?" My answer, which I never said aloud, was to stop exercising.

Dr. Rosenbaum assigned me a stress test. I rode a bicycle with a breathing mask attached to my face and EKG wires all over my chest. When the technicians asked me why I'd been assigned the test, I told them I really didn't know. When I asked them, after the test, how I had done, they said, "Okay. No real evidence of heart disease." I wanted to take their words and wave them in front of Dr. Rosenbaum's face.

He looked over the results of the stress test and my latest echocardiogram. He said he wanted to do a cardiac catheter exam. He wanted to admit me to the hospital for the night, run a wire into my heart, test its pressures, and see how that right ventricle was doing.

I refused to take the test.

He sighed. He swiveled in his chair. Marlon's a phlegmatic guy, with a manner so calm he can sometimes seem sleepy. "Okay," he said. "But next year I might twist your arm a little."

I hated him for saying that. I called my friends. I called my family to complain. I didn't want a doctor who wanted to *twist my arm*.

"Maybe you should get a different doctor," people told me.

I came back for my next appointment. I lay on the bed in the dark room of the echocardiology lab. The woman who performed the exam, very attractive, businesslike, thin, and of south Asian descent, had me take off my shirt and lie on the table. She squeezed the clear jelly on my chest. She told me to lie close to her, and she sat on the table, and my naked skin was pressed close against her skirt. The room was dark. Her perfume smelled good. We were alone in the dark, but at that moment my eyes and attention were not on her body but on the monitor of her echocardiogram machine, on the pictures of my right ventricle, on the mysterious patterns of leak and blood flow.

I went back from the echocardiogram lab to Dr. Rosenbaum's examination room and waited for him. He entered with a file in his hand and a frown on his face. He was the frustrated detective. I was the squirrely criminal. He wanted to get a closer look at my heart. He wanted me to spend a night in the hospital. He wanted to guide a wire into my heart and to measure its pressures. I was twenty-eight years old. I did the only thing I was capable of doing. I ran from him.

11.

GALEN'S VISION OF the heart held until the age of discovery. While sailing ships explored the globe and telescopes charted the skies, the knives of anatomists mapped the body. In Italy, Gabriele Fallopio identified the tube that ran between the ovary and uterus. He also named the placenta, which in Latin means "cake." Bartolomeo Eustachi located the canal in the ear that is named for him. In 1559, Realdo Colombo claimed to discover the clitoris. Colombo's teacher, Andreas Vesalius, was one of the great translators and editors of Galen's works and one of Galen's sharpest critics. Vesalius shook medical knowledge free of classical authority.

Before Vesalius, dissections and anatomy lessons were always carried out in reference to Greek and Roman works. The body of an executed convict was laid out for the medical students to see, and a *sector*, a local barber or surgeon, cut into the corpse. An *ostentor*, often one of the senior medical students, pointed out the body part to be discussed. The *lector*, the professor himself, sitting in the cathedra above, read from a text, usually Galen, to describe what the students were looking at. Vesalius's great innovation was *autopsia*, literally, "see for yourself." He did the cutting, he did the pointing, and he did the describing—based on what he observed and not on a text. As the great medical historian Roy Porter puts it, "Vesalius interrogated Galen by reference to the human corpse." What Galileo did for the skies, Vesalius did for the body, moving authority from the ancient text to the living eye.

He was born in Brussels and educated in France, when medical school was a quasi-religious institution. (Medical students in Paris in the early 1500s had to remain celibate over the course of their studies.) Vesalius did not confine his interest to books; he was interested in bodies. He snuck out of school to examine the bones of the plague dead in the Cemetière des Invalides. In 1536, war chased Vesalius out of Paris and back home to Louvain, but he continued his investigations. One day, walking outside the walls of the city, he came upon the body of a thief "which had been partially burned and roasted over a fire of straw and then bound to a stake." The skeleton had been picked clean by birds, and so "the bones were entirely bare and held together only by the ligaments." Then he did something extraordinary:

> Observing the body to be dry and nowhere moist or rotten, I took advantage of this unexpected but welcome opportunity. . . . I climbed the stake and pulled the femur away from the hipbone. Upon my tugging, the scapulae with the arms and hands also came away. . . . After I had surreptitiously brought the legs and arms home in successive trips—leaving the head and trunk behind—I allowed myself to be shut out of the city in the evening so that I might obtain the thorax, which was held securely by a chain. So great was my desire to possess those bones that in the middle of the night, alone and in the midst of all those corpses, I climbed the stake with considerable effort and did not hesitate to snatch away that which I so desired. When I had pulled down the bones, I carried them some distance away and concealed them until the following day when I was able to fetch them home bit by bit through the outer gate of the city.

In Padua, Vesalius became a professor, a translator, and an editor of new editions of Galen's works, and he began to notice some of the master's errors. "There is no truth," he wrote in 1539, "in what others say about the five lobes of the liver." In the 1543 edition of his great work *De humani corporis fabrica libri septem* (*Seven Works on the Structure Human Body*, usually called the *Fabrica*), Vesalius denies the existence of the *rete mirabile* in the human body, those great vessels at the base of the brain that turn natural spirits to animal spirits. Vesalius stuck with Galen's idea that blood was manufactured in the liver, but on the subject of blood passing through the septum of the heart, he wrote that he was "greatly driven to wonder at the handiwork of the Almighty by which the blood sweats from the right to the left ventricle through passages which escape the human vision." In his revised 1555 edition of the *Fabrica*, Vesalius expresses his doubts more directly: "In considering the structure of the heart ... I have brought my words for the most part into agreement with the teachings of Galen, not because I thought that these were on every point in harmony with the truth, but because I still distrust myself. But the septum of the heart is thick, dense, and compact as the rest of the heart. I do not therefore know, in what way even the smallest particle can be transferred [through it]."

Realdo Colombo, Vesalius's student and later his adversary (and, yes, the guy who discovered the clitoris), went further: "Between the ventricles of the heart ... is the septum, through which nearly everyone thinks that there is a way open for the blood to pass. ... But those who believe this err by a long way." In his lectures, Colombo described the movement of blood from one ventricle to the other via the pulmonary artery and the lungs. "Blood is carried to the lung by the pulmonary vein ... and in the lung it is refined, and then together with the air it is brought through the pulmonary vein to the left ventricle of the heart."

In 1600, William Harvey arrived in Padua to study. Harvey was the son of a wealthy yeoman from Kent. He was short, fierce, ruddy, ambitious, and always well armed. In England as a young man, he had witnessed no public dissections of human corpses or vivisections of animals; his Cambridge anatomical education had focused on the classics, but he had read Vesalius and Colombo. Harvey's professor in Padua, Girolamo Fabrizi, worked under the name Fabricus; he was an older man whose anatomy lessons were celebrations of the human body intended to "display the glory of nature no less than did the circus games and gymnastics of antiquity."

Everyone came to the theater to see Fabricus perform: "teach-ers, tailors, shoemakers, sandal-makers, butchers, salted fish dealers, porters, basket-bearers . . . money-lenders, and barbers," according to Harvey's biographer, Thomas Wright. The rectors of the city and the university wore ceremonial gowns, as did the professors of anatomy. The body was dissected in a chamber underneath the anatomy theater and, at the appropriate time, raised up through a trap door, while musicians played on the lute. Fabricus, seated and wearing purple and gold robes, read from classical anatomical texts, while his assistant, his *ostentor*, pointed at the relevant body parts with a rod. The performances began in early morning and went on late into the day. No one was allowed to chat or laugh, especially not during demonstrations of female anatomy. Porters tried to keep the peace. After the body was examined, the lesson would continue with vivisections of animals, the howls of the dogs accompanied by music.

Harvey returned to England with his prestigious Italian medical education. He married rich and rose up the ranks of London doc-tors, becoming president of the College of Physicians and physician to the king—first James I, then Charles II. He was sworn to uphold Galen's teachings and to prosecute physicians who contradicted them. Publicly, Harvey was intellectually conventional. Privately, he was something else.

He came home from days as a London doctor and performed experiments by candlelight. He brought home dogs and cats and deer and calves, tied them down to his dissection table in his li-brary, gagged the animals, and cut them open to examine their naked beating hearts. In the candlelight, with the blood and the squirming of the panicked animal, it was hard to see. Harvey found that he was able to observe the heartbeat more closely when viv-isecting cold-blooded animals, fish, snakes, and lizards. He was able to observe how the heart relaxed in diastole and squeezed in systole. He filled a right ventricle of a heart with water, squeezed it, and proved that no liquid could travel through the septum. In vivisections of mammals, he punctured the aorta, which burst like a balloon. With each contraction, he saw a massive, explosive spurt. By measuring the outflow, Harvey was able to calculate how much blood was moved by every heartbeat. He multiplied the quantity in each beat to determine how much blood moved each minute, each hour, and came up with a massive quantity of blood, too large to be produced by the liver every day. Where would all that blood come from? Where would it go?

Harvey had caves dug in his garden, and alone at night he crawled into these caves and meditated on the structure of the heart. He encountered a patient with a hole in his side—the young nobleman had had an accident as a child, and the wound had healed to leave a cavity in his ribcage. Harvey brought his patient to the king. He reached his fingers inside the young man and touched the beating heart. He had the king do the same. It shook them—the heart, the center of human feeling, the place where the soul resided, could be touched, just like a face or a hand.

Back home, he called his servants into his study and experimented on them, ligating their arms, watching their fingers and hands go bloodless. He saw that the blood could only run in one direction, away from the heart through the arteries and back to the heart through the veins. It became clear to him: there was a fixed amount of blood in the body, and it went around in a circle, from the heart to the lungs, back to the heart, out to the body through the arteries, then back to the heart through the veins.

Harvey's conclusion verged on the unspeakable. As everyone had understood it to that point, the blood of the hand stayed in the hand, and the blood of the feet stayed in the feet. Harvey's notion was almost as shocking as if he were arguing that the bones of the skeleton were slowly moving around in a circle, exchanging parts with each other. It was also illegal, a violation of the professional code Harvey had sworn to uphold. The statutes of the British College of Physicians explicitly forbade its members from contradicting Galen in any way—and Harvey was its president. He published his findings as *Exercitatio anatomica de motu cordis et sanguinis in animalibus* (*An Anatomical Exercise on the Motion of the Heart and Blood in Living Beings*, usually referred to as *De motu cordis*). He coined a term for this new movement of the blood, "circulation." He said, "I do not believe that my theory destroys Galenic medicine, rather it enhances it." His colleagues did not concur.

If the blood was circulating around and around in the body, then the humors would be confused all the time—and according to Galen the confusion of the humors was the essence of disease. Furthermore, if the body maintained a constant supply of blood, then bleeding as a medical treatment made little sense. To bleed an infected leg could cause no relief; the blood from the rest of the body would move there. Harvey was cautious. He insisted he was making no challenge to bloodletting at all: "Daily experience satisfies us that [bleeding] has a most salutary effect in many diseases." Skeptics made larger, empirical challenges. Harvey could not explain how the blood got from the arteries to the veins; the capillaries would not be discovered until 1661, so there was a gap in his circulatory system. He also could not explain the purpose of circulation—what Aristotle called its "final cause." In Harvey's time, no one knew what oxygen was or what cells were.

For decades, his theory faced resistance. Doctors would not relinquish their devotion to Galen or to bloodletting. For 150 years after he died, Harvey's vision of the heart and blood had little effect on the work of the ordinary physician. As Thomas Jefferson wrote in 1806, "Harvey's discovery of the circulation of the blood was a beautiful addition to our knowledge of the animal economy, but on a review of the practice of medicine before and since that epoch, I do not see any great amelioration which has been derived from that discovery." Doctors kept on bleeding their patients to cool fevers or reduce swelling or mitigate what was diagnosed as a plethora of blood. When in 1799 George Washington had a fever and a sore throat, he got the same kind of medical treatment that would have been delivered to a European patient in the time of Michael Servetus during the Middle Ages. Washington's doctors blistered his throat with Spanish fly, and it swelled up so he couldn't swallow or breathe. They drained two pints of his blood before bed and a quart more in the morning, taking out nearly half the blood in his body. They killed him. The great seventeenth-century anatomists mapped the heart and circulatory systems, but it would be years before doctors could learn to navigate these charts. The word "cardiologist" would not appear until the 1920s.

This book recounts my particular struggle to come to terms with my particular heart—my defect, my surgeries, and the risks to my life—but when I look at the history of medicine, my experience feels like the whole in miniature, a tiny, revealing example of a great historical reckoning. It seems human nature not to want to look too closely at the function of the heart.

12.

I N THE FALL of 2017, I saw Dr. Jamil Aboulhosn, head of the
UCLA adult congenital heart disease (ACHD) program, speak
to doctors and medical students at New York–Presbyterian. He
was there to talk about single-ventricle heart conditions, but very
early in his talk he was careful to address what he called the psy-
chosocial aspect of care for ACHD patients. Many of them, Dr.
Aboulhosn cautioned, have undergone multiple open-heart surgeries before the age of ten, and so as adults they have developed
a fear of medicine, what Aboulhosn called almost a posttraumatic
stress disorder.

"This is the reason so many fall out of care," he said.

Most adult congenital patients go years or even decades avoid-
ing the care they require. In the first visit with such a patient, Dr.
Aboulhosn warned the assembled doctors, "Don't bring up the
T-word, 'transplant.' That's one way to make sure they won't come
back and see you."

His audience laughed in recognition.

Why do so many patients fall out of care? This is the deep ocean
of my subject. I asked Mark Roeder, president of the Adult Congenital Heart Association (ACHA), if there were some geograph-
ical, economic, or educational factors determining who stayed in
care and who fell out, and he only shrugged. There's little solid
data. Most US numbers on patients lost to care are approximations
based on statistics garnered in Canada, where because of the national health system, doctors can accurately keep track of patients

with congenital heart disease. In the United States we can only project those ratios onto our population.

Some patients lose their medical insurance and simply can't afford a hospital echocardiogram. Others are geographically distant from the right doctor. If you live in Idaho, you have to fly to the Mayo Clinic in Minnesota to reach the closest ACHD center. If you're feeling well and money is tight, you might not want to pay for a ticket every year. But a lot of us avoid doctors because we simply don't want to think of ourselves as sick.

"This is one of my interests as a physician, but also as a human being," said Dr. Ali N. Zaidi, an adult congenital cardiologist working at Montefiore Hospital in the Bronx. "I see patients who haven't seen a physician for twenty years, and I say, How are you feeling, and they say they're feeling fine. They don't grasp the gravity of the situation because they've been living like that for so long. That's their normality." Patients like me don't know the meaning of the word "healthy."

Dr. Zaidi is tall and thin, with a neat gray beard and a boyish, enthusiastic smile. He grew up in a family of physicians, moving from London to Karachi to the United States, and he works with pediatric and adult congenital heart disease patients. Dr. Zaidi has a particular concern for patients who are lost to care—who, as they grow up, stop seeing the appropriate cardiologist. I came to his office after meeting one such patient, Bridgette Ratliff, whose case Dr. Zaidi described as "adult congenital heart disease in a nutshell."

Bridgette, a tall, glamorous, chocolate-skinned woman, is about my age but looks younger. A dean of a public middle school and the proud mother of a charming adult daughter, Bridgette plans to retire soon from the New York City public school system and start a faith-based nonprofit helping teenaged girls in the Bronx. She is a delightful person, and she is doing great. But when she met Ali Zaidi in March 2015, she was in florid heart failure and unaware of it, and she came to the doctor almost against her will.

The first time he met her, Dr. Zaidi told me, as soon as he walked into the examining room, he could see her deteriorated condition, the fluid buildup in her belly, the fluid buildup in her legs. He knew right away she was in right-sided heart failure. But Bridgette would have none of it.

"She was like, 'I have ten minutes. My car is parked out there, and I'm going to get a ticket. I don't know why I'm seeing you.'"

She was working full-time and raising her daughter, and though she was in heart failure, Bridgette kept up a rigorous exercise routine. Every day after a long day of work she walked up three flights of stairs to her apartment. When she got home, she put on a Jillian Michaels exercise tape and jumped up and down in front of her television and did leg lifts and thrusts and stretches.

"Working out," Bridgette told me. "Working out hard."

Her coworkers could see her health was in decline. Bridgette, usually vivacious and energetic, was lethargic and tired. One day she was so exhausted after work that she parked and fell asleep for two hours in the driver's seat. But then she got up, climbed three flights of stairs, changed clothes, put on her Jillian Michaels exercise tape, and began her routine, her planks and her step aerobics.

She had fits of lightheadedness. Her memory became compromised. She could not think up words or phrases. She developed a cough typical of heart failure, a constant, wheezing cough like a smoker's cough, a sign that she wasn't getting enough oxygen, but when people asked her if she had a cold, Bridgette got angry.

"I got an attitude," she told me. "Like, *no*, I do *not* have a cold."

Ali Zaidi put a stethoscope to her chest. He could hear the top chambers of her heart running fast, way out of time with the bottom chambers.

"You're in atrial flutter right now," he told her.

Bridgette demurred. "No, I'm not."

Atrial flutter, right-sided heart failure—this was, as Dr. Zaidi explained, her normal. She didn't know what sick was because she had never experienced health. For Bridgette, this was the story of her life: trauma and denial and pushing through all her difficulties with willpower and faith in God.

She grew up in North Carolina, and for the first eight years of her life, Bridgette's heart condition was a mystery. She lived with blue lips and heart palpitations but no diagnosis. She was attended to by pediatricians and family doctors who did not understand her heart and were afraid of it.

"The doctors I saw were always in panic mode," she remembers. They were terrified when she got a cough; they feared that coughing would strain her heart. They didn't want to give her shots and vaccinations for fear of breaking her skin. "They were afraid of infection," she told me. "They said if she gets an infection, it's going to go to her heart, and she's going to die."

Once as a kid she showed up for an appointment with earrings. The doctors were aghast and made her mother take the studs out of her ears. She was forbidden from exercising. At the park, she had to sit on a bench and watch the other children play. It wasn't until her family moved to the Bronx that she started seeing a pediatric cardiologist.

"I had to go to the doctor twice a year," Bridgette remembered. "They still didn't know what was wrong. As I got older, I began to get really scared. Everyone else had a name for their disease. If they had asthma, they could explain it. But for me?" Her lips were dark. She got tired easily. She suffered palpitations. "The teachers would ask, What is it? And my mother would say, We don't know. That was the roughest part."

Finally, when she was ten years old, she got a name for her condition: Ebstein's anomaly, a congenital heart defect in which the right side of the heart develops as if it were upside down. The big pumping chamber is at the top, and the little chamber is at the bottom. The valves are abnormal. In 1973, there was nothing that could be done for a heart like Bridgette's. Her future, according to the doctors, would be one of slow, unavoidable decline. She learned to compensate for her condition and to do the best she could.

She lived in an apartment with her mother and her three older sisters. In the streets, kids played baseball, dodge ball, running bases, and volleyball. Bridgette joined them. When her heart went wonky, she'd take a break and sit on a stoop, and another kid would take her place in the game. Her friends would come over. They would touch her shirt to feel the panicked heart and call to the other children.

"Look! Look! Her heart is beating really fast!"

Bridgette could feel her heart beating in her ears, beating, she said, "like it was going to beat out." She never called an adult. She never went upstairs to her mother. She knew that if she drew attention to her condition, she would not be allowed to play, and so she developed habits of stubbornness and secrecy.

"I got used to it," she explained. "It became my identity. That's who I was in the neighborhood. Like, there was the kid with glasses. And I was Bridgette, the skinny girl with the heart condition." She did well in school. She was smart. She loved to read. And she was feisty. When other kids picked on her, she stood up for herself. She got in fights. "I had a bad heart," she told me. "There was no way I was going to be weak on top of that."

As she got older, her palpitations became more extreme. She had to stay home for college, when she really longed to go away. Though the doctors predicted that she would not live long, she pursued her career. She got a master's degree and a teaching license. When she was getting near what the doctors described as the limit of her life expectancy, she got pregnant. Her physicians felt her pregnancy might kill her. They told her that even if she brought the child to term, she would not live long enough to see it grow. Bridgette defied them.

"I wasn't going to let the doctors play God," Bridgette told me. "I figured, I'd trust their medical expertise on certain things, but when it comes to what's really important, I'm going to live my life. Twenty-eight years I'd been living with this heart condition. I'd been able to do a lot of things they said I wasn't going to be able to do. I was going to have a baby. I trusted God."

Bridgette's was a high-risk pregnancy. She was monitored carefully by a medical team. She developed difficulty breathing and was admitted to the hospital. Her daughter, Rachel, was born by caesarian section, a five-pound, beautiful child. The baby was healthy. Bridgette, though she didn't know it at the time, was not.

"The pregnancy did something to the heart," she told me. "It strained it."

One morning in 1993, when she was at work as a fifth-grade teacher, her heart went into an extreme and new kind of palpitation,

a powerful thumping in her chest that began at the start of the
school day. It was 8:30 a.m. Her heart was running a race, even
when she was standing still. She was alone in a classroom with
twenty-five students. She told the students to get to their lessons.

She's a good, experienced teacher. "A strong teacher," she told
me. With her life in the balance, a single mother with a three-year-
old daughter at home, Bridgette set the children at a task at their
desks, doing math worksheets. For hours, her heart continued its
panicked thumping. When the kids got noisy, she said, "I don't
want to hear a sound!"

At 11 a.m., it was time for lunch. She lined the children up by
size and marched them to the cafeteria, her heart firing BANG
BANG BANG all the while. She left the kids with the lunchroom
monitors and climbed the stairs back up to her classroom, her heart
pounding bloody murder.

"What was wrong with me?" she asked, as she told me her story.
"With a three-year-old daughter at home! How could I do that to
my students? From childhood, I was always like that. Very stubborn.
I was born with this heart condition, so I wasn't afraid of it. I had
no fear because it had been with me all my life. I kept saying to
myself, it's going to be fine. It's going to stop."

But it didn't stop. Alone in her quiet classroom, Bridgette sat
down at her desk. She tried to stand. She almost fainted. Finally,
when she was slipping off the edge of consciousness, Bridgette
called the principal's office. The principal came up to the classroom
and saw ashen, blue-lipped Bridgette exhausted at her desk. He
offered to call an ambulance.

"No," Bridgette said. "Let someone drive me."

In the emergency room, she collapsed. When the doctors revived her, she told them the story of how she had gone to work
and stayed at work, while her heart beat murderously in her chest.

"Two and a half hours?" they said. "You could have died!"

In 1999, Bridgette and her daughter and mother went back to
North Carolina. For a year, Bridgette took a job as an elementary
school teacher. That spring, she took her students on a class trip
to the James K. Polk historic sight in Pineville, in the suburbs of

Charlotte. She was leading the children off the buses toward the cabin in which the former president was born, when her heart finally let her down. She could not breathe. She could not walk. Her lips were so blue as to be black. But Bridgette, as was her habit, refused to admit that she was in danger.

"Somebody else would probably have gone to the hospital right away," she told me. "I just didn't. It's weird. I thought I had a summer cold."

When she finally did get to a clinic, she told me, her oxygen level tested at an impossible 67 percent. Normal blood-oxygen saturation is 95 to 100 percent; 90 percent is considered low and 80 percent dangerous. The doctor panicked.

"Oh my God!" she screamed. "You're blue!"

Bridgette, so insistent, so capable, and so seemingly strong, convinced the doctor that she was okay. She left the clinic with some antibiotics.

That was a Friday. Come Sunday, Bridgette was unable to get off the couch. She couldn't stand. She couldn't go to church. She told her mother that she was fine, but her mother insisted and called an ambulance. Bridgette was admitted for emergency heart surgery, and she left the hospital with a new heart valve.

At this point, the reader who is not an ACHD patient will assume that Bridgette must have reconciled herself to her condition and, back in New York City, must have found an appropriate doctor and submitted herself to appropriate care. The reader would be wrong. After a lifetime of terrifying crises with her heart and a recent heart surgery, Bridgette went back to her old habit: pretending everything was just fine. I can only say in her defense that she is my twin—that her story is my story. You will see, in the coming pages, that in crisis I have always behaved in much the same way that she did. We are typical of our kind—we deny weakness, defy it, and try to imagine it away. Bridgette continued to ignore her symptoms even when they were acute and crippling. Dr. Ali Zaidi was the first adult congenital cardiologist she had met in her life, and it was nearly her fiftieth birthday. There he was, offering to help her, and Bridgette did what she had done all her life. She refused his attentions.

Siddhartha Mukherjee has written eloquently about how hard it is to help a patient confront her own death. "It is a task almost impossibly difficult to describe," he writes, "an operation far more delicate and complex than the administration of a medicine or the performance of a surgery." This is what Ali Zaidi faced as he looked at Bridgette.

"I could tell she was leaning out the door," Zaidi told me. "I just very gently said to her, 'Listen. I think you have Ebstein's anomaly. I think a valve is leaking tremendously. I really think you need to come back. We need to sit and talk. I need to explain to you what is going on with your heart.' It took me at least two clinic visits to really walk her through the process. Eventually, when we did the MRI and sat her down, we said, 'Bridgette, we can really help you, and if you don't do it at this stage, we might get to a point where we can't reverse things.'"

She was facing a heart transplant, but Bridgette insisted on finishing out the school year, going to work all through March, April, May, and June. Like so many patients, she could reconcile herself to living with heart disease but not to any intervention. The very strength of character that allowed her to overcome so much in her life had become a weakness that almost killed her. Colleagues remember how frightening it was—how they worried she would fall down the stairs as she was climbing them, how she worried they would have to take the defibrillators from the wall and shock her to life again. For Bridgette, heart transplant surgery was strangely less stressful than the valve replacement she had had in the 1990s.

The day after the operation, a doctor put a stethoscope to her back and asked her to exhale. She took in a breath. All her life Bridgette had had trouble blowing out birthday candles. Now, as she blew out, the empty Styrofoam cup at her bedside fell over. Nothing like that had ever happened before.

"The only way I can describe it," she told me, "is if I were an athlete, I would have been Serena Williams."

13.

IT HAD BEEN five years since I'd finished an MFA degree in writing at Columbia University. I watched my friends and classmates publish their books. I attended their publishing parties and their weddings. I sublet a cheap apartment in downtown Brooklyn. I supported myself with part-time teaching jobs. Every day, first thing, I sat down at my desk with a cup of coffee. I used the belt of my bathrobe to tie myself to my desk chair so I wouldn't wander off.

The novel I was writing had a decent premise. After college Arno Fein moved with his girlfriend, Naomi, into an East Village apartment and became fascinated by the crack house next door. She went to work. He read the newspaper, scanned the classifieds, and drank coffee with his friend Jack Gottlieb.

But I could not move my novel to action. Arno Fein didn't get a job. He didn't have an affair. While Naomi was out of the apartment, he sat at the window and watched the scene on the street. He didn't buy crack. He didn't smoke crack. He didn't sell crack. He didn't sleep with whores or work with undercover agents. I could not manage his leap into the dangerous world. When I met strangers at parties and they asked me what I did, I said, "I write." I was not yet a writer. A writer was the thing I would become, I hoped, when I published my novel, won the National Book Award, and in my acceptance speech noted that awards were no true measure of any writer's art.

Of course I was incapable of dealing with Marlon Rosenbaum's news: that I needed to have a test on my heart, that maybe my heart was failing, that maybe I needed to have heart surgery again. Heart surgery! Again! My parents were aghast. For five long years, from 1966 to 1971, almost the length of the entire Vietnam War, it had haunted them, and they had shielded their little child from the knowledge of the lurking danger. Now the thing we had all buried had crawled up from underground.

Some ancient deep response was triggered, and we went into formation, fingers into a fist. My mom was in a panic. My old dad rose up onto his hind legs roaring. He was Poppa Bear, and he was going to rip Marlon Rosenbaum's head off. My dad called up an old acquaintance, let's call him George Lloyd, a retired heart surgeon who had once worked at Columbia Presbyterian. All the things that had baffled me about Marlon Rosenbaum baffled George Lloyd. If I was asymptomatic, why were they talking about heart surgery? If my cardiologist didn't want to do heart surgery, why send me overnight for a catheterization? What on earth could Marlon Rosenbaum mean by "prophylactic" heart surgery?

"It's bullshit," said my dad. "Catheterization is low risk, sure, but you don't let people stick things in your heart just because. You could get an infection, you could have bleeding, you could die. Don't do it."

Though he worked all his life as a psychotherapist, my dad is an MD, good with his hands, generally conservative in his medical judgments, and a strong diagnostician. He can get jumpy about the small details of life, packing a car or wrapping a package, but in a crisis he is focused, cool, and determined. He's well-read, and his experience is wide. When my dad was in his prime, friends, neighbors, and family stopped by the apartment all the time for advice. Even now that he's old and in decline, former patients call him when they're in trouble. By the time I'd gone off to college, I'd stopped consulting him, but now, in crisis, I turned to him again.

"No," he said over the phone. "Not unless you know why he really wants to do this. Don't let him do it just for research of his own."

I went to Marlon Rosenbaum's office in the spring, and I read him the questions I had in my notebook. Each of his answers seemed to make his position more obscure.

Say that I took the catheter exam, I said, and it showed that my right ventricle was weakening. Did that mean that I would get sick anytime soon?

Not necessarily, said Dr. Rosenbaum, uncomfortable in his chair.

If I underwent the proposed surgery, would that guarantee that I would stay healthy?

He shook his head. There were no guarantees. His desk was cluttered with files.

I asked, had he ever seen a patient like me go into heart failure?

No. But patients had come to him after their hearts had fallen apart.

What did that look like? I asked, departing from my script. Marlon winced and gave me a quick précis of heart failure: immobility, swollen limbs, decline.

Okay, I said, changing the subject, but what about the surgery: How many patients of his had undergone it?

None, yet.

None?

But there were some good results, he said, in Europe.

I mentioned my dad's old friend George Lloyd, who had said that there was no reason, as far as he could see, for me to undergo a cardiac catheterization.

"George Lloyd? But he's a *heart surgeon.*" Marlon pronounced this as if George Lloyd was an air-conditioning repairman.

Okay, I said, confused. So not George Lloyd—but weren't we talking about heart surgery? And wasn't there someone else I could talk to about this, someone who might give me a second opinion?

Marlon shrugged. He raised his palms slightly. He said, "Not really."

I told him I wasn't going to consider undergoing a cardiac catheter exam unless I could see someone for a second opinion.

"There's one guy," Marlon relented. "Michael Freed. But he's in Boston."

"Fine," I snapped. "So I'll go to Boston."

"Okay," he tried to calm things down. "Why don't we do this? We'll schedule the catheter exam for the fall, and you go to Boston before then. If Dr. Freed says to cancel the catheter exam, we'll cancel."

Boxed into a corner, I scheduled the test, but privately I suspected that he was on a fishing expedition, looking for data for a paper, like my dad said.

The truth is, my father was not entirely wrong: Marlon Rosenbaum did want data on me and on people like me. But there was nothing remotely dishonest in his research. There were no data. There was no conventional course of treatment. He couldn't give me statistical likelihoods on surgical success, because there were not enough people like me, tetralogy patients in their late twenties with big leaks and big right ventricles. He'd seen failed hearts, and he'd heard about successes in Europe, and he thought I was a good candidate for a new kind of surgery. He was the only person within hundreds of miles who dealt regularly with adult congenital heart patients. There was no second opinion in the New York area. I could go to Boston, I could go to LA, I could go to Mayo, or I could talk to Marlon.

Now it's become standard operating procedure. Almost all the adult tetralogy patients I've met have had their pulmonary valves replaced in a second surgery when they were in their twenties or thirties. For some patients a couple of decades younger than me, the surgeries were expected, part of the long-term plan, but in 1994 Marlon Rosenbaum was going out on a limb. He was going against consensus. His textbook on adult congenital cardiology, published in 2002, has a chapter on the subject, and whenever Marlon talks about it with me, he gets slightly chagrined: he had to temper his language about pulmonary valve replacement in tet patients.

For him, catheterization was a no-brainer. It was the only way to get a good sense of the pressures in my heart, and it was relatively safe: 99 percent of people who undergo cardiac catheter exams suffer no ill consequences whatsoever. On the train home from the hospital, with the echocardiologist's jelly still sticky under my shirt, I rehearsed those odds. If there was a 1 percent chance, on every subway ride, that I'd end up bleeding, infected, or dead, I would never go underground. I would always ride the bus. I made the appointment with Dr. Freed for a second opinion.

I had decent health insurance through my part-time work. After rent, health insurance was my biggest expense. But otherwise, socially, spiritually, and psychologically, I was totally unprepared. I had friends with whom I watched basketball and drank beer and friends with whom I traded drafts of my chapters. But I didn't feel comfortable talking about my heart, not even with my brothers.

"You can't do this alone," my old friend Anne warned me.

But doing it alone was my way of doing things. I could not afford a psychotherapist, and I didn't want a support group. "What I want people to see," Bridgette Ratliff told me about her own story, "is that there is a God, there is a purpose in life." But I don't believe in God the way that she does, and I had no access to her kind of faith. I was engaged in a willful struggle not to see the truth of my condition. My heart was an unspeakable thing dwelling inside my chest. My heart was my mortality, and I didn't want to look at it.

April came and with it my visit to Boston to see Dr. Freed. I was late, running underground from the 34th Street subway to the Amtrak hub at Penn Station, down that long nightmare arcade of beggars and commuters, fluorescent lights, and TGI Fridays. That way was New Jersey Transit. The other was the Long Island Railroad. I checked my watch. My backpack jerked on my shoulder. Past the stinking men's room, I found myself in the big sunless Amtrak ticketing hall. It was almost 10 a.m. My train to Boston left at 10:03. If there wasn't a long line at the ticket counter, I might make it.

I pulled out my credit card. I got to the sales counter. Would I make my train, I asked the guy behind the bulletproof glass. He shrugged. He moved his microphone to his left, away from his mouth.

I bought my ticket. I looked up at the big departures sign, with its clattering placards.

Fast as I could, I hustled across the hall, past the rolling suitcases and young Euro tourists with hiking packs and businessmen in suits. There was the gate, and the stairs down to the platform, and the last few passengers like me rushing to make it. At the landing halfway down stood a trembling woman in sunglasses. She held a ticket in one hand and a long white cane in the other.

"I am in need of assistance!" She held out her white cane with its soft rubber tip. "Please!" She wore a stodgy schoolmarm plaid suit. She was frightened. Her hair looked like a wig. All the New Yorkers rushed past her.

"All aboard!" called the train conductor. A woman in heels shoved me, galloping for the train, black skirt vanishing into its doors.

"I am in need of assistance," the blind woman cried.

I stopped. The conductor said it again: "All aboard."

I took her ticket from her hand. I told her she was on the wrong track if she wanted to go to Baltimore. I gave her back the ticket and took the last flight of stairs in a leap, and made it through the doors as they shut. The train floor started rolling under my feet. I found an empty seat and collapsed into it, breathing hard. My heart was pounding, like I'd just won a race. I raised my face to the ceiling and shut my eyes. Please God, I prayed, for the good deed with the blind woman, save me from heart surgery. Please God, let the doctor tell me everything is fine.

Funny thing is, in retrospect, if my prayer had been granted, if Michael Freed had told me what I wanted to hear—that my heart was as strong as I hoped it was—I'd be dead now.

14.

THE FIRST PERSON to describe my particular birth defect was Nicolaus Steno, the great Danish polymath. He made that description early in the history of cardiology, roughly forty years after William Harvey published *De motu cordis*. In 1665, in a' Paris salon, Steno dissected a stillborn baby and anatomized what would come to be known as the tetralogy of Fallot.

Steno's contributions to human knowledge are extraordinary and wide-ranging. He wrote impressively on the glands, demonstrating that the tongue was a muscle and not a gland and that tears came from the lachrymal glands and were not (as was widely believed) watery secretions of the brain. He proved that the heart was made of muscle and showed that bones, after centuries, became fossils. Steno invented geology: he was the first person to see that the earth developed in stratified layers and that the strata indicated different epochs in time. The observations he made on the female reproductive glands were crucial in the development of the so-called ovist school of thought—the notion that women's gonads produce eggs.

Long before such ideas were common, Steno saw that hearts were made of butcher's meat, that people reproduce in the same way chickens do, and that the ground we stand on is not fixed but changing. However, he's most striking not for his discoveries but for his later abandonment of them. Though his observations led in a straight line toward Charles Darwin, Steno gave it all up. Just as his career was hitting its peak, he quit the study of nature, converted to Catholicism, and became a priest, a bishop, and finally a saint. He shut his eyes to all he had understood and intuited.

In his worship, Steno was as radical as he had been in his anatomy. When summoned to the Vatican, he walked barefoot from Pisa to Rome, and his bleeding feet horrified the pope. As a bishop in Germany, he gave his cathedral over to the poor, letting them sleep there, and he so enraged the town burghers that they threatened to cut off his ears and nose and drive him out of town. After Steno's death, Gottfried von Liebniz, the greatest mathematician on the continent, ran all over Europe seeking the promised dissertation that Steno had said that he was writing. Liebniz never found any of Steno's final papers.

I first stumbled on Steno because of historical coincidence—he was the first to describe my heart defect. But as I read about him, I found something more: a story that weirdly echoes the ones told to me by Ali Zaidi and Bridgette Ratliff. What do we mean by healthy? How do we deal with the problem of mortality? To me, Steno's life reads like a parable of knowing and not knowing, of perception and denial. He looked deep into the nature of hearts and time and material being—maybe deeper into the existential void than anyone in his century—and at a certain point he snapped and turned his eyes toward heaven. Steno is my hero and my opposite. I've never in my life been as brave or committed or observant as he. I've always wanted to be normal, and I've never been able to look directly at my heart.

———

Steno was born in Copenhagen on January 1, 1638, according to the Julian calendar, January 7, according to the Gregorian. He was called Niels Stensen in Danish, but he signed his name Nicolas Stenon in French and Niccolo Stenone in Italian. In scholarly Latin, he called himself Nicolaus Stenonius. His last name was shortened when his papers were read at the Royal Society in London after his death, and so that's how he's known in English: Nicolaus Steno.

His mother was a widow, his father a widower, both on their second marriages. Denmark was in decline, in a world of medieval violence, pestilence, and famine. His father was goldsmith to the king but to make a decent living had to sell wine out of his cellar, and the family lived upstairs from his father's workshop. The street outside was fetid with rats and sewage. The family attended a church without a roof. It had been blown off in a storm and never repaired.

At three years old, Niels became mysteriously crippled— "morbis satis difficiles," as he wrote. He could not run. He could not play. "When I was very small," he wrote, "I took little pleasure in talking with other children. Because for three whole years, from three to six I was ill, I became accustomed to the company of older persons and formed the habit of listening to adults talking about religious matters rather than playing with my contemporaries."

His disease lifted in 1644. That same year, his father died. His mother married her third husband, Peter Lesle, another goldsmith. Lesle died the next year. She married a third goldsmith when Niels was twelve. The boy worked with all these fathers. He polished lenses, fixed the gears of watches, changed the colors of metals, and examined the properties of mercury, all obsessions of seventeenth-century physics. His fingers became extraordinarily nimble.

In 1654, the plague hit Copenhagen and wiped out roughly 9,000 people in a town of 28,000. The students in Steno's school were enlisted to cart away the bodies. About half of them died. Steno's Lutheran education was heavy on the classics and religion. He was taught Latin in the early years, Greek in the fourth and fifth grades.

Entry into Copenhagen University involved a ceremony in which the applicant dressed in blackface, wearing a peaked hood, a hump back, horns on his head, and a giant nose. He was attacked by a trustee wielding sticks, pliers, and a knife. After the beating, the boy appeared in ordinary clothes and begged for admission. A dean poured wine over the accepted student's head and put salt on his tongue.

At Copenhagen University, the dominant cosmological plan was the one devised by Tycho Brahe, the school's most famous alumnus and the last of the great naked-eye astronomers. Tycho had coined the word "nova"—he had seen one explode in the sky. He wore a gold nose because he had lost his own in a duel, and rumor had it that he was later murdered by Johannes Kepler, who wanted to steal his notes and library. Tycho's geoheliocentric astronomy was a compromise between Copernicus's and Ptolemy's, proposing that the sun revolved around the earth and the other planets revolved around the sun.

At school, Steno kept a journal, which he called *Chaos*. In it, Steno rejected medicine as he saw it practiced around him. "I would fear that someone might define medicine," he wrote, "as: The art of standing with furrowed brow in front of the patient, uttering inanities." He read Paracelsus, the sixteenth-century mystic who burned the books of classical physicians and believed in chemistry, that the body's health lay in a proper balance of sulfur, salt, and mercury. He also studied the works of Althanesius Kirchner, the most popular intellectual of the day, who had mapped Atlantis, who claimed to be able to read hieroglyphs, and who had himself lowered into Vesuvius to see its roiling insides.

After reading Francis Bacon, Steno became devoted to experiment. "From now on," he wrote, "I shall spend my time, not on musings but solely in investigation, experience and recording of natural objects." He studied water as it turned into ice—proving that it changed not in weight but in structure. Steno used mathematical rules to study the permeability of skin and muscle membranes: "This should be investigated more carefully and systematically according to Descartes' method, or by considering directly what enters the pores of the blood, what its particles are, how they move, what is expelled from there and how." He scolded himself for his laziness: "Almost the whole day my disturbed mind, being preoccupied with various reflections, could do nothing else than skim lightly over everything, then immediately to leave the causes of everything aside, but I pray, thee, o God, take this plague from me and grant me the power to free my soul from all distraction, to work on one thing alone and to make myself familiar with the tables of medicine alone." For him, the study of nature was the study of God: "One sins against the majesty of God by being unwilling to look into nature's own works."

The winter of 1660 was brutal. Sweden invaded Denmark, and the troops burned the suburbs around Copenhagen. The seas around the city froze solid, and the invading army laid siege. The citizens starved. Steno was enlisted in the city's defense. Skinny, small, and studious, he manned the battlements, and in his journal he kept notes on snowflake formation, setting out principles of crystallography. No one knows how he did it, but with his journal in hand and carrying letters of recommendation from his professors, Steno snuck out across the frozen sea, through the besieging troops, down into Germany (also war-torn) and from there to Amsterdam. He was twenty-two years old. From a walled, isolated town of 20,000 half-starved and sickly people, he came to the center of the modern world.

Amsterdam was ten times the size of Copenhagen, clean, peaceful, and prosperous; the shipbuilding, banking, and whaling capital of the Dutch Republic; the seat of the world's most powerful mercantile empire. The city was cosmopolitan, with refugees from all of Europe's religious wars: Jews from Spain, Quakers from England, Baptists, Walloons, and French Huguenots. Hundreds of printer-publishers produced tens of thousands of titles, more books than the rest of Europe combined. Steno presented his letters of recommendation to Gerald de Blaes, known as Blasius, professor extraordinary at the Athenaeum of Amsterdam. Blasius accepted him and allowed him to work in his laboratory, but he didn't think much of the homely young Dane. The contempt was mutual. Steno watched Blasius lecture on chemistry and dismissed the master's work as vulgar and messy.

After he saw Blasius perform a five-day dissection on the head and neck of a convict, Steno bought the head and neck of a sheep at a butcher's stall and brought it back to Blasius's workshop. He investigated the sheep's neck and mouth. He introduced a probe, examining "the course of the arteries and the veins." Delicately, he poked the membranes. His probe slipped. "I felt that the point of my knife, no longer confined between the membranes, more freely moved in a wide cavity, and as I pushed the iron further, I even heard it clink against the teeth."

Steno showed his discovery to Blasius. Blasius did not believe that Steno had found anything novel. Maybe he had made the hole with his knife, Blasius suggested. Steno demonstrated that was not the case. Then, Blasius continued, Steno must be confused. This was not a new salivary duct, but one already discovered, probably—he said—Wharton's duct. No. Steno knew where Wharton's duct lay. He showed it to Blasius in the mouth of the sheep. The duct that Steno had found was in a different spot. Maybe it was a freak, Blasius suggested. Again, no. The duct occurs in all sheep, in most mammals, and in every human being.

"I seem to have discovered a little salivary duct," he wrote in a letter home. Steno's former professor, Thomas Bartholin, wrote back expansively: "The learned men of our country join me in not finding enough words to praise . . . the success you have attained. All rejoice that their fellow citizen, and I trust my disciple, is making such strides in the study of glandular systems. Proceed, my dear friend. Proceed with great steps toward immortal glory."

The duct would be named the *ductus stenonius*, also called Steno's duct and Stensen's duct. Blasius became enraged and accused Steno of plagiarism. He, Blasius, should get credit for the duct that had been discovered in his lab and not that "wretched boy" from Denmark. Steno had to leave Amsterdam. He headed for the University of Leiden, the leading center of anatomical study in Europe. Blasius sent letters ahead of Steno's arrival, trying to destroy the young man's reputation, but to no avail. Steno devoted the next two years to the study of the glands, discovering seven new ones in a single ox head and writing on the production of saliva, tears, and breast milk. As he built his own reputation, Steno raged at Blasius, pointing out how little Blasius knew about glands and how obvious it was in his writings that Blasius couldn't distinguish between the different ducts of the mouth.

The public fight between the two anatomists, as well as his discoveries about the glands, made Steno a prominent man. He began lecturing, performing anatomy publicly. The anatomy theater in Leiden, built on the model of Vesalius's famous one in Padua, held two hundred people, the audience packed tightly in concentric, rising rings around the central table in which the anatomist worked on the corpse. Relics were on display in the hall, including the penis of a whale and a skeleton rider on a skeleton horse. Public dissections were held in the winter months so the cold could keep the corpse from rotting and keep down the stink. Steno performed on January 1, 1661, anatomizing a male corpse. On January 5 to 7, he vivisected a dog, examining the animal's lymphatic, pulmonary, and vascular systems. On January 14, he vivisected a pregnant dog and its unborn puppies. On February 7, he anatomized the body of a man named Janicke Jansen, recently dead of syphilis.

The students were rowdy. The university gave them a tax-free annual allowance of 194 liters of wine and 1,500 liters of beer. In taverns, they liked to play a game where they threw clubs at a cat hanging in a cage from the ceiling. When the cage broke, they all gathered around and beat the cat to death. Another popular game was "Head in a Lap." One student would put his head in a girl's lap, and he would try to guess which other girl was spanking him. Most of these women worked in the fabric mills around the university, and as one English traveler reported, "The women are said not much to regard chastity whilst unmarried." Steno stood apart from all this. His Jesuit biographer, Raffaelo Cioni, draws him as celibate: "He was of fine appearance, gentle of disposition, and one whose modesty was evident. An object of interest to the young women of Holland, he was no more beguiled by them than he had been by the girls of Copenhagen."

All his life, Steno never had a romantic attachment to a woman. In Leiden, his circle of friends were all men, most of them unmarried, all of them scientifically, aesthetically, and philosophically inclined. In the summer of 1661, after the anatomy season was over, he and his new friends took a tour of northern Europe. They took walks and boat rides, visited musicians, writers, and chemists. They looked at old castles and churches, toured gardens and market-places. They spent a lot of their time at libraries and feasts.

The penalty in Holland for sodomy was execution by strangu-
lation, burning, and then drowning. But in the 1660s, there was a
thriving gay male culture both in Amsterdam and in Leiden, with
secret meeting places and secret codes. The men called each other
nicht, or "niece." They met in private houses, in parks, and in particular taverns, like one in Amsterdam called The Serpent. Steno, a
solitary child in Copenhagen, a monkish student in the university,
and a visiting scholar in Amsterdam, seems to have discovered a
home for himself in Leiden, intellectually, socially, and perhaps ro-
mantically as well.

15.

I WAS FIDGETY ON the train, going over the questions I had for the doctor, rehearsing my anxieties, drinking coffee, and unable to read. Around noon, I ate a Hebrew National frank on a gluey bun that had been stuck in the snack car's microwave. I looked out the window at the wide marshy Hudson, and as we traveled north, I was on the wrong side to see the Atlantic and the buoys and marinas of Rhode Island.

I got off at Back Bay Station with a couple of hours to kill. It was April. I had no luggage, just a backpack. I strolled from Copley Plaza to the Fenway Gardens and stopped at the Museum of Fine Arts. I don't have any particular memories of what I saw or thought while I walked those streets or which paintings I looked at in the museum. I remember the warm weather and a kind of lightheaded sense of the surreal. I always like walking alone and anonymous in a city, a city whose monuments don't hold any memories for me, but this time I felt like I was undercover, pretending to be somebody I wasn't. I was sweaty inside my healthy-person disguise. The lobster shell of my denial hadn't cracked, but it trapped me.

The pediatric cardiology waiting room at Boston Children's is a cheerful place, a big open space with lots of bright colors and sunlight, soft couches and toys on the floor. While Columbia Presbyterian has the busy polyglot feel of Washington Heights, Boston Children's feels clean and dignified like Harvard. Most of the patients were babies and toddlers. There were mothers everywhere and the occasional dad—a guy my age with a mustache, a job, a marriage, and a child in trouble. Tables were stacked with copies of parenting magazines and books for kids. *Highlights for Children* and *Clifford the Big Red Dog*. A woman beside me asked what I was doing there (Was she suspicious? Do child molesters hang out in the pediatric cardiology waiting room?), and when I told her I was there to see Dr. Freed, her eyes brightened. What was my kid's defect? Hers had been born with tetralogy of Fallot. There was the baby, bundled in a bright car seat, sleeping. I had to explain it was me—that I had been born with tetralogy. Her eyes welled up, and I saw how she saw me, tall and looking healthy, a sign of what her own child might grow up to be. She asked how I was doing, and I told her I was doing great—teaching at a college, feeling strong, and repaired completely.

After the nurses weighed and measured me, Dr. Freed came out and introduced himself. He was tall and slightly stooped, bald with a walrus mustache around an O-shaped mouth. We shook hands. He had cleared some time for me, he said, since I'd come in from out of town. He walked me to his office. Late afternoon sun fell through the windows across his big wooden desk.

"Did you enjoy your trip to the Museum of Fine Arts?" he asked.

I was startled. How did he know I had gone to the museum? A dreamlike thought came to me, the kind of thought a small child might invent about the magical powers of a teacher or a parent. Dr. Freed was that kind of cardiologist, I decided: the kind who kept track of his patients on the days they visited him, who knew where they traveled and what they did, the kind who knew everything. My wonder must have read on my face. He chuckled and pointed to the MFA pin on my lapel, the one they gave me at the museum after I paid admission. I took off the pin and put it in my pocket.

I was expecting a battery of tests in Boston, but Dr. Freed said there was no need. He had the results from Columbia. In his office he asked about my work, my teaching, and my writing. He felt my neck with his cool and gentle hands and warmed his stethoscope before he touched it to my back. He felt my hands and my feet and ankles. He watched my chest rise and fall as I breathed. We talked about diet and exercise.

In very broad terms, Dr. Freed described the problem I was facing. He drew diagrams on a piece of paper, explaining the basics of my heart as no one had ever done for me before. As a result of surgery, I didn't have a pulmonary valve, he explained, crossing out one part of the heart. The blood leaking backward had enlarged my right ventricle. He drew arrows in magic marker and plumped out one side of the box marked "RV." For the first time, I could visualize my condition.

"What does it mean?" I asked.

He was silent and then spoke carefully. I seemed to be tolerating the situation well, and the history of patients after tetralogy correction suggested both that right ventricles, over time, tend to expand and weaken and that most people like me tended to do well despite that.

"Should I get the catheter exam?" I asked.

He asked me how I felt about the exam. I told him.

He nodded. He needed time, he said. He wanted to look over the information that had been sent to him by Columbia. I was in no immediate danger, he assured me. He promised to give the case some thought and get back to me with a letter. I left the office. I stood out on Longwood Avenue and tried to hail a cab. I stepped like a New Yorker into traffic and raised an imperious hand. Every cab slipped by me. That wasn't how it was done in Boston.

I took the train back home feeling calmed. I had taken some kind of action. I had seen the oracle, and now I had to wait for the oracle's report. This warm, gentle Harvard professor doctor was going to take care of me. I was sure of it.

16.

IMAGINE STENO AT the dissecting table in the anatomy theater in Leiden. It is 1663, winter in the Netherlands, cold, salty
air. He is performing a three-day exploration of the brain. The
corpse on the table has been disemboweled to reduce its odor.
The audience is packed in rows. Light flows from the big windows. Candles burn close by the body. Steno dresses elegantly but
simply. He wears a smock. Packs of drunken students fill the back
rows. In the front row sit the university professors, chief among
them Sylvius, the leading doctor in all of Holland, a large, bearded,
darkly handsome man who makes twice the salary of any physician in the Netherlands. Beside Sylvius sits a foreign dignitary,
Melchisédech Thévenot, an aristocrat, a scholar, and a spy, whose
inventions included both the spirit level and ipecac as a cure for
dysentery. (Thévenot's book, *The Art of Swimming*, would later be
a favorite of Ben Franklin's; Thévenot advocated the breaststroke.)
He was librarian to Louis XIV. The salons in his Paris home were
the beginnings of the French Académie de Sciences, and from his
collections of books and maps grew the Bibliotèque Nationale.

Behind the faculty and the dignitaries sit the more advanced
anatomy students, among them Jan Swammerdam. Swammerdam
will become the greatest entomologist of his time, but right now
he's studying respiration, conducting loud, messy vivisections of
dogs in rented rooms above public houses (he's had to move four
times in the last year). No one really knows what Swammerdam
looked like. There's a Rembrandt portrait of a man said to be him,

but its authenticity is in dispute. So let's make him small, handsome, and blond. He and Steno are inseparable.

Beside Swammerdam stands Regnier de Graaf, twitchy and ambitious, a few years older than Steno and his great rival. After Steno has given up natural philosophy, de Graaf will claim Steno's observations on the ovary as his own, and the follicle that releases the egg during ovulation—which Steno discovered—will be called the Graafian follicle. Steno, having abandoned science, will not protest. In the back row of the crowded room, incognito, stands Baruch Spinoza, who has recently been driven out of Amsterdam after being excommunicated by its rabbis. Spinoza is living not far from the university, among the Mennonites, making his living as a lens grinder. He has a high forehead and enormous brown eyes, and it's never clear if he's smiling or frowning.

The dead man on the dissecting table has a neck that's marked and twisted by the rope that hung him. "When the soul is in its own house," Steno says, to open his discourse on the brain, "it cannot describe it and does no longer know itself." From within the mind, Steno argues, we cannot understand the brain.

He is elegant in his work with the saw, scalpel, scissors, and probe. He's much stronger than his small frame lets on and cuts through the skull without much effort. After sawing a line on either side of the head, he asks for a hammer and chisel. He smacks the chisel smartly, removes it, and delivers a blow to the other side. He frees the top of the head, which he hands like a bowl to his waiting assistant.

Steno directs his audience's attention to the brain and how little can be viewed from the outside. "All you can say is that there are different substances, one grayish, and one white, that the white substance is continuous with nerves which are distributed all over the body." His lecture is less about the anatomy of the brain than about the impossibility of knowing it. Slice it in pieces, unravel its folds, still you cannot see how it functions. "Personally I assert that the true dissection would be to follow the threads of the nerves through and where they arrive at. It is true that this manner meets so many difficulties that I do not know it could ever be completed."

He shows how the substance of the brain can be manipulated, how different anatomists mold it to support their various arguments and explanations.

Steno reviews the history of brain science. He dismisses those philosophers who have opined on the nature of the brain without ever practicing anatomy. "One can read them only as amusement." Finally, at the end of a long day, after having displayed the organ in all its detail, Steno praises the example of his mentor. He describes "the simplicity of Sylvius, who speaks to this matter only with uncertainty though he has worked on it more than anyone I know." This is his conclusion: to be careful in one's studies and modest in one's claims. Steno bows.

Sylvius congratulates him. Thévenot insists that Steno must come to France, to his salon, to lecture. Swammerdam, dazzled, cannot look Steno in the face. A banquet awaits, but just as Steno reaches the exit, a stranger accosts him and asks what implication his lecture has for René Descartes, for the posthumously published *Treatise on Man*, which scandalously proposes that the human body is a clockwork thing.

Steno has been reading and rereading the *Treatise on Man* all week. He is obsessed with Descartes's backward anatomy (Descartes has the heart working like a furnace, heating up the blood) and his scandalous theology. (If a person is like a clock and has no free will, then the whole moral order is thrown into question; if the person is built to sin, like a clock is built to tell time, then what point is there in repentance?) Steno has yet to meet anyone so interested in Descartes as he is. He and the stranger gesture excitedly as they talk. They finish each other's sentences. Swammerdam tries to hustle Steno out the door.

"You must come visit me in Rijksberg." The stranger has big brown eyes and a long, delicate nose.

Swammerdam is pulling at Steno's arm.

"I would be delighted," Steno says. As he says it, he realizes who he's talking to: the excommunicated Jew Spinoza, the famous heretic—talk to him and you will burn in hell! But Steno is open to everything.

It takes him an hour to walk from Leiden to Rijksberg, past canals and windmills, farms and pastures, and hothouses full of tulips. Steno has been studying circulation, muscles and blood and hearts, and as he walks, he imagines the blood flying up his carotid artery and bathing his brain in light. He imagines the newly discovered blood vessels, the microscopic capillaries that run finely beneath the skin of his fingers. He can feel his heartbeat, he can feel his legs moving, muscles getting warm and sore, but he cannot, cannot feel a single fiber of his brain, a single function inside his mind. Will Spinoza have horns? Will the house smell of brimstone? There is an anxious moment as he approaches the door. But the room is bright. Steno is impressed by the simplicity of the place. The door is shut, and it's like Steno has stepped into another world.

They speak in Latin, a language that Steno has understood as long as he can remember and that Spinoza has only recently taught himself. They talk at first cautiously but then excitedly about Descartes and the nature of God, the relation between the divine and the physical. It is in the close study of nature that one sees the works of God, Steno avers, and it enrages him how Descartes fails to grasp the natural world's complexity, a complexity much more baffling than any simple cuckoo clock. A question of mathematics, Spinoza says, and he argues that the divine is demonstrably inherent, logically, in all things: in the brain, in the heart, and in the cuckoo clock. We are all, all made of God. Steno leaves Spinoza's house, and it's like he's stoned.

Watching the windmills turn, and the sunset, and the cows, it comes to him: he knows how to destroy Descartes. In Leiden in 1663, William Harvey's theory of circulation was as controversial as global warming is in any university environmental studies program today, which is to say, circulation was accepted fact. There was a professional class, physicians, who opposed the theory of circulation because they feared it would undermine their business, and in the general population the notion of circulating blood was too spooky to be believed, but anatomists knew it was true: the blood moved around the body. As to the nature of the heart, anatomists were less unified. Descartes, in his *Treatise on Man*, described the heart the same way Shakespeare had—as a furnace, a warming engine. Steno doubted this was accurate. And he wondered how someone like Descartes, who didn't understand the workings of something as simple as the heart, how such a person could claim to understand something as complex as the nature of God.

Steno returned from Rijksberg and in his laboratory began to investigate the heart of a deer. He boiled the heart so as to firm it up before he looked more closely at its structure. He stripped off the pericardium. He examined the fibers strip by strip, strand by strand. "The first fibers of the heart which I touched, led me to the lower tip and from the tip upwards again," he wrote, "a truth explaining the whole structure of the heart which up to that moment neither I nor anyone else had ever known." His observations demonstrated that the heart was a muscle, shaped like a muscle, with fibers that worked like the fibers in other muscles. He compared the muscle fibers in his deer heart with those in the leg of a rabbit and found them to be identical.

He had made his breakthrough. The heart, Steno wrote (emphasis his), was "*not* the seat of a determined substance like fire or innate heat or of the soul; also *not* the creator of a determined liquid, like the blood; also, *not* the producer of certain spirits like the vital spirits." Everything Descartes had said about the heart was wrong. If Descartes could not know the heart, how could he presume to know God? "I knocked down all the constructions of these finest heads without words, only evidence," he wrote. "The ancients did not know what is obvious every time meat is brought to the table." Steno proved that the heart was made of meat and did so with holy purpose, to destroy the arguments of a heretic.

After the publication of this discovery, Steno took up Thévenot's invitation and left for Paris, bringing with him his companion Jan Swammerdam and a few other friends. They visited the Sorbonne together, and the Louvre, and the menagerie at Versailles. In the Tuileries, they saw Louis XIV bless and touch a crowd of scrofula patients, whose necks bulged with tumors. They attended a party where the Sun King led the dance. For Thévenot's guests, Steno explored a calf's head and showed the tear ducts, the salivary glands, and the *ductus stenonius*. He cut into the brain and pointed out the Sylvian fissure. Vivisecting a dog, Steno demonstrated circulation by ligating its abdominal aorta and paralyzing its legs. To refute Descartes's claim that animals felt no pain, Steno touched the dog's sciatic nerve. The dog writhed and howled.

He performed an autopsy of a dead, deformed child. Windows were open. The smell of the corpse mixed with the stink of the street. The Frenchmen wore wigs and heavy coats, jewelry and high heels. They carried canes. The baby had a hand like a flipper, with all the fingers fused, and a ghastly harelip that the mother blamed on her own fondness for eating carrots.

The stillborn appeared to be a hermaphrodite, but Steno showed that what looked like a penis was in fact a clitoris. His hair was long. He had a thick, drooping mustache between his big nose and fleshy lips. Andre Graindorge, a doctor who saw Steno perform at Thévenot's, wrote, "To say it straight, compared with him we are like pupils." According to another Parisian physician, "In this field he leaves behind him the ancients and the moderns."

The infant chest was almost entirely cartilaginous. The heart, the liver, and the spleen, Steno reported, "all adhered to the stomach." What interested him most was the heart. He entered it and noted odd absences. The pulmonary artery was narrowed, narrower than the aorta. Steno opened the right ventricle and introduced his probe. Where he expected to find the solid muscle wall, he found a hole. There were "three orifices [leading] into the ventricle." He saw that "the same canal" came from both ventricles into the aorta.

Three hundred years before I was born, Steno saw it all: the ventricular septal defect, the overriding aorta, the stenosis of the pulmonary artery, and the thickened ventricle wall, the birth defect that has come to be known as the tetralogy of Fallot. Why God would form a child like that, Steno restrained from speculating. He declared, "I have nothing to say about the cause of this phenomenon."

That summer, he and Swammerdam moved to Thévenot's country home to collaborate in their studies of reproduction. Picture the young men running through the high grass after specimens: chasing butterflies, catching tadpoles and frogs, examining the eggs of chickens, witnessing the sex of invertebrates, a summer of delight in the natural world. Swammerdam wrote sexy descriptions of the coitus of snails:

> After all is finished, the little creature, having wantonly consumed the strength of life, becomes dull and still, rests quietly without much creeping, until the furious lust of generation gathers new strength and effaces the memory of weariness suffered after the former coitus.

The summer ended. Swammerdam went back to Holland to complete his studies and to be with his family. Steno had been turned down for a professorship at the University of Copenhagen and had no official position in Leiden or in France. Thévenot used his connections with the Medicis to secure Steno a position at the Pitti Palace, where the students of Galileo had formed a new scientific society, the Academia del Cimento. The couple parted. Steno walked all the way to Tuscany, sometimes with company and sometimes alone, more than six hundred miles. Decades of war and plague had left the roads dangerous, with roving bandits and desperate refugees. Steno wore a sword, but he didn't really know how to use it.

One disassembles a machine to understand its construction, he thinks. One knows the artificer by knowing his designs. The heart is made of tiny fibers, the same kind of fibers as the muscles in the legs, but those muscles in the heart are twisted into a powerful ingenious knot, clenching and unclenching for a lifetime. Yet a heart can be formed imperfectly; a heart can be a monstrous thing. At night he dreams of Swammerdam, and in the morning he repents. He watches a procession of pilgrims: "The thought came into my mind: either this Host is a simple piece of bread and those who render it such honor are mad, or else truly it is the body of Christ."

At the Abbaye Royale de Frontevraud, Steno met with the abbess in her private chamber, where she prayed every day from 5 to 9 a.m. In Montpellier he performed an anatomy lesson, dazzling his audience, among them traveling English scientists. Over dinner, the

Englishmen discussed the work of one of their colleagues, Robert Hooke, who was investigating the strangely shaped stones found in mountaintops and fields, with shapes in them like sea animals. The Frenchmen at the table mentioned Guillaume Rondelet, a naturalist who worked in Montpellier a century earlier, who had argued that the so-called tongue stones, or *glossopetrae*, found on local beaches were once the teeth of ancient sharks.

Steno arrived in Pisa. In Tuscany, the viscera of the earth are exposed, and he runs his fingers across the lines of sandstone, examining the strata. *Provando e reprovando*, test and test again, is the motto of the Academia del Cimento. The Medici dukes show Steno Galileo's instruments: his telescope, his astrolabe, and his armillary sphere. Here, convicts are strangled gently to death so as not to disturb the anatomy of their necks before dissection by anatomists. The grounds of the Pitti Palace reek with the experiments of Francisco Redi, who has been investigating the way that maggots rise from rotting flesh. At the dukes' palace, a strange, thin woman is shocked by Steno's Lutheranism. This is Sister Maria Flavia, a nun and the daughter of a senator. She has enormous bulging eyes. What is it like to live unconfessed, she asks, to live outside the possibility of redemption? Steno tells her, shyly, that it is not his custom to dispute matters of faith, but he will listen to all arguments.

Then a monster is discovered!

Fishermen have caught an enormous shark, the largest anyone has ever seen. The behemoth is decapitated and its head brought to the palace. Steno measures the jaws: they are so large a man can walk right through them. The skin is tough. The brain is tiny. But what really impresses him are the teeth, the ones easily picked from the jawbone. They are exactly the same shape as the *glossopetrae*, the tongue stones he discussed with the Englishmen at Montpellier. He thinks of the hills all around, the crags in the landscape, the seashells discovered on high ground.

He travels to the coast, to Livorno and Piombino. He visits marble quarries in Carrara and salt mines in Cecina, studying the formation and history of the earth. "How the present state of anything discloses the past state of the same thing," he wrote, "is made abundantly clear by the example of Tuscany above all others."

Even as he investigates the nature of the planet, he is being drawn into discussions of the ineffable. Sister Maria Flavia introduces him to Lavinia Arnolfi, a married woman and devout penitent who wears spikes inside her stockings and a hair shirt under her court clothes. The women take Steno to see Paolo Segneri, a charismatic orator who prays naked in cold weather and every day whips himself until he bleeds and faints. Steno falls in with religious cultists.

In 1667 he publishes a short three-part book. The first part, *Elementorum myologiae specimen*, examines the geometry of muscles and the way animals move. In the second part, *Canis carchariae dissectum caput*, Steno describes how sharks' teeth turn to fossils, and he describes the stratified layers of the earth. The last section is nine pages long, focusing on the dissection of dogfish, and after examining the ovaries of a fish, Steno by analogy concludes that the ovaries of women contain eggs, a radical reimagination of human reproduction. As the historian of science Matthew Cobb describes it in his book *Generation*, in this short, three-part book, Steno upended the world's knowledge. According to Cobb, Steno found "a mathematical explanation for one of the most widespread living phenomena—movement." He laid out "the basis for scientific study for earth and its history," and finally he proved that "human eggs were like the eggs of other animals."

As Steno forged forward in his studies, penetrating the layers of material reality, his religious crisis deepened. He visited the Biblioteca Laurenzania, poring over Greek and Hebrew manuscripts, running through gospels and translations. In 1671, he published *De solido*, his last great work, which outlined the basic principles of geological study, principles that still hold true today. Two centuries would pass before the great Scottish geologist James Hutton teased out the implications of this work and described what Hutton called "deep time," the eons and eons it would take for the earth to form itself according to Steno's principles, but careful seventeenth-century readers understood where Steno was heading. Liebniz hoped that Steno might be able to "draw from [*De solido*] conclusions regarding the origin of the human race."

Steno was verging on unspeakable conclusions, things no one in his world would dare to think. Walking in the night on a dark street in Pisa, he heard a voice cry, "Come over to the other side," and something inside him broke. Steno never knew where the voice came from, but he knew what it meant, and even as the censors were reviewing the manuscript of *De solido*, he converted to Catholicism. Almost simultaneous with Steno's conversion, Swammerdam in Leiden suffered a breakdown. Like Steno, he had never married, and like Steno he was at the summit of his career. And shortly after Steno did, Swammerdam gave up his research. He fell under the sway of a mystic named Antoinette Bourignon, a wealthy lapsed Catholic who had a grotesque harelip and who preached the incipient arrival of end times. Steno and Swammerdam never met again.

In 1675, Steno was ordained a priest. In 1677 he was made a bishop. The church sent him to Hanover, where the population was largely Protestant. Steno sold his bishop's ring and silver crucifix and gave away the money to the poor. He wore rags, alienated his parishioners, and wrote to Rome, begging to be relieved of his duties. He was, he said, like "a dead man who feels nothing." On November 21, 1686, gripped by intense abdominal pain, he wrote,

> To my usual ailment, colic, it seems now that the stone has been added. Last night, I had the most terrible pains in the *os sacrum*. After an enema, they have shifted to below the *os pubis*, and from this morning it seems as if they are increasing, as if an inflammation is forming there. Not a drop of urine comes. I believe that the stone has embedded itself in a fold in the bladder, and that there, besides causing pains, it is causing inflammation of the mucous membrane of the bladder and will be the cause of my death.

Four days after writing those words, Steno was dead.

Jacques Lacan, the French psychological theorist, once defined trauma as "a missed encounter with the real." Steno approached the abyss, the blank material underpinnings of life. He saw, more than anyone around him, the base material nature of life, the *real*— and the effect of this vision was like trauma. He had to look away.

His description of the muscular structure of the heart would have no medical utility until three hundred years after his death. The heart defect he discovered would not be named for him. No doctor would attempt to diagnose and treat a child with tetralogy of Fallot until Helen Taussig did in the 1940s. It would be centuries after Steno's death until the Western world could grapple seriously with the formation and malformation of the human heart.

17.

I GOT HOME FROM my visit to Dr. Freed, and I got the news that my sublet in downtown Brooklyn was done. In July, I taught a college prep class at the New School. In August, I spent a long weekend at my parents' house in Vermont. I still hadn't heard back from Dr. Freed. I still hadn't decided about the cardiac catheter test. It was scheduled, but I wasn't committed to it, and any conversation with my parents that touched on any of this led to yelling and screaming. Then, at the end of the month, I went to visit my friends Jeff and Anne in Nantucket. They were getting married, and we toasted with champagne, and I confessed that I was getting kicked out of my apartment. Anne and I played another round of "Gabe, What Are You Doing with Your Life?"

I took a ferry and a bus and then a train home from Boston. Summertime in New York, late August, and it stank. My mailbox was full of rejections from literary magazines and bills, and buried in there, something from Boston Children's. I fumbled for my keys, got my bags inside my apartment, and opened the letter, sitting on my bed. I remember the smell of suntan lotion that was still on my face, the feel of my shirt collar on my sunburned neck. Dr. Freed's letter was three-pages long, single spaced. It was addressed to Dr. Rosenbaum. I was cc'd on the bottom. I must have read it three times, sitting there on my fold-out futon, without opening the windows of the apartment or getting myself a glass of water. I still have the pages, and they're filled with my scribbles and penciled marginalia, diagrams, underlining, and notes.

Next to *dyspnea*, I wrote, "trouble breathing," next to *cyanosis*, "discoloration of the skin," and next to *orthopnea*, "feet swelling (?)." According to Dr. Freed, I had none of these. He wrote, "He's done very well, but recently has been noted to have increasing right ventricle dysfunction on echocardiogram." Never had I read such a thorough discussion of my own condition.

In the group [of adult tetralogy of Fallot] patients that has significant symptoms, we have started to replace the pulmonary valve with a homograft in an attempt to restore competent pulmonary valve function. This is, however, a temporizing measure since the homografts eventually become regurgitant and thus the children or adults end up with significant pulmonary regurgitation again and occasionally stenosis when the homografts calcify.

My doom was spelled out right there, but I took comfort: he didn't seem to want me to have surgery! On top of the second page, there's one sentence I underlined thickly. "I suspect that Mr. Brownstein is somewhere along the path of tolerating the pulmonary regurgitation very well to becoming significantly symptomatic." But where was I on the path? How fast was I traveling? "It may be years or even decades before Mr. Brownstein becomes symptomatic from right ventricular dysfunction. Since we know RV is dispensable from our Fontan experience, I suspect that Mr. Brownstein will have no difficulty as long as the tricuspid valve is competent." By "RV" I knew he meant right ventricle. "Fontan experience" refers to a treatment of infants born with a single ventricle: blood can be rerouted to the lungs, and the left ventricle alone can keep a child alive.

The idea that I would be fine without a pulmonary valve and then without a right ventricle was the very idea that Marlon Rosenbaum's research, and the research of adult congenital cardiologists, was challenging, but as yet there was insufficient data to support it. Dr. Freed was weighing the danger of heart surgery against the danger of waiting and tentatively leaned toward the latter. Had I read more carefully—had I been able to listen to both doctors objectively—I might have intuited the two doctors' basic agreement and Marlon Rosenbaum's as yet unsubstantiated belief: since treatment couldn't be adequate after the heart failed, the surgeons might have to attack before there was heart damage, which was to say, prophylactically, which was to say *now*. But I didn't think like that.

"Years or decades," I read through the scrim of my denial. Who can say they will be healthy longer than that? On the bottom of the second page, Dr. Freed came to his conclusion:

> Since we don't have a great solution, since he's unsymptomatic, and since the operation is likely to be a temporizing procedure rather than a permanent cure, I think we should be conservative at this point. . . . If surgery would not be considered at this point, then I'm not sure that it's necessary to do a cardiac catheterization to determine the degree of pulmonary regurgitation. This would be semi-quantitative at best, and I don't think it would alter the decision to be conservative.

I put down the letter. I believe I may have pumped my fist. It was the reprieve I had longed for. I didn't have to take the test! I called Jeff and Anne, and they were happy for me. Jeff thought it was a nice pun, the doctor's name being Freed. I'd been freed, hadn't I?

It was Sunday, late August. Tomorrow was the first day of school, and I was teaching an introductory English class at Barnard College. Tuesday, I was scheduled for my catheter exam. After that, I had to move to my new apartment. There was no reason to call Dr. Rosenbaum's office now. I would do it first thing in the morning, and I would cancel.

So I did that. I left a message on his answering service before I sat down to my cup of coffee at my desk, turned on the computer, and reread, for the umpteenth time, the first sentences of my novel.

I lost my troubles for a moment in my coffee and my writing. I was stepping out of the shower when the phone rang. I let the machine pick up.

"It's Dr. Rosenbaum," said a glum voice. "Calling about your heart."

I didn't pick up the phone.

18.

S O LONG AS I shut my eyes to my troubles, they weren't there. This was how I had always lived my life. I had heard Dr. Rosenbaum's advice; I had read Dr. Freed's letter. Where it said "years or decades" on the page, I emphasized the second word, "decades," but in the back of my mind, I heard the first, "years." In some ways, Rosenbaum's position was much more optimistic than Freed's, whose letter, read in its darkest, starkest terms, spelled out my doom. Once my heart started to fail, Michael Freed seemed to be saying, there was going to be no way to save me. I shoved that idea away, but it leapt out at me, in the middle of the night, in rides on the subway, attacks of anxiety that made it hard to breathe. A couple of years of health might be all I had left.

Rosenbaum had described to me his patients in heart failure, and Freed had described the regurgitant hearts, the leaking, stenotic homografts, but I swallowed those thoughts as quickly and as forcefully as I could. I continued drafting and redrafting my static novel, teaching my adjunct courses, and rooting for the New York Knicks. My leaking, failing heart was the monster under the bed. To do the cardiac catheter test would be to face it, which I was too afraid to do. I wanted to be safe under the blankets. I wanted to be normal. As a heart patient, I was in the closet, and I was repressed—I was closeted most profoundly to myself. This point— this connection between trauma and self-delusion—was made for me most forcefully by Alan Sabal, a congenital heart patient a decade older than I am.

"Your body holds the reactions to the invasiveness of surgery," said Alan, who had an operation to repair subaortic stenosis in 1962, when he was ten years old. "The body doesn't understand, particularly at that age; as a young child, you don't know where this stuff is coming from."

Sabal is ebullient and youthful in his early sixties, chubby and charming, quick to laugh, and easy with intimacies. He has a neat goatee and a warm smile, and at our first lunch together at the café near the Stuyvesant Town apartment in which he lives, he confided in me the twin struggles of his early life. Speaking rapidly and seriously, he explained to me that in his childhood in the 1950s and 1960s, both his sexuality and his heart condition were unspeakable. His homosexuality was categorized by the psychiatric establishment as a mental disorder, something he could not express. His cardiac condition, similarly, in a middle-class Jewish home in the Bronx, was something that dared not speak its name.

In the café, screaming children sat to the left of us. Alan, in hushed and urgent tones, described his struggles to repress both his sexual desire and the trauma of his health condition. Both haunted him. Both were secrets. When he was little, no one had told him anything about his heart. No one had prepared him for his invasive treatments. He knew something was wrong, and the doctors were concerned, but no one explained anything.

"My parents didn't tell me why I was coming back to the hospital," he said of the heart surgery he had when he was ten. "They said I was going for more tests."

Spooked, little Alan threw a tantrum. His parents packed him in the car anyway and took him to Manhattan. In those days, parents didn't stay with their kids before surgery. His mother and father said good-bye. No one mentioned the operation. Alan was left in a room over night for pre-op. There was another boy in the bed next to him, and the two kids began whispering.

Nowadays, the family of a ten-year-old going in for surgery on his aorta would get a lot of coaching. There would be a meeting with a social worker and maybe even a psychologist. Doctors would follow established protocols and offer specially printed brochures, describing the procedures in careful, age-appropriate language. A number of good kids' books are available for children with heart conditions and their parents, to help them make their way through surgery. There are beds for parents in patients' rooms so they can keep their children company through the night.

Alan Sabal got none of that. His parents couldn't bear to mention what was going to happen. (This seems to me like a dark variant on an old Jewish joke. Of course, his parents didn't want to talk to Alan about surgery. They didn't want to upset him.) He was in the old Flower Fifth Avenue Hospital up near Central Park. From the window of the shared room, he could see the tracks of the trains heading north to Westchester. He couldn't sleep, and neither could the kid in the bed next to him, a twelve-year-old.

What was he there for? The other boy asked Alan.

Alan didn't know.

The kid explained that this was the room they kept you in before surgery.

So in the middle of the night, Alan learned of the surprise that awaited him in the morning. He guessed it would be surgery on his heart.

Nurses arrived before dawn. At 5 a.m., terrified and confused, Alan was washed down. They shaved his hairless chest. They used stinging antibiotic soap, affixed the suckers of the heart monitor to his skin, and rolled him on a gurney into a tiled and busy operating room.

"The last thing I remember before going under, I got an enema," he told me. "It must have had anesthesia in it. All I remember is getting something up my butt and getting taped."

Subaortic stenosis is a narrowing of the aortic valve and in many cases involves a narrowing of the aorta. Alan's chest was sawed open, he was connected to a heart-lung machine, and surgeons reworked his valve and his aorta so more oxygenated blood flowed out to his body and his brain. He awoke in a ward full of postoperative adults, all of them groaning and stinking and half-alive. Alan wavered in and out of consciousness. His parents were allowed only short, intermittent visits. For the most part, he was alone. Initially, he did well in his recovery, but he was moved from post-op to the pediatric wing too soon. Orderlies wheeled his bed in the middle of the night, IV tubes swinging and rattling around him. The door to pediatrics was too narrow for his gurney, and so Alan, with his sawed chest, was lifted and manhandled and passed to a new rolling bed. He developed postoperative pneumonia. His fever spiked. The surgeons returned and stuck a tube down his throat and suctioned Alan's lungs. He spent three weeks in the hospital. He remembers the nights, his only comfort a little transistor radio he kept in the bed with a single headphone he stuck in his ear, listening to the hits of 1962: "Roses and Red" by Bobby Vinton, the Four Seasons singing "Big Girls Don't Cry."

As a man, Alan learned to express his sexuality comfortably. He lived through the AIDS crisis. But the horror of his early surgery was something silent and buried deep down, and the reality of his heart was something he could not face. After his childhood cardiologist retired, Alan didn't see another doctor to monitor his heart, not until 2011. But the trauma kept coming back to him. He recounted to me a time, during those years lost to care, when he was in the mountains in California at a retreat, lying on a table, getting his back massaged, when the childhood surgery burst into his mind.

"The pre-op came flashing back." He remembered the violation of his anus, the doctor's taping him shut. "All of a sudden I was screaming, 'Get away! Get away!' I was bawling. I was crying. All of this emotional stuff of the heart coming out of me." When, in his fifties, he was told he needed heart surgery again, Alan, like me, panicked.

I suppose we all seem a little crazy—Bridgette, Alan, and me—refusing to face our problems and risking our lives as a consequence, but when I consider our collective reactions, they don't seem to me entirely neurotic. It's perfectly reasonable to want to avoid heart surgery. Having had the experience once, it's natural not to want to have it again.

Nobody wants to be sick. These days, *healthy* is a synonym for *normal*, whereas sick means *crazy*, *evil*, or *unkind* (or, I guess, for a skateboarder, *gnarly*). In one of my favorite novels, Don DeLillo's *White Noise*, there is a comic-sage, Murray Siskind, a sportswriter turned Elvis scholar, whose words are intended ironically but seem to me absolutely true. "Fear is unnatural," Murray opines. "Lightning and thunder are unnatural. Pain, death, reality, these are all unnatural. We can't bear these things as they are. We know too much. So we resort to repression, compromise and disguise. This is how we survive in the universe. This is the natural language of the species." I was only doing what everybody does. I knew there was something wrong with my heart. The problem was engraved on my body by the big scar right down the middle of my chest. But I couldn't face it. The only available options were repression, compromise, and disguise. I didn't run from my doctor out of ignorance. I ran because I knew too much.

You can call the heart "just a pump," as the great cardiac surgeon Denton Cooley does in his memoir *100,000 Hearts*, and that phraseology can give you a confident and macho feeling, but everyone knows you're just shutting your eyes to the mystery of the strange beating within you. Some internal organs are silent. It's easy to forget about the liver, the kidneys, or the spleen. Other organs make explicit demands. I'm hungry, says the stomach. The bladder says, I need to pee! The heart makes itself heard constantly, but it does not address you. It does its ba-boom, ba-boom, ba-boom thing on its own, like Miles Davis turning his back on the audience. In the middle of the night, you wake up, and you eavesdrop on that intrusive little tenant in your chest practicing its scales, and this is frightening because you know that the minute your tenant stops playing, you're going to die.

Another memory from seventh-grade biology (which I experienced at the time as crushingly boring, my boredom relieved only by immature sex fantasies, but which seems in retrospect to have made a deep impression): Mrs. Sturbenz told us that respiration was not something we could control, and the whole room full of us twelve-year-old junior Nicolaus Stenos began to experiment, hyperventilating and holding our breath. The lungs are spooky— but the heart is spookier still. The heart has a mind of its own.

In the late nineteenth century, scholars of the heartbeat divided themselves into two camps: those who supported the neurogenic theory, that the heartbeat was controlled by the nervous system and ultimately the brain, and those who supported the myogenic theory, that the heartbeat originated in the organ itself. The myogenic theorists won. Your heart does its thing without you. Your brain is not really involved.

At the top of the heart, above the right ventricle, lies a cluster of cells, the sinus node, that sends out an electric impulse every second or so. This is the heart's brain. The electric impulses from the sinus node travel through a network of beating muscle tissue. The heart doesn't use nerves; heart cells are the only muscle cells that conduct their own electric impulses. The electricity travels through ionic exchange, countless molecules of sodium and potassium traveling across hundreds of thousands of cells. The electrical impulse routes first around the upper, smaller chambers, the atria, and, compelled by that impulse, the top chambers beat. Then the energy collects again at a second node—the atrioventricular node—that lies between the right atrium and ventricle. A second burst follows, down the septum of the heart, through pathways called the Purkinje fibers that run the outsides of the ventricles. The ventricles contract. The blood flows.

When we exercise or get excited, our heartbeat accelerates. When we sleep or relax, it slows. In the early nineteenth century, French physiologist François Magendie demonstrated through vivisection that all the sympathetic nerve connections could be cut from the heart and that the organ would continue to beat on its own. In contemporary transplant surgery, all the patient's necessary blood vessels are attached to the new heart, but the nerves are not, so the sympathetic connection between heart and brain is severed—after transplant, the mind conveys excitement to the heart only through blood-borne hormones like adrenaline. Should the heart get damaged by infection, injury, or heart attack, the electrophysiological system can adapt. If a circuit is blocked, a new circuit will develop. If the sinus node fails, the atrioventricular node will take over. The broad outlines of this system are well understood by modern medicine, but the subtleties of molecular conduction and adaptation remain mysterious.

"No one knows," Michael Freed once told me, "how the heart communicates with itself."

The heart is its own creature, a second secret intelligence obscure to the one in the brain, and this is essential to the heart's mystery and metaphorical import. This is why it makes you cry when W. B. Yeats writes, "I feel it in the deep heart's core." The deep heart's core is unfathomable.

In researching this book I had the pleasure of talking with Dr. Abraham Rudolph, the first doctor to perform a cardiac catheterization on an infant. He did it at Boston Children's Hospital in 1956, when most of his patients were babies, dying in the first year of their life, untreated. Rudolph began catheterizing babies in the hopes that they would be treated and cured. According to my sources, he is the most historically significant pediatric cardiologist still alive.

Dr. Rudolph, in his mid-nineties, has thin, dark hair and a somber, lined face. His long fingers have swollen knuckles, and he gestures with them expressively as he speaks. His words are precise and measured out carefully with a bit of a South African accent (as in "heart etteck" or "cet sken"), and he tells wild stories with a charming, self-deprecating giggle. What were you thinking the first time you catheterized a baby? "Well," Abe Rudolph said, "I was scared." Why were you scared? "I was scared," he giggled, "that I'd kill the baby with the catheter."

I spoke with Dr. Rudolph about the history of pediatric cardiology, about the struggle to understand and to treat the heart and to grasp the effects of new treatments. We discussed the complex relationship between new technologies, new diagnoses, and new interventions—for instance, how his early catheterizations helped doctors to understand and operate on the heart. Sometimes his answers were opaque.

"There is unquestionably a relationship," he explained to me regarding catheterization and surgery, "but it is not a direct relationship."

I tried to get him to talk to me about the mid- and late 1950s, the birth of open-heart surgery, and the fears that Welton Gersony had described to me. My questions seemed to frustrate Dr. Rudolph.

How did he feel when he learned about C. Walt Lillehei's two-patient bypass? "Oh, we were very excited," he said, and there was that giggle again, "because now we could do ventricular septal defects." As I pressed him more closely, his responses seemed to grow more general. "In those days we made our decisions based on poor information," he told me. "You base your decisions on what current medical dogma is." He turned rueful about what seemed historically some of his greatest successes. He wondered if some of the riskiest breakthrough heart surgeries he had participated in—in the 1950s, on atrial septal defects—had been necessary. Many atrial septal defects, he told me, close up on their own.

Not until our conversation was over, when I was typing up my notes and going over it in my mind, did I realize what he was trying to tell me. It was difficult for him to explain what those days in the 1950s and 1960s felt like—heady though they were, with their complex calculations of risk and reward, balancing current patients against future patients and developing new technology—because that's what medicine is always like. There is always an area of well-established practice, and then, at the outskirts of that solid ground, an unlit, uncertain wilderness.

In an email exchange after our conversation, Dr. Rudolph surprised me by quoting something Salman Rushdie had originally said about the magic realism of his novel *Midnight's Children*: "Facts are hard to establish, and capable of being given many meanings. Reality is built on our prejudices, misconceptions and ignorance, as well as on our perceptiveness and knowledge." I couldn't decide if Dr. Rudolph was quoting Rushdie to describe my bumbling attempts at history or his early attempts at treatments and diagnosis, and I decided in the end that he meant both.

It's a cliché that medicine is as much an art as a science. ("If we wanted art, Doc," says a character in that Lorrie Moore story, "we'd go to an art museum.") But it's important for patients to understand how much medicine, particularly experimental medicine, is a discipline of the imagination. "We work in the dark—we do what we can—we give what we have": these are Henry James's most famous words about novel writing. "Our doubt is our passion, and our passion is our task." Apparently, Dr. Abraham Rudolph feels much the same about pediatric cardiology.

PART TWO

Etherized Upon a Table

19.

OCTOBER 1931. IMAGINE that you're riding a southbound train from Montreal to New York City. The woman across the aisle smells strange, a mix of rose water and formaldehyde. She has packages everywhere, on the seat beside her, in the rack above, bags, boxes, some wrapped in twine, some in brown paper. The paper looks stained, as though what's inside is leaking. She's got a portfolio full of prints and drawings. She keeps knocking over a big striped umbrella.

She's an older woman, her hair bobbed like a boy's. Her coat is a horrible shade of purple, its velvet patchy and worn. She never takes it off during the length of the ride. She wears a polka-dotted blouse with a stiff collar and a long black skirt with mustard stains from the sandwich you saw her eat at lunchtime. She has glasses and deep lines on either side of her mouth.

You would take her for an eccentric housekeeper or unemployed schoolteacher if not for her masses of papers: journals, manuscripts, and notebooks. She's indefatigable and seems to spend the whole eleven-hour train ride at work. You have a drink, you take a nap, you wake up, and she's still at it, brow furrowed, mouth set, pen working. You find yourself staring at her, and she catches you, and you're embarrassed, but when she smiles, her face turns grandmotherly and childlike, and she makes an odd self-deprecating apology for all the space she's taking up with her packages.

You both get out at Penn Station. She puts on an absurd wide-brimmed hat. She's hardly able to manage her umbrella and handbag. The papers crammed into and protruding out of her briefcase threaten to fall everywhere, and you have no choice but to offer to help her. Even as her boxes clog the aisle of the train and the stairs down to the platform, she's telling you and everyone else who is helping that their assistance is unnecessary. She blushes and stammers and apologizes.

You call her a redcap. The redcap straps it all down on a trolley, but there's still one stinky, fragile box left for you to hold, and you walk with her to the Eighth Avenue cabstand. You accompany her through the packed crowds, and you've got that box in your hands, jars inside clanking, something sticky on the bottom—you wish you'd never picked it up. To relieve the awkwardness, you ask what she is bringing with her to New York, and she begins to talk fast and fluently about the history of the human heart, how it forms in the womb and how it can malform—you didn't know that could happen!—and her eyes are watery and blue and super intelligent, and you're trying to keep up as she discourses about lizards and turtles and ventricles. You walk under the station's huge ironwork columns, the big cathedral ceiling with its enormous panes of glass, and she seems to pay no attention to what's behind or in front of her. When she goes up or down stairs, it's a miracle she doesn't topple, and as you leave the station for the street, you try to get the answer to the first question you asked: What have you been carrying for her?

Oh, she says, laughing, "That box of fetal hearts!"

She snatches it from you. She tips the redcap in Canadian money. The cab door slams. She lowers the window to say something more. She introduces herself as Dr. Maude Abbott, and she invites you to see a display of her work at the Graduate Fortnight at the New York Academy of Medicine. She is still talking as the cab pulls away, and her words are swallowed up by the city.

——

The history of pediatric cardiology begins with Maude Abbott. She was the first doctor to devote her career to the study of congenital heart disease, the first to describe the varieties and pathologies of cardiac birth defects, and the first to publish a book on the subject.

In 1869, two hundred years after Steno, Abbott was born in a small town in Quebec, not far from Montreal. Her mother, Elizabeth Abbott, was the daughter of an Anglican priest and one of eight children, seven of whom ultimately died of tuberculosis. Her father, the Anglican clergyman, was a murderer. On a wintery night in 1866, Maude's father, Jeremiah Babin, took his crippled sister Mary to the Du Lieve River and drowned her there in the icy water and snow. Jeremiah Babin fled Quebec before Maude was born, and seven months after Maude's birth, Maude's mother, Elizabeth, died of tuberculosis.

Maude and her sister Alice were raised in the rectory of the church in St. Andrew's, a small town north of Montreal, by her grandmother, Frances Smith Abbott, a sixty-two-year-old widowed immigrant from Great Britain and a descendent of the Marquis of Hereford. The Abbotts were a prominent family, and the orphaned girls' last names were changed from Babin to Abbott by an act of the Canadian parliament.

In the rectory at St. Andrew's, Maude lived a childhood out of *Anne of Green Gables*. A penknife for Christmas was a wonderful gift; so was a bit of bright ribbon. She was a bookish girl. In her teenage diary she wrote, "One of my day-dreams, which I feel to be selfish, is that of going to school. . . . And here I go again: once begin dreaming of the possibilities and I become half daft of what I know will never come to pass. Oh, to *think* of studying with other girls!" Her grandmother, when Maude was seventeen, indulged her and sent her to a girls' school in Montreal. That same year, McGill University opened its doors to women; Abbott applied a couple years later, and she was admitted. The university became the great love of her life. For the most part, that love was unrequited.

"Very enthusiastic we all were," she wrote of those first classes of women to attend McGill. "But I think perhaps I, who was country-bred, and had not had my fill of school or directed study before I entered Arts, felt our new advantage most acutely of all. I was, literally, in love with McGill, and I have never really fallen out of love with her since." This was Abbott's lifelong romance, with a university that would never take her seriously. She entered McGill dreaming of a career in the arts but graduated with her heart set on medicine.

It was an exciting time to be a physician. Throughout Abbott's childhood, medicine had been changing, emerging, and becoming increasingly rigorous, scientific, and professional. The English doctor Joseph Lister had published his first accounts of antiseptics in the *Lancet* in 1867, just two years before Abbott's birth. Lister used carbolic acid on the dressings of his patients' wounds, and he demonstrated statistically that infection rates dropped. When he came to the United States in 1876 to promote germ theory, his ideas faced doubt and resistance. "People say there are bacteria in the air," said Alfred Loomis, president of the New York Academy of Medicine, "but I cannot see them." Loomis and his colleagues worked in unwashed wool coats, going straight from operating rooms to morgues to delivery rooms, unwittingly spreading sepsis and death. Hospitals were as dangerous as battlefields. (The denial of germ theory among so many doctors, like the denial of blood circulation 250 years before, makes one wonder about how reflexive the denial of science is; no matter how seemingly obvious in retrospect, any new theory will face contradiction.) Germ theory changed medicine, and concordant with its advance, medical education changed.

The father of modern medical education, William Osler, taught at McGill from 1876 to 1884 and in 1893 helped found Johns Hopkins Medical School, the first medical school in America to require that its entering students have four-year college degrees. "The future belongs to science," Osler said. For him, laboratory technicians were "essential to the proper equipment of the hospital. . . . They are to the physician just as the knife and the scalpel are to the surgeon." Osler's 1892 *The Principles and Practice of Medicine* was the modern, turn-of-the-century physician's bible.

Abbott wanted to enter this new world of scientific medicine, but because she was a woman, she was not permitted. Though she graduated valedictorian of her class, McGill rejected Abbott's medical school application. The idea of a woman doctor was laughable. Her application was a scandal covered by Montreal newspapers. "Can you think of a patient in a critical case," wrote Dr. F. W. Campbell, a member of the McGill faculty, "waiting for half an hour while the medical lady fixes her bonnet or adjusts her bustle?" Abbott was forced to attend the much smaller Bishop's College Medical School, which accepted women, Jews, and blacks from the Caribbean. There, she distinguished herself. She won prizes. She did postgraduate work in Europe. Abbott was the first woman ever to have her work read at the Montreal Medico-Chirugical Society—the same paper was presented overseas in England in 1900, the first by a woman given before the Pathological Society in London. She had hoped, initially, to become a gynecologist, but her success in diagnosing rare conditions of the liver led her to consider a career in pathology.

She needed to stay in Montreal—her sister Alice was mentally ill; Maude had to take care of her. While Maude worked in Montreal, Alice rested in the rectory at St. Andrew's. Abbott was offered a position at the Verdun Protestant Hospital for the Insane, a residency in neuropathology, but all she wanted was McGill. She petitioned Dr. George J. Adami, who ran the pathology lab there: "If you could do for me what you suggested, and allowed me to work in your laboratory on a scholarship in neuropathology . . . I would be extremely happy, which is nothing to the point, but I think I could do better work than I have been able to give evidence of yet." He did not offer her a scholarship to work in his lab. The best he could offer her, Adami said, was the part-time job of assistant curator of the medical museum.

"I would infinitely prefer to work anywhere else," Abbott wrote back.

She didn't have an office. Her desk lay in a curtained space at the end of a hallway. The museum itself was a mess. It contained records of all Osler's early work—he had performed some 750 autopsies there and kept everything that seemed interesting. Adami was devoted to expanding the collections, but his zeal for collecting was unmatched by any organizational genius. In 1900 there was no standardized way of cataloguing pathology specimens. All the material was boxed and bottled and shelved almost at random.

Abbott traveled to Washington, DC, to see how the Army Medical Museum sorted its specimen collections. While there, she went to Baltimore to see Osler lecture. When the great man left the hall, Abbott approached him, but the door closed on her hand and took off a fingernail. Osler himself attended to her wound.

She revered him. Her devotion was to scientific medicine, her Parthenon was McGill, and Osler was the god of her temple. Now he stood before her, big, bearded, brilliant, authoritative, and taking care of her bleeding finger. He was interested in her work on his specimen collections. He invited her to his home for dinner. "I wonder, now," he said, "if you realize what an opportunity you have?" He sent her a letter, urging her to look up an article, "Clinical Museum," in the *British Medical Journal*. "Pictures of life and death together—wonderful," wrote Osler. "Then see what you can do." He set before her the prospect of building something that did not yet exist in North America, a great medical museum, a living resource of pathology.

Back in Montreal, Abbott was overcome. The task ahead of her was stultifying. "Promising drudgery," she called it. The sheer volume of work was overwhelming. Abbott suffered a nervous breakdown. She stopped working for six months. But then she began again—labeling and sorting every specimen in the McGill medical museum. The museum secretary had to remind Abbott of the end of the workday, and Abbott would apologize for holding the secretary and then stay there late into the night. She worked for hours on end, forgetting to eat, forgetting to sleep, completely consumed by her task. Maybe she had some of the same mania that possessed her murderer father and invalid sister.

She traveled back and forth to Europe to learn about medical museums. At home in Montreal she lay in bed surrounded by letters from all over the world, writing furiously back to doctors, pathologists, and curators. She organized an international society of medical museum curators and became editor of its bulletin.

In sorting out the McGill collections, Abbott was inventing a profession.

The most intriguing of all the items in the collection, for Abbott, was a heart with one ventricle, the Holmes heart. In a letter, Osler explained to her that this was a rare congenital deformity, discovered at McGill in 1834. In 1901, Abbott wrote a biographical sketch of Andrew Holmes, the doctor who had first reported the heart, for the *Montreal Medical Journal*. This was her first contribution to the study of congenitally deformed hearts.

At the turn of the century, the heart was beyond medicine's reach. Understanding of it hadn't advanced much since Steno's time. Doctors had a poor sense of the organ and few tools for looking at it. For the most part, they thought of the heart in the same way that William Harvey had described it in 1618, when he coined the term "circulation." In *De motu cordis*, Harvey wrote,

> The heart, consequently, is the beginning of life; the sun of the microcosm, even as the sun might be designated the heart of the world; for it is the heart by whose virtue and pulse the blood is moved, perfected, made apt to nourish, and is prevented from corruption and coagulation; it is the household divinity, which, discharging its function, nourishes, cherishes, quickens the whole body, and is indeed the foundation of life, the source of all action.

Theodor Billroth, the most prominent European surgeon of his time, was reported to have said in 1883, "A surgeon who tries to suture a heart wound deserves to lose the esteem of his colleagues." In 1886, Billroth's British colleague Stephen Paget wrote, "Surgery of the heart has probably reached the limit set by Nature to all surgery: no new method, and no new discovery, can overcome the natural difficulties that attend a heart wound." Osler himself, in 1892, described adult heart disease as "relatively rare."

The earliest recorded cardiac surgeries were not on the myocardium, the heart muscle, or the great blood vessels on the top of the heart but on the pericardium, the tough, triple-layered sac that surrounds the heart, and these first surgeries were practiced in obscure corners of the medical world and soon forgotten. In 1815, Francisco Romero, a Catalan doctor in the French army, described a technique for treating pericardial effusion, or fluid around the heart. Romero believed the cause of pericardial effusions were the south wind, gazpacho, and tobacco rolled in paper. For treatment, he made an incision at the curve of the sixth rib, then used a pair of small scissors to cut the pericardial sac and let the fluid drain. For the patient in recovery, Romero recommended a diet of partridge broth, wheat bread soaked in red wine and sugar, and small doses of absinthe to drink. Romero performed seven of these surgeries, without antibiotics or anesthetics, and remarkably only one of his patients died, but when he presented his findings before the society of medicine in Paris, the authorities did not receive his paper favorably, and his contribution to medicine was lost.

Nearly a hundred years later, in 1893 in Chicago, an African American doctor named Daniel Hale Williams III repaired a stab wound that had reached his patient's pericardium. It was the summer of the World's Fair. The original Ferris wheel rose above the city, and facsimiles of the *Nina*, the *Pinta*, and the *Santa Maria* floated in Lake Michigan. Exhibitors displayed new products: Pabst Blue Ribbon beer, Juicy Fruit gum, and Quaker Oats. In a bar on the south side, a railroad worker named James Cornish got into a brawl. Someone carved a hole in Cornish's chest, and he was taken to Provident Hospital, a three-story, twelve-room, brick building on 29th and Deerborn, run and founded by Williams and the Chicago black community. (Frederick Douglass was one of the original supporters and fund-raisers.) Williams was one of just four African American doctors in the city.

Pictures of Williams show a man with close-cropped hair, a big bushy beard, and the light skin and sharp features of his Shawnee ancestors. Many of his patients were workers from the nearby Armour Meatpacking Plant, who came to him bleeding and mangled by the slaughterhouse machinery. Cornish, drunk and dying, arrived at the row house hospital on the night of July 9. Dr. Williams felt his pulse, listened to his breathing, and put a long tubular wooden stethoscope to Cornish's chest. Initially, Williams diagnosed the wound as superficial, sewed it up, and let the patient rest, but overnight Cornish's condition worsened. The heartbeat got weak and slow. Williams could hardly feel a pulse in Cornish's neck.

In a hospital room hotter than one hundred degrees, six of his colleagues gathered around. They opened the windows to ventilate the space. Williams cut a six-inch incision into Cornish's chest. He retracted the ribs and siphoned away the blood. There was the beating heart, something that no one in the room had ever seen. The hole in the muscle was tiny. Williams let the heart be and sewed up the rip in the pericardium with catgut. The patient recovered. It took two months, but Cornish left the hospital as a new kind of thing, a survivor of cardiac surgery. But the work of a black doctor at a small black-owned hospital didn't get much attention at the time.

The first person to demonstrate to the medical establishment that a wound to the heart muscle could be repaired was Ludwig Rehn, the chief surgeon at Frankfort City Hospital, already famous for his surgeries on cancer and his pioneering thyroidectomies. Rehn's patient was (like Williams's) stabbed in a bar fight. In the early morning of September 8, 1896, Wilhelm Justus, a gardener's assistant, had been discovered behind a park bench, bleeding and clutching his chest. Blood was oozing from him when Justus was taken to the hospital, and in the morning Rehn found him lying in a corner, waiting to die. Rehn listened to Justus's breathing and examined his skin. He palpated the chest wound. He opened the chest and found Justus's pericardium swollen like a balloon, blown up to twice its normal size, stretching toward Justus's armpit. Rehn picked up his scalpel and made his incision. There was an explosion of blood and then a trickle. When Rehn suctioned the mess away, he got a good look at the right ventricle and the blood that with each beat of the heart came leaking from a half-inch gash. He put his finger on the hole, and then he did something that no one had ever recorded doing before. He sutured the wound in the muscle, and the patient survived.

Rehn expanded on this operation, recommending a surgery for pericardial effusions that was in many ways quite similar to Romero's (less the partridge broth, etc.). Theodor Billroth, Rehn's eminent colleague, called these repairs of pericardial effusions "prostitution of the surgical art" and "surgical frivolity." Despite Rehn's success, the heart retained its holy aura in 1899 when Abbott went to Europe to do her postgraduate studies, but diagnostic technology was improving, and as it did, so did medical understanding.

From a single wooden tube, the stethoscope became the two-ear device we know today. Early machines called sphygmomanometers traced and measured the movement of the pulse, and by the 1880s French physician and inventor Etienne Jules Marey had adapted these devices to measure systolic blood pressure. Wilhelm Röntgen invented the X-ray machine, and it became possible to picture the size and placement of a patient's heart. The first electrocardiograph machine was Willem Eintoven's string galvometer, invented in the Netherlands in 1901. The machine filled three rooms in Eintoven's lab. The patient sat with a hand and a leg each in a separate bucket of water, and these buckets conducted the impulses of the heart to a tiny, sensitive filament—Eintoven's first filaments were made of molten glass, spun fine by shooting a bolt from a crossbow and catching the trailing strings, then covering the strings with silver. The slight tremblings of these silvered glass threads were magnified by a Zeiss lens and made decipherable. It took decades after its invention for the EKG to become a commonplace clinical tool, and even with all these new technologies, heart disease remained mysterious.

In 1901 doctors focused less on heart function than on morbid pathology of the heart—the scars on the valves left by syphilis, rheumatic fever, and diphtheria. Doctors weren't interested much in the aging heart or how it worked. It wasn't until the 1920s that doctors agreed on a clinical diagnosis for heart attack—acute myocardial infarction—and this came, according to the historian of medicine Roy Porter, "only after huge debate and negotiation over the meaning of clinical and machine-readable signs." In the 1920s, "cardiology" was a newfangled word, and if adult heart disease wasn't a real concern of the medical establishment, congenital heart disease was still more neglected. In *Principles and Practices of Medicine*, Osler discusses "congenital affections of the heart" briefly, and his section on the subject begins, "These have only a limited clinical interest, as in a large proportion of the cases, the anomaly is not compatible with life, and in others nothing can be done to remedy the defect or relieve the symptoms."

In 1904, Osler, now a British peer and an Oxford don, paid a visit to Maude Abbott at McGill. "I shall never forget him as I saw him walking down the old museum toward me," Abbott wrote, "with his great dark shining eyes fixed full upon me."

They sat together, reviewing his collections. Based on her work on the Holmes heart, he invited her to write the section on congenital heart disease for his forthcoming *A System of Medicine*, an encyclopedic work on medical subspecialties. Of the 104 medical authors he selected, Abbott was the only woman. Her contribution would be a small essay in a huge encyclopedia, but, characteristically, Maude Abbott threw herself into the subject. She reviewed the records of 412 autopsies. She developed large charts of features and symptoms. She began to systematically imagine and organize the pathology of congenital heart disease. The writing took two years, and when she sent it to Osler, he was delighted. "I knew you would write a good article, but I did not expect one of such extraordinary merit. It is by far and away the best thing ever written on the subject in English—possibly in any language. I cannot begin to tell you how much I appreciate the care and trouble you have taken."

Abbott was now the world's foremost medical museum curator and expert on deformed hearts. In 1910, McGill awarded her an honorary medical degree, but it turned down her application to join the medical faculty, even though the pathology courses she taught were now a compulsory part of medical education at McGill. As her colleague Dr. Harold Seagall later recalled, "The mood at McGill was rather provincial. In certain circles it was acceptable to regard Dr. Abbott as an inferior character, someone to be tolerated and humored—a 'hen medic.'"

Outside McGill, women were increasingly advocating for their own rights. As the historian Jill Lepore tells it, "The word 'feminism,' hardly ever used before 1910, was everywhere by 1913. It meant advocacy of women's rights and freedoms and a vision of equality." In 1911, Abbott delivered a lecture at Harvard titled "Women in Medicine." The lecture is a sixteen-page epic, a tight little demonstration of erudition. It moves from the medical skills of "Antiochis, daughter of Diodotos," for whom a statue was raised in the ancient city of Tlos, to "Fabiola, the founder of hospitals in Italy, AD 380," to Allessandra Giliani of Periceta, a fourteenth-century anatomist, to the Countess of Cinchona, "who, in 1640, introduced the use of quinine bark" for the treatment of malaria, and Lady Mary Wortley Montagu, who brought vaccination to Europe in 1718. Abbott was claiming her place in history—asserting, contrary to her colleagues, that there was nothing extraordinary about her doing so, that women had always been a part of the development of medicine.

In 1900, there were about 7,000 female doctors in the United States, comprising about 5.6 percent of American physicians. (England, by contrast, had just 258 women doctors, and France had only 95.) In Boston, the numbers were considerably better: almost a fifth of the doctors there were women. But at McGill, Abbott was still seen as something of a freak, like a dancing bear—the wonder not that she knew a great deal about medicine but that she knew anything about it at all. At the outbreak of World War I, McGill Medical School was reorganized, and administrators wanted to get rid of her and to dismiss her from her position at the museum. Threatened, she wrote to her superior, George Adami, in a panic, finally expressing her rage and asking McGill to take her seriously:

> The cure is surely to treat me with the decency that I deserve and that the facts demand. To acknowledge *me* as the museum expert, the one who really does know most about the work and its needs . . . to give me on the basis of my museum teaching, and my lectures on congenital cardiac disease, the Associate Professorship that is my due . . . to raise my salary to a real

'part-time' salary corresponding to what I do, or else a real 'full-time' one; and to give me an assistant at $1,500 a year. . . . I *am* on the breaking point financially and in other ways.

The response she got was dismissive: "Take the world cheerfully and do not worry. . . . I think every true friend of yours must see that your wisest policy is to 'Do your duty in the state of life to which it has pleased God to call you.'"

Abbott fell ill. She had major abdominal surgery for the removal of ovarian tumors. Soon after her recovery from that operation, Osler died. She undertook to edit a special Osler memorial volume of the *Bulletin of the International Association of Medical Museums*. It took her six years to put together and in the end ran to over six hundred pages. The year before it was published, Harvey Cushing came out with his two-volume biography of Osler, which won the Pulitzer Prize. Abbott's memorial volume left her $1,000 in debt. She set out to write a history of her beloved institution, *McGill's Heroic Past*, only to discover, just as she was about to publish, that the university had hired an art history professor to write a similar book. She was finally made assistant professor at McGill, but her museum was taken away from her.

Maude Abbott was an eccentric woman. She looked at the ground as she walked and muttered to herself. She had trouble crossing streets and climbing stairs. She got lab samples all over her clothes. Friends called her "the beneficent tornado" and the "big chief of heart." Enemies mocked her. She was offered jobs elsewhere, at the University of Texas and at the Women's College of Pennsylvania. All she wanted was McGill, but McGill would not have her. By the time she came to New York City to present her work in a display at the Graduate Fortnight of the New York Academy of Medicine in the fall of 1931, her career seemed at a dead end.

———

In the exhibition hall of the grand building on 103rd Street and Fifth Avenue, she set up a long piece of gray millboard, about four feet high by thirty-two feet long. Her exhibit gave an overview of 1,000 cases of congenital heart disease, set into three large categories and some dozen subcategories, illustrated by photographs, paintings, models, and EKG readings. There were fetal hearts and turtle hearts and lizard hearts. The exhibit reviewed the heart's development in the womb and in evolutionary terms. It was huge, cluttered, and complex but a marvel of comprehensive study, and for the first time in her life, Abbott gained a wide audience for her work.

English doctors invited her to include her exhibit in the centenary meeting of the British Medical Association in London. The display was praised by the *British Medical Journal*, and Abbott shipped it back across the Atlantic and showed it again in Atlantic City in 1935 at the joint meeting of the American and Canadian Medical Associations, and then again before the Ontario Medical Association in 1936. The American Medical Association published the exhibit's contents in a single volume, *The Atlas of Congenital Cardiac Disease*. Abbott was nearly seventy.

The volume is a large, thin, beautiful book, 110 pages long including its index, and the first comprehensive book ever published on the subject. The left-hand pages are dense with small type and Latinate phrases; the right-hand pages are cluttered with complex collages of line drawings, photographs, diagrams, and EKG prints.

There's something eccentric and homemade about the atlas. It's a portrait of congenital heart disease but also of the mind of Maude Abbott. Each page has the concentrated force of a lifetime of intellectual labor crammed into a narrow space. Plate 1, a single 11- × 14-inch page, "Development of the Reptilian and Mammalian Heart," has sixteen illustrations sorted into four subsets: a pig heart, the hearts of two turtles, a sand lizard heart in nine stages of development, and the developing human embryotic heart. A short paragraph gives a terse history of the evolution of the human heart, a summary of the development of the fetal heart, and a theory of the etiology of heart defects: "The critical period in the human subject lies between the fifth and eighth weeks of embryonic life, i.e., before the cardiac septa are formed, and while the complex processes of torsion, involution, readjustment and fusion are taking place at the base, interruption of which is the source of most of the graver anomalies." All her expertise is boiled down into paragraphs short enough to fit on a wall of a traveling exhibit.

Plate XIX is tetralogy of Fallot. Eleven images are squeezed onto a single plate: two schematic line drawings, two diagrams demonstrating the results of medical tests, a couple of EKG readings, an X-ray, and four delicate illustrations of cross sections of the deformed heart. The facing plate includes a short introduction, two or three inches of knotty prose, and then annotations of all eleven images. Between the introduction and the annotations runs a band of smaller text, a list of sixteen references for further study. Tetralogy of Fallot, she says, "is also the most important [defect] from the clinical stand point" because of its frequency and also because patients suffering with it can survive into their teenage years.

"The whole appearance," she writes in her dense, rapid-fire prose, "is highly suggestive of the relationships that would result from the uncovering of the right reptilian aorta and obliteration of the left in the delayed torsion of Spitzer's theory (his types I and II of transposition) and is of great interest in this connection." There's little room for elaboration. This book wants to be a museum, a museum that wants to be an encyclopedia, and it seems to carry its own delayed torsion, its own power, and a sense of embattled growth of intellectual life, an intelligence overflowing the arbitrary boundaries that try vainly to restrain it.

These knotty sentences are the beginnings of pediatric cardiology. With her atlas, Maude Abbott brought congenital heart disease out of obscurity and into serious study—carrying kids like me out of darkness and into the light. Her book (no exaggeration) saved my life.

20.

S O, AFTER I got the letter from Dr. Freed and canceled my catheter exam, I stepped out of my morning shower and heard that message on my answering machine: "It's Dr. Rosenbaum, calling about your heart." I went to work without calling him back.

Barnard College had been nice to me, and while I taught there on an adjunct basis, I was given use of the office of a distinguished professor currently on leave. So on the first day of school, I had the key to a beautiful book-lined room, and a big desk with framed black-and-white photographs of the distinguished professor's children, and a leather swivel chair and windows overlooking the quad. I sat in the well-appointed office and picked up the phone. I told Dr. Rosenbaum's secretary that I was returning the doctor's call. Then I went to the photocopier. I looked like an academic. I wore a blazer, and I carried a notebook and a copy of Emily Dickinson's poems. Photocopies made, I went back to my borrowed office and stared hard at the telephone, waiting for it to ring. I drank an entire sixteen-ounce bottle of seltzer, and then I was late to class.

In the hall, I ran into the novelist Mary Gordon, someone whose books I'd read and admired but whom I'd never before spoken to. She stopped to chat and introduce herself. She wondered what books I'd assigned for my class. She ooh-ed and aah-ed at my choices. She asked after my writing, and I asked after hers, and then I was so distracted and insecure that I didn't stop at the bathroom to urinate.

Around the big seminar table sat sixteen bright young women, all ready for their first day of college. I went through the syllabus with them and asked them to introduce themselves.

"Say your name and something you'd want the class to know about you," I said. "Something interesting or funny or just something you feel okay telling us all. Let's go around the room."

I heard the sighs. Everyone hates to *go around the room*. The nervous ones announced their hometowns. The cute ones talked about their pets. The pretentious ones mentioned Fyodor Dostoevsky. Then it was my turn.

"I'm Gabe," I blurted, "and I'm not a real professor."

Before the words came out, they seemed reasonable—or at least honest: their families were paying tens of thousands of dollars for the privilege of their sitting in that room with me. But once spoken, the words hung in the air like a fart.

"What do we call you then?" one student asked.

"Gabe?" I suggested. "Gabriel? Mr. Brownstein?"

"How about Comrade Brownstein," said my new favorite. Let's call her Olivia. Olivia had tiny features, freckles, a wide face, and a gigantic smile.

"Comrade Brownstein," I agreed. She had rescued me. We got to the Dickinson poem "I like to see it lap the Miles." We read it aloud, a student for each stanza. I asked for vocabulary questions.

Once all the words were nailed down, we read the poem a second time. I kept spacing out, thinking of the big, black Bakelite telephone on the distinguished professor's desk, imagining the ring and, on the other end, Marlon Rosenbaum. Also, I had to pee.

The students got to work on the poem's famous riddle. They wanted to know what the "it" was that lapped the miles and licked the valleys up. Some kind of monster? God? Jesus? Sex? I urged them to go slowly. What would "neigh"? What would have a "stable door"?

"A horse!" someone cried.

"Why is she writing about a giant, angry, valley-destroying horse?"

I threw out a question in return: "What's a 'horrid, hooting stanza'?"

"It's a train!"

Bingo! Elation!

And then for an awful moment I felt there was nothing left to say. All sixteen ounces of soda bubbled in my bladder. I reminded my students that in the mid-nineteenth century, the train was a new, anomalous thing. I asked about the words "I like" at the start of the poem.

"It's not a train," said Olivia, intently, big smile gone from her freckled face. "Or it's a train but it's not a train. If it was a train, she would just say it was a train, but the whole point of the poem is that she can't speak it. It's the thing you just can't say, and when she says she *likes* it, she doesn't mean she likes *it* at all. She likes to *watch* it. Or that's what she says."

I stood. Sixteen pretty expectant faces looked up at me, as if I could extend or explain Olivia's point.

"I gotta go," I said.

I handed out the assignment sheet and dashed out of the room, down the hall for a toilet. When I closed my borrowed office door, I was sweating. I sat down in the big chair. I stared at the phone. When it rang, it startled me.

"You can't cancel today," said Dr. Rosenbaum. "We've got the cath lab set up. Everything's scheduled. You can't call up the day before and say no."

I just got Freed's letter, I explained. How could I have called earlier when I just got that letter Sunday?

"Dr. Freed wrote a long letter." He sighed.

"He said I should wait. I don't want to take the risk."

Dr. Rosenbaum assured me the procedure was safe. "We do this on people who are moribund, Gabriel. *Moribund.*"

I was getting frustrated. "I can't do it if he said no."

"What do you want?"

"I want time to think about it. To talk about it."

His patience snapped. "We have talked about it a lot."

I hung up. As a patient and doctor, we seemed done.

That night, I went to a party for a colleague who taught with me at my other adjunct job, at Parsons School of Design. The chair of my department at Parsons was there, along with the rest of the liberal arts faculty. There was a stack of handsome volumes of poetry and an open bar, and I started on gin and moved to whiskey. I flirted recklessly with a redheaded actress/model and got so drunk I vomited in the toilet. The redheaded actress/model took pity on me and helped me into a cab, and when I got home, I knew that I would never see her again.

I woke up with a dry mouth and a head like an egg whose yolk had been replaced with mercury, an egg that had to be held very carefully because at any moment it might split, and the goop within would go spilling all over the place. I drank water and coffee and took Tylenol and ate eggs, and my head swelled and shrank. There was a message on my answering machine, the same one I had heard the morning before.

"It's Dr. Rosenbaum," it said, "calling about your heart."

21.

HELEN TAUSSIG ENTERED the lab carrying a small cage with a cat in it. She turned on the lights, put on a smock, and tied up her hair. There was no one in the room but her. It was 1923. In US medical schools and hospitals, congenital heart diseases were not being studied or diagnosed, let alone cured. Taussig was twenty-six years old.

She had been loaned this laboratory at Boston University. She was not a student there, or a doctor, or a technician. She had no assistants. She had no salary. She was working in a purely amateur capacity.

She set out her instruments: her scalpel, scissors, flasks, lever, saline solution, digitalis, adrenaline, and oxygen tanks. She prepared a syringe, filled it with the necessary dose of chloretone, and opened the cage, gripping the mewling cat by the nape of its neck and murmuring to it sweetly. She jabbed her needle into the animal's belly, careful not to hit the liver or any other major organ. The cat convulsed. It kicked and flashed its claws. Twenty minutes later, it was deeply anesthetized. Thirty minutes later, it was dead. Taussig jotted down the time of death in her notebook: 2:40 p.m.

She took out her scissors and snipped open the cat's belly, cutting through the blood-matted fur. She excised the heart. With her scalpel, she cut it free from the great arteries. Then it was in her hands, a cat's heart, the size of a plum. She placed it in a warm bath of 75 ccs Tyrode's saline solution and marked the time: 3:40 p.m.

As the heart lay in its bath, the dead ventricle began slow, definite contractions.

Carefully, Taussig segmented off a strip of muscle fiber. She held it with a clip specially covered with paraffin and attached the clip to a glass hook. She attached the hook by fine threads to her lever and then gently lowered her strip of muscle fiber into a new flask of saline solution, this one mixed with cat blood. The muscle strip began to contract in strong, alternating pulses. The beating continued for nearly fifty minutes. When the beating stopped, at 4:40 p.m., Taussig administered a solution of 1:1000 P&D adrenaline chloride to the flask. One tiny, calibrated squeeze from the glass dropper, and the muscle beat in short, jerky rhythms. Five minutes later, the effects of the adrenaline passed. Now, Taussig administered five drops of digitalis and watched the muscle fiber work for a full half hour more. Then she looked at the clock. It was 5 p.m. She bundled and disposed of the cat corpse and soaped and sponged down the tables. At 5:15 p.m., when she had to leave the lab, the little strip of ventricle muscle was still beating.

Taussig had tried to gain admission to Harvard Medical School, but because she was a woman, she had been refused. She'd tried to attend the School of Public Health and was told a woman could attend classes but could not receive a diploma.

"Who is going to be such a fool as to spend four years studying and not get a degree?" she asked the dean.

"No one, I hope," he replied.

"I'll not be the first to disappoint you," said Taussig. "Good afternoon."

At lectures at Harvard, she was forced to sit in the back row of the auditorium. When the medical students examined slides, Taussig and her microscope were put in a separate room.

"So I wouldn't contaminate the other—male!—students," she remembered.

She set out on her independent research through the help of a friendly professor at Boston University and began investigating the beat of the heart muscle. She prowled the morgue and the hospital for subjects. A patient died at 2:30 p.m. one afternoon, and by 5:30 p.m., Taussig had the man's heart in her lab. By 5:50 p.m., a strip of his ventricle was on a glass hook, tied by a linen thread to a lever. In 1924, Helen Taussig's first academic article was published, "Rhythmic Contraction in Isolated Strips of Mammalian Ventricle," in the *American Journal of Physiology*.

Taussig, unaffiliated with any medical institution, was the first to discover that "isolated strips of mammalian muscle" could "give spontaneous rhythmic contractions after simple immersion in oxygenated solution." This was the level of achievement required, in 1924, for a woman to get into medical school. Johns Hopkins, at the time of its founding, had accepted a large donation from a group of wealthy women and in return accepted ten female applicants each year. ("In effect," as historian Paul Starr puts it, "American women were forced to buy their way into elite medical education.") Taussig went off to Baltimore and began her career.

In 1924, there were no organized descriptions of congenital heart defects. It was a decade and a half before Maude Abbott published her atlas. In 1924, no one was interested in diagnosing children with defective hearts because no one believed those children could be cured—least of all Helen Taussig. But she was a remarkable woman, born to a remarkable family.

Her paternal grandfather, William Taussig, a Jewish immigrant from Prague, had been a chemist who became a doctor, and a mayor, and a judge. He was a friend of Ulysses S. Grant, and during the Civil War, Judge Taussig served in the Union Army. When a band of Confederate terrorists led by Bloody Bill Anderson overthrew an insane asylum in Fulton, Missouri, Judge Taussig got on his horse, guns and medical supplies in his saddlebags, and rode a hundred miles. Arriving in town, he organized a volunteer posse, and he gathered the lost patients together and loaded them into farm wagons. Without military escort, he led the wagon train through a territory wild with guerrilla warriors—Quantrill's raiders were out there and men like Frank and Jesse James, murderers and rapists and sadists whose most grotesque exploits were celebrated in the rebel press. Taussig guided his patients to Mexico, Missouri, and loaded them on a train for St. Louis.

William's son Frank was a large, handsome boy who played basketball and rowed crew at Harvard, graduated a year early at the top of his class, completed a PhD in economics, and married Edith Guild, a wealthy New England girl with two degrees in botany from Radcliffe. They bought a big Victorian house in Cambridge, a few blocks from the university. You can still see it, painted white and gray with high hedges that surround its generous lawn. Except for the satellite dish, it probably looks like it did in 1898, when Helen Taussig was born, their fourth child and third daughter. Frank Taussig was the chair of the economics department at Harvard, one of the most influential economists in the country—he helped settle the terms of surrender in the Treaty of Versailles.

Helen's first scientific interest was botany. She examined the pistils and stamens of the gladioli in her mother's flower garden and used a magnifying glass to look into the parts of the geraniums. With her father, she planted seeds and tended a vegetable garden. Frank Taussig taught all his children German and music. They took picnics in the countryside and had a summer home in Cotuit in Cape Cod. When Helen was three, her father suffered a nervous collapse. Frank Taussig left his wife and children and spent two years in Europe recovering. Not long after his return, Edith Taussig came down with tuberculosis.

For two years, she coughed up blood. Frank Taussig had an elevator installed in the house, with big rope pulleys so servants, nurses, and doctors could heft his wife up and down between the second and first floors. Young Helen found herself struggling at school. Letters played tricks on her. They reversed themselves, *p*'s turned into *q*'s, *b*'s into *d*'s, *d*'s into *q*'s and back again. The orders of letters dissolved and reorganized. She saw no difference between the words *dread* and *bread* and *beard*. Dyslexia was not a common diagnosis then. To her teachers, Helen seemed slow and stubborn. They forced her to stand and read in front of the class, and she suffered panic attacks, sweats, stomach cramps, and trembling. She'd get it wrong, and they'd ask her to do it again, and she would burst into tears and go running home, where her bed-bound mother was coughing up blood. Her father would tend to Helen.

The chairman of the Harvard economics department sat with his youngest daughter night after night, going through her homework, helping her with her French verbs, reading with her slowly and carefully, while his wife lay dying upstairs. When Helen was eleven, she became tubercular too. She had to sleep on the porch of the house—the fresh air was thought to be good for her lungs. From the upstairs open windows came her mother's coughing, and from all around, the sound of Cambridge at night. Edith Taussig died. Helen, after two and half years of sickness, recovered.

As an adult, she liked to sleep on porches. She liked to say that childhood sickness had taught her "a sound lesson in how to economize one's strength and an understanding of those who did not have it." At Radcliffe, she played basketball and volleyball. When her father remarried, Helen moved across the country to California. She finished school at Berkeley. She liked to hike in the hills and look down at the harbor.

Although Johns Hopkins admitted ten women each year, it only awarded one graduate internship per graduating class. In 1927, a competing female student had a GPA two-tenths of a point higher than Taussig, and that was it: no internship for Helen Taussig. Her career had hardly started, and on a second important occasion she had been knocked to the side on account of her sex. After graduation, she left Baltimore for a period of wandering, part-time positions. She went to New York and to Boston.

Dr. Edwards Park, one of her professors at Hopkins, wanted to hire her for a position that interested no one else: running the dispensary at the Harriet Lane Home, a new clinic for the study of children with heart disease, mostly kids with scarred valves due to rheumatic fever. Taussig seemed to prefer no job at all to a job looking after those heart-sick babies.

"The field does interest me," she wrote Park, politely declining his offer, but "my experience in dealing with acute cardiac conditions in children is virtually nil." And "I do appreciate the opportunity that it offers to me, but my feeling is that I do not offer it enough to make it the success I want to see."

Though she wasn't interested in taking care of sick babies, she was interested in research on the heart. In Boston, she wrote to Park, "they have very kindly introduced me to another group of 'cardiologists' who meet one evening a week at Dr. Paul White's laboratory." That she put the word "cardiologists" in quotation marks begins to describe her skepticism but also the state of cardiac medicine at the time.

Cardiology wasn't a recognized medical specialty. In 1911, in Osler's suggested list of hospital units, there isn't one devoted to the heart. It wasn't until 1914 in London that the first clinic specifically devoted to the heart opened. By the 1920s, new technologies—the EKG, the X-ray, and blood pressure measurement—were being used by doctors like Thomas Lewis in London, who was beginning to consider heart function and cardiac efficiency in clinical terms. Harvard's Dr. Paul Dudley White brought this new cardiology to the United States. At one of White's weekly meetings in Boston, Helen Taussig encountered a strange old woman: short, plump, rumpled, with her hair a mess, her dress stained with food, carrying various odd packages. At least one of those packages contained a very interesting specimen. A single-ventricle deformity? A tetralogy of Fallot? We'll never know. In a letter to Edwards Park, Taussig wrote, "Last night there was a most interesting informal meeting in Dr. Paul White's laboratory at which Dr. Abbott showed a most extraordinary heart." Soon after, Taussig accepted the position at the Harriet Lane dispensary.

Initially, the majority of the pediatric cardiology patients at the Harriet Lane Home were children not with congenital heart defects but with rheumatic heart disease. Before the widespread use of penicillin, strep infections frequently spread from the throat to the heart, and in children this could cause scarring and lifelong dysfunction of the heart valves. The devastation was widespread. A Depression-era study in New York City surveyed forty-eight schools and found sixty-eight special-ed classes devoted specifically to kids with scarred heart valves—at least 7,000 students in the New York public school system suffered from rheumatic heart disease.

"Congenital abnormalities were the last thing in the world I expected to be interested in," Taussig once explained. "I started with a busy rheumatic clinic. . . . It [congenital heart disease] fell on me—or I fell on it."

Abbott had published her much-praised encyclopedia article on congenital heart disease in Osler's *A System of Medicine*, but not much else had been published on the subject. In the late 1920s, the literature on congenital heart disease was both ancient and foggy, going all the way back Steno, but still no one was trying to cure kids with defective hearts.

Park invested in the clinic. He made sure it had access to X-ray and EKG equipment, and he procured a fluoroscope, the latest in diagnostic technology: a fluoroscope projected a continuous X-ray image of the heart onto a fluorescent screen, providing a rudimentary movie of the heart.

"Dr. Taussig," Park told her, "you are now going to learn about congenital heart malformations."

Taussig remained ambivalent. She told Park that she didn't particularly want to learn about them.

He said, "It doesn't make any difference how you feel, you are going to learn about them."

In an interview, she remembered, "I vowed then and there not to get trapped in this 'narrow' field."

The congenital defects were incurable, but Taussig treated those patients as she did the ones with rheumatic heart disease. She did EKGs and X-rays. She fed them pudding containing barium, set them in the fluoroscopy machine, and ran the machine herself. She became intrigued, intellectually, by their conditions. Taussig called her patients the "crosswords of Harriet Lane": they were little puzzles that no one else could solve. In the 1930s, there was no system for diagnosing children with congenital heart disease—which child had transposition of the great arteries, which had tetralogy of Fallot, which had a septal defect, which had a stenotic valve. There was no clinical reason to get an accurate diagnosis, because the children could not be cured. In 1931, when Abbott first presented the exhibit that would become her atlas at the Graduate Fortnight at the New York Academy of Medicine, Helen Taussig was there. (They were two of only four women's names I found in a program that includes at least a hundred doctors.) Taussig traveled to Montreal to look at Abbott's collection of hearts.

She began to notice patterns. She began learning about the size and shape of the hearts. She learned to distinguish between the babies with transposition of the great arteries—they had essentially two separate circulatory systems—and the other babies who were not getting enough oxygen in their blood.

But just as she was committing herself to a lifelong study of congenital heart defects, something awful happened. Taussig's hearing, compromised all her life from a case of whooping cough when she was two, began to desert her. Birdsong was lost to her. She found herself turning up the volume of her radio and then creeping closer to hear it. She still played her music, pressing her fingers to furniture to feel the vibrations of symphonies. Soon, she couldn't hear other people's voices. She started wearing a hearing aid—in those days a bulky vacuum tube device that hung on a chain like a necklace. She struggled to hear her patients' heartbeats. She tried to use a specially amplified stethoscope, but it was unsatisfactory.

Frustrated, she approached the children's chests as she had the sound of the radio. She came closer. She pressed her hands to their skin. She touched each patient gently, sensitively, from head to toe. She taught herself to listen to their heartbeats with her fingertips. Eventually her touch became more effective diagnostically than a stethoscope. She learned to lip read. She sat up front at conferences. Names and numbers were the hardest things for her to follow, so she asked people to write them down. Neither her deafness nor her dyslexia got in the way of her accumulation of knowledge.

Her focus in the mid-1930s was on the cyanotic children, the blue babies, the ones who did not have enough oxygen in their blood. She was particularly fascinated by the children with tetralogy of Fallot. She noticed that some tet kids did better than others, and strangely it wasn't the kids with healthier hearts but the children with an additional cardiac deformation, yet another hole in their circulatory system, something called a patent ductus arteriosus (PDA).

In the womb, the fetus swims in amniotic fluid. It doesn't breathe. Its lungs are closed. The placenta is highly vascular, and oxygenated blood comes in through the umbilical cord. This is why a fetus can survive with the most grotesque heart defect. Right up to birth, babies depend on the mother's cardiopulmonary system for oxygen. Every child is born with two holes in the heart, conduits that divert blood from the useless fetal lungs. As the infant breathes, the heart matures, and these holes close.

One of these holes is at the top of the heart, between the two atria, and it's called the Foramen ovale. In most infants, the Foramen ovale closes in the first weeks of life, but a substantial minority (about 25 percent of the population) live with a patent, or open, Foramen ovale. According to the American Heart Association, a patent Foramen ovale is not a serious concern: "It causes no adverse health effects."

The second conduit is the ductus arteriosus. This runs between the pulmonary artery and the aorta. In most people, this closes in the first fifteen hours of life, but in some babies it can take as long as three months. A patent (or open) ductus arteriosus is common in premature babies. Most children with small PDAs live without symptoms until the ductus closes. On the other hand, a large, chronic, untreated PDA—one that never closes—means a slow, painful death.

Some kids were born with both a tetralogy and a PDA. Taussig followed these cases closely. She felt the children from head to toe to see how their hearts were beating, how their bodies were swelling, and how poor their coloration was. She noted their heart rates and blood pressures. She took EKGs and X-rays. She fed them barium pudding, set them in the fluoroscopy machines, and took movies of their hearts. Then she put them in their cribs and described their worsening conditions.

There are two available book-length biographies of Helen Taussig. One, *To Heal the Heart of a Child* by Joyce Baldwin, is a book for intelligent young readers. The other, *A Gentle Heart* by Geri Lynn Goodman, is a scholarly dissertation available through Yale University's website. Both writers interviewed Taussig when she was older, and both present her as a sweet and kindly woman with a soft spot for kids. This is not how the people I interviewed remembered Taussig.

Dr. Eugenia Doyle, a student of Taussig's at Johns Hopkins and later Michael Freed's mentor at NYU, found Taussig forbidding: "Not the kind of person you'd like to wrap your arms around, not a warm person, very cerebral." Doyle's abiding image of Taussig is of a doctor looking at corpses, "poring over the autopsies" of kids with congenitally deformed hearts. For her colleague Abraham Rudolph, Taussig was "an interesting character, very proud of herself, somewhat isolated, someone remote." I asked Dr. Rudolph if he thought this remoteness had something to do with her deafness, and Rudolph agreed that probably it had. To Sylvia Griffiths, Taussig was a New England aristocrat. "Think Barbara Bush without all the makeup," she said. Taussig was famous for her devotion to her patients, her students, and her discipline but not for her personal warmth. This was a formidable woman, as determined in the face of incurable disease and male-dominated medicine as her grandfather Taussig had been in riding out into the Missouri wilderness alone, ready to face down roving gangs of bandit terrorists in order to rescue a bunch of mental patients in need.

Through relentless analysis, Taussig discovered that the tet kids with PDAs did better than tet kids whose patent ductuses had closed. They had more energy. Their skin was a healthier color. Some of them were nearly asymptomatic. She watched her patients over long periods. Taussig was famous—even to the point of being resented by other doctors—for her persistent attention to her patients, her possessiveness of them, and her fascination with their cases.

As the tet babies grew, some of them grew out of their PDAs. The ductuses closed naturally. When this happened, the kids didn't get better. They got worse. They got bluer. They got less energetic. With an open ductus, a tet kid had a heart murmur but good coloration. With the ductus closed, the kid got very sick. Kids with tetralogies *or* chronic PDAs didn't do well. Kids with tetralogies *and* chronic PDAs did better.

Taussig saw that the PDA was in some ways compensating for the tetralogy. She speculated that the diversion of blood from the aorta back into the pulmonary artery meant that more blood was going to the lungs, and this in some ways made up for the oxygen deprivation that came from the hole in the center of the tet kids' hearts and for their pulmonary stenosis. The tet kids with PDAs were getting more oxygen in their blood than the tet kids without.

In 1938, about the same time that Taussig was collecting the data about her tet patients with PDAs, she learned that a surgeon in Boston, Dr. Robert Gross at Boston Children's Hospital, was beginning to put his scalpel in places no one had ever dared. He was not operating on the heart itself but right above it. He was curing children with PDAs. He was sewing shut the ductuses.

So Helen Taussig made a wild leap of imagination: she imagined a surgeon cutting into the chest of a dying baby, a baby with a tetralogy of Fallot, and she imagined that surgery giving the infant yet another defect, a man-made PDA. When she first began to describe this idea to people—giving a dying baby one more birth defect—they thought it absurd. They thought that Helen Taussig had gone out of her mind. She went to Boston to see Gross to see what he would say.

22.

ON SUNDAY, JUNE 14, 2018, I drove out to St. Stephen's Lutheran Church in South Plainfield, New Jersey, to see Pastor Chris Halverson at work. He's in his mid-thirties, very blond, very fair, and physically quite small. His face is triangular, and his manner is reserved. He's balding and youthful, and he has bright blue eyes. His church sits on Park Avenue in South Plainfield, a long stretch of two-lane blacktop lined with modest houses and square little lawns. St. Stephen's is set back from the road. The main building of the church complex was built in 1960, and it has a Jetsons-era swoop to its roof, high on the sides and low in the middle (stylish, said Chris, but a nightmare, drainage-wise). The church interior is simple, with an open bare-beamed vault. The unpainted wood shines a golden yellow. The low windows of the clerestory fill the room with light. Cheerful green and white banners hang at the back walls of the chancel.

I first visited on a cold Sunday during Martin Luther King Jr. weekend. One musician in a camel hair coat moved from the organ to the piano and back. A choir in purple robes gathered to the pulpit's right. Some families brought their children, and some middle-aged folks came alone. There were a lot of older women in cardigans, trifocals, and short hair. When I'd first met Chris, months before, he'd been wearing a shirt celebrating the NPR program *The Moth*, but now he was in his vestments. His hair had grown long in the back, and his pale beard was big and bushy, the beard of a nineteenth-century American preacher.

That weekend, the sexual assault scandals that had been sweeping the nation had hit the Lutheran Synod of New Jersey. A colleague of Chris's had recently been disbarred, and as pastor Chris took the news to his flock. The day's readings were from 1 Corinthians, Samuel, and John, and Chris's thoughts went to the apostle Paul. As Chris explained to his quiet, conservative, suburban congregation, body and soul were inseparable. The violation of the body of a child was not just a crime but a blasphemy against God. "Bodies matter," he said, and he reminded them of the surgeries he had been through on his heart.

Chris shut his eyes. His childhood surgeries had been traumatic, he explained, but beneficial. His doctors had cared for him. He tried to imagine—he said he could not—what such a violation would have been like had it been malicious. His congregation became still and very somber. I thought of the scars on his chest, underneath his robes.

Chris was born in Fargo, North Dakota, in 1983 and turned blue soon after birth. Surgeons put a shunt between the great arteries above his heart, allowing blood to flow into the pulmonary artery and to the lungs, and so he was able to survive until the age of three, at which point he had surgery at the Mayo Clinic. Chris's diagnosis—pulmonary atresia with ventricular septal defect—is different from mine. Though we were both born with a hole in the middle of our hearts, people with Chris's condition lack a pulmonary valve entirely. For Chris, a conduit had to be implanted between his right atrium and right ventricle, and the surgery when he was three years old was successful, a "complete repair" like mine. His parents assumed that meant Chris was all better, and off they went, out into the world.

Chris had a poor sense of his body's strength, so typical of patients with congenital heart disease. When he was little, between the ages of three and nine, his heart condition posed few difficulties for him. "I felt like I was in really good shape," he told me. "I was doing everything you do as a kid." His grandparents lived in Minnesota, and each year his parents went for a visit; then after the family gathering, Chris and his mom and dad would head to Rochester, to Mayo. The phlebotomy lab was always torture. Chris's veins are small, and they tend to roll. They're hard to puncture. The technicians would show him Disney movies while they took his chest X-rays and did the EKG and the echocardiogram. When he was nine years old, the tests revealed a crisis.

"I never have a sense that there's anything wrong with my body," Chris told me, "until they're cutting me open and doing their thing."

Before he really understood what was happening, he was waking up from surgery with an IV dripping into his arm and urine flowing out through his catheterized penis, the world a fog of painkillers and antiseptic smells. As the tubes were pulled out from deep within his chest, they felt like long balloons in a magician's trick. The split bones of his sternum hadn't yet knit as he and his parents drove back through the days and nights to Wyoming. His little chest had surgical tape covering the stitches of the incision. There were bandages and sutures in his groin and bruises on his arms.

They got back home to Cheyenne. Chris, haunted by his near-death experience, was asking profound questions of his mom and dad. What was life all about? After he died, what would happen to him? His parents, both agnostic, refused to give an answer. Could be Buddha, they said, could be Krishna, could be the Culligan Man. So as soon as his bones knit and he was able to walk by himself, the boy began to look for answers. He prowled the bookshelves of the Salvation Army in Cheyenne, dipping past the clothes and cookware to the rows of yellowing paperbacks, squeezing his way through the book sections until he got to religion, and then picking up anything that looked interesting.

"Some pretty weird shit," he told me, "in retrospect."

Religion, among the kids on the school bus, meant fundamentalist Christianity. "Fundamentalists," Chris told me, "really love selling answers, even when you're not asking questions." Without his parents, he started attending a Nazarene church. The Nazarenes urged Chris to renounce his mother and father as heathens. Chris's father's response to this was simple and brilliant. He gave the boy a Bible, which Chris began to read. What he saw there was far different from what the kids on the school bus were telling him.

"I simply read the book," Chris said. "It was weird. I fell in love with the Bible before I realized there was a community attached to it."

He kept attending the Nazarene church, despite the gap he felt between what was preached there and what he saw in the gospel. He felt strong and well. Then, when he was eleven, his mother enrolled in a program in San Antonio, Texas, to get a public health degree to complement her expertise as a pharmacist. The Halversons' plan was to drive to Minnesota, visit the grandparents and check out Chris's heart, and then drive from there down to San Antonio. At Mayo, Chris was scheduled for a cardiac catheterization.

"I felt the pressure in my groin," Chris wrote in a semiautobiographical short story that he kindly shared with me. "It was a strange, outward, inward, upward sensation, and then I felt the heat rumble around my chest, the heat right there in the pumping lifeblood, a mellow heat, increasing as the object stayed there, radiating unnaturally."

The doctors discovered something there in the catheter lab, and when Chris awoke, it was from deep anesthesia. He was surprised to find that his chest had been split again. "I tried to move my hands," Chris wrote in his story. "My limbs were of lead, and the back of my head felt heavier still. My whole body had a pulled back feeling, like some invisible force more powerful than gravity had exerted its own special pull on me." He was attached to a breathing tube. He was in the cardiac ICU again, on his back, his body chopped to pieces.

In San Antonio, when the family finally got there, Chris was a broken, frightened boy. "I made the conscious decision not to make friends, and I tried to hole up with books for a year." Some Sundays, his mother drove him to the local Presbyterian church. Other Sundays, Chris got a ride from a fellow parishioner. On account of the fragility of his chest, Chris wasn't allowed to lift more than thirty pounds. He could not participate in the ordinary life of a Texas middle school student.

When the family returned to Cheyenne, Chris was more isolated still. His minister, Chris's best friend's father, had been kicked out of his Nazarene church because, as the church put it, he could not control his wife. This was Chris's best friend's mother—she was mentally ill, Chris knows in retrospect. Her illness dynamited her family and also Chris's world. He was separated from his best friend, his minister, and his church.

Every trip to Mayo now felt like a game of Russian roulette. The scars inside his chest were growing, he knew, constricting openings, narrowing the flow of blood to his lungs. He had to sit in waiting rooms full of small children and their mothers. The other patients were reading *Highlights for Children*. Chris carried *The Brothers Karamazov*. In echocardiology, strange women inspected his body. They were sweet to him. In the dark, quiet rooms, the technician rolled the transducer wand across his scars, and Chris felt shy and ashamed of his body and of his own desires.

All the disconnections in his life were growing, between his mind and his body, between himself and his friends, between himself and his family. He knew what he wanted in Christianity: close attention to the Bible and purposeful engagement with the world. One day in tenth grade, he came to Christ Lutheran Church, a box of a building on a highway toward the southern edges of Cheyenne. He saw a thin young woman with long dark hair in the pulpit.

"She was kicking ass and taking names, preaching the love and the mercy of Christ," said Chris. "Everything about her exuded grace."

This was Pastor Sarah Moening. Chris was moved by her sermon on racial justice but also by her closeness to the Bible. All the other churches in Cheyenne had asked him to reject his parents. Pastor Sarah did not. Chris was enraptured by the Lutheran theology of the cross.

"God is in the last place you look," Chris told me. "What saved my life? Not butterflies and unicorns, but a piece of Gortex, a piece of cadaver. God is with you in the pain, with you in the suffering. When God shows up, he shows up not in a castle, but in a manger."

Chris was feeling okay in the last year of high school, as the family drove to his annual visit to Minnesota. The pediatric cardiology ward was familiar to him, and he gave directions to the parents of the other patients, this way to the X-rays, that way to the echocardiograms. He carried a copy of *Black Nationalism: The Search for Identity.* "I couldn't stop listening to the pounding in my chest," he wrote in the story he showed me. "I was waiting to hear a missed beat. I was waiting not to hear it at all. I was waiting to die." There was another crisis.

Chris was rolled into the operating room. His mother held onto his hand; his father held hands with his mother. The anesthesiologist put the mask to Chris's lips, a taste Chris described as tangerines and iodine. Then he was waking up, or not quite waking up, from surgery. His vision was blurred. His body was unfreezing. The breathing tube was pulled from his mouth—I know what that feels like: it goes intolerably far down one's throat, and it comes out with a dry saliva like epoxy. Chris wrote,

Cocooned in the white bed I knew I was safe. I gathered that the heaviness and lightness were both unreal. I felt the pain, perhaps paradoxically, more strongly because of its morphine mask. It felt like the breathing tube—something lodged in my chest. The morphine mask felt like I should be able to cough it up, or puke it up, but my body couldn't react in this way. The pain I knew was real. My body knew it was real. But the unreal contraptions around me made that reality disappear. The man was the shadow and the shadow was the man.

All he was allowed to eat on the long ride home was McDonald's salad without dressing. His parents bickered and fought with hotel clerks. His mother hovered over Chris. His father became disengaged. In the car, they listened to NPR and to the rock band Rush. Every half hour they had to stop so Chris could walk and cough to make sure he didn't develop blood clots. He took a shower in a hotel bathroom and, under the unforgiving lights, looked at his chest in the mirror. There were the incisions healing where the chest tubes had been. Chris felt like he could stick his fingers in the holes. He felt he could see his insides. When he got home to Cheyenne, he knew what he had to do with his life. He went to college in Oregon and finished in three years. Before he was old enough to drink, he was a Lutheran seminarian.

When I saw Chris in his church in January 2018, giving his sermon on sexual harassment and the #MeToo movement, I felt anxious for him, and I felt anxiety throughout the room—not disapprobation of their pastor but a sense that he was skating near subjects on which he and his congregants might disagree. I looked at a solitary old white man across the aisle from me. He was the only fellow there in a suit and tie, a thin man, his hair neatly parted. I imagined he was a widower and had been attending this church since its founding. In my mind, he had married and mourned his wife here. This was where all his children had been baptized. What would he make of this long-haired, bearded kid in the pulpit, talking sympathetically about a feminist movement that had started with a hashtag on the internet?

I was a fool to think protectively of Chris Halverson, here in his church. He had made—even as he stood there, he was making—his vulnerabilities into his strengths. His sermon was based so clearly on the liturgy, so powerfully on his own experience, so forcefully within his own synod, and had such moral clarity that the very discomfort around the subject seemed to draw his flock closer to him and closer to each other.

"Peace be with you," we all said to each other after the sermon was done. Every member of the church shook hands with every other, and some embraced, and some were too ill to shake hands or embrace but nonetheless were touched by their fellow congregants. Even I, a stranger there, an unbelieving Jew, was moved and welcomed and comforted.

When it was all over, Chris stood at the door shaking hands. The woman who was serving coffee and cookies behind the counter stopped him. "You know," she said, "I was sexually assaulted when I was young." She and Chris conferred privately, along with her son. Later Chris told me that her boy had had corrective heart surgery as a kid and was facing another operation soon. Chris was shepherding them through it.

———

I guess there are several ways to deal with something like a congenital heart condition. One way is through understanding the science, by facing one's condition objectively. This is something that in my teens and twenties I had trained and conditioned myself never to do—never to face the hard facts of my own heart defect and never to think of myself as sick or in danger. Another way is through religious consolation, through trust in a higher power. I don't have the gift for this, not the way Chris Halverson or Bridgette Ratliff do. I pray, but my prayers are spasmodic, there and gone, and of little continuing consolation. A third way is through community, through emotional connection with other people, which is maybe something I am trying to do now, even as I write this book, but in my late twenties, I was incapable of that kind of connection.

In my childhood, denial and independence had been a powerful adaptation to my condition. I think my parents were right in raising me not to think of myself as crippled. Mike Freed once talked to me about patients who were brought up to dwell on their heart conditions and to carry themselves as invalids. "They never grow up," he said. But in refusing to acknowledge my condition, I had constructed a little prison for myself.

There I was in my late twenties, adjunct to my life, shackled to my ambition, and in profound denial about my state of health. I had no capacity for intimacy. I kept my fear secret. I didn't like to talk to my friends about my heart. With my family, the subject was taboo. The result was a stunted, shuttered emotional life. Romance was fleeting. There were flirtations and one-night stands. A beautiful, kind, intelligent woman lay in my bed after sex, and she told me she loved me, and I said, "I'm not ready to build my life around a relationship." I lived alone; I wrote alone; I worked alone. I was solitary. But back home from Boston that fall when I was teaching at Barnard, after I left Dr. Rosenbaum's practice, I was exhausted.

The cracks in my shell were giving way. I quote William James, one more time:

> There are only two ways in which is it is possible to get rid of anger, worry, fear, despair or other undesirable affections. One is that an opposite affection should overpoweringly break over us, and the other is by getting so exhausted with the struggle that we have to stop—so we drop down, give up, and *don't care* any longer.

Maybe a couple weeks after I got that letter from Dr. Freed, I bumped into Marcia Lerner, a woman I'd known for years and in front of whom I'd always been intimidated. She was so beautiful. She was so funny. She'd always been a little bit haughty around me, something that turned me on and made me play the ass, blurting out the weirdest things, always boasting and pretentious. (I'd attended Columbia's MFA program, I told her once [oh, do I really have to write this?], because of "the high publication rate among its graduates." [GAHHHH!!!!]) That fall, somehow, when I saw her, I was free of bullshit. I was relaxed. I asked if she'd have a cup of coffee with me.

We sat together in a café. We talked, and I liked her even more. We walked together through the West Village. Down by the Hudson, we watched trash bob in the river. I turned to look at her face in profile. I just wanted to be with her.

The first time we were alone together in her bedroom, I did something I had never done. I warned her before I took off my shirt. Every time, with every other girl, I'd just pretended it wasn't there. But I said, "I have something to show you." I was really nervous that she would be frightened by my scar, but Marcia didn't seem at all frightened or even bothered so much as interested. She asked me about the operation I'd had as a kid. And I explained to her, as I really hadn't to anyone before, all about my heart.

23.

I N THE LATE 1930s, while Helen Taussig was working in Baltimore and beginning to measure the effects of patent ductus
arteriosus on children with tetralogy of Fallot, the first-ever
pediatric cardiopulmonary surgery was performed several states up
the East Coast by Dr. Robert Gross at Boston Children's Hospital
on a little girl named Lorraine Sweeney, who had been born with
a defect not to her heart but to the great arteries above it: she
had a ductus arteriosus that would not close and that—if it stayed
open—would kill her.

Lorraine was the eighth and youngest child of Irish immigrants.
The Sweeney family lived in a crowded apartment in South Boston. Lorraine's father played accordion, her mother Mary Ellen
sang, and "music came on with the kettle in the morning," Lorraine
remembered. Some Gaelic was still spoken in the home. Lorraine
had seemed to be a healthy baby when she was born. There was no
cyanosis in her first weeks of life—no blue fingers or lips—and no
edema, no swelling of any part of the body. But as she got older,
she got weaker. Her breath grew noisy and labored. She easily grew
fatigued. She was diagnosed with a PDA. Though she was otherwise healthy, in 1931 nothing could be done for her. Lorraine sat at
the window as a child, doomed to die slowly, watching other kids
play in the street.

Her father drove a streetcar for the Boston Elevator Company.
His route ran between Brighton and Cambridge. One day, when
he and his wife were crossing the street in front of their church,

St. Columbkille's, an automobile struck him down and killed him. Lorraine's mother—now a widow with eight children, the youngest dying of heart disease—was devastated. In despair, Mary Ellen Sweeney took seven-year-old Lorraine again to see the doctor—was there really nothing to be done?—and she was referred to Dr. Gross at Boston Children's.

When Gross met Lorraine Sweeney in the summer of 1938, he examined her carefully. The girl told her doctor that she knew she had "something wrong in the chest." Her mother said she could hear "a buzzing noise" whenever she was close to her child. Gross's notes run as follows, directions on how to diagnose PDA with nothing but a stethoscope and a blood pressure gauge:

> At the time of admission, the patient was slender and under-nourished. The pulsations of the carotid arteries were abnor-mally forceful. . . . The veins over the chest were somewhat prominent. There was a precordial bulge. The heart was defi-nitely enlarged by percussion, the enlargement being for the most part to the left. Over the entire precordium there was a prominent coarse thrill which was most intense in the third interspace to the left of the sternum. This thrill was contin-uous but was accentuated during systole. There was a rough "machinery" murmur heard with maximal intensity of the pulmonic area to the left of the sternum in the second and particularly in the third interspace. It was continuous through the cardiac cycle but like the thrill was greatly accentuated during systole.

Robert Gross was a short, broad-chested, narrow-eyed young doctor, well-dressed, formal in bearing, and somewhat reserved. Childhood cataracts had left him blind in one eye, a fact he hid from his patients and colleagues. As a boy, he was mechanically inclined, and his father encouraged young Robert to take apart and put together clocks and watches—perhaps to help the one-eyed boy improve his depth perception. Gross could disassemble and reassemble a car engine. He could mend his own clothes. In his operating room, he had a special toolkit, painted gold by his nurses. He took an interest in the machinery of the operating room, later inventing pumps and gauges, and he was an innovative, creative surgeon, if not an especially deft one. He knew that Lorraine Sweeney was suffering a PDA, and he knew he wanted to operate.

PDA surgery had been attempted before Gross, but not successfully. The year before, at Massachusetts General Hospital, Dr. John William Strieder had performed an emergency patent ductus arteriosus ligation on a twenty-two-year-old woman who then died of a blood stream infection after surgery. Gross himself had been running experiments, working on PDAs in dogs. He created artificial PDAs in his laboratory dogs, and then he shut them. He saw an opportunity—to be the first ever to close a PDA, to perform the first-ever surgery on a cardiac defect, and to save a little girl.

He went to his supervisor, Dr. Charles Ladd, for permission. Ladd turned Gross down: it was too risky and too early in Gross's experiments to try to operate on a human being. Then Ladd went off on vacation.

Ladd was a Boston Brahmin, the child of generations of Harvard men, and the preeminent pediatrician in the world. Gross's father had built pianos in Baltimore.

While Ladd was away in Europe, Gross went back to Mary Ellen Sweeney, the widowed immigrant with the dying daughter. He wanted to operate on her daughter. He explained that it was an experimental procedure but that he might be able save Lorraine's life. Mrs. Sweeney went to her church, St. Columbkille's, the same church in front of which her husband had been run down. She sought council from the priest. "Well, Mrs. Sweeney," said Monseigneur Tracey, "if God wants her, he'll take her either way. You let her have the operation and God be good to her."

In 1938, there was no pretty patients' waiting room at Boston Children's, nothing like the warm pediatric cardiology lounge where I waited in 1995. There were just cold, wooden benches. Parents were not allowed to accompany their children into the hospital. Lorraine's mother was so racked with grief and terrified that she could not take her daughter to the hospital. Mary Ellen

Sweeney was sure she'd never see her child again. The family lied to seven-year-old Lorraine and told her she was going to the hospital to visit her niece. Lorraine's big sister took her in a streetcar and walked her to Longwood Avenue. Lorraine went up the steps and into the hospital alone. The doors closed, and she was abandoned.

On the morning of surgery, she sat by herself on the big wooden benches in the surgical waiting area, listening for her number to be called. She was number ninety-nine.

———

Gross was the first to perform pediatric cardiac surgery, but he had important predecessors, most significantly, Alexis Carrel, the father of vascular surgery and among the first to hypothesize a heart-lung machine. While Maude Abbott, devoted to congenital heart disease, was toiling in obscurity at McGill, even as she was riding a taxi uptown from Penn Station to put up the display of her late-career work in the halls of the New York Academy of Medicine, Carrel was blocks away at Rockefeller University. He was a celebrated genius but also a mystic, and a madman, and a reactionary who called for the slaughter of those he deemed genetically undesirable.

In 1902, when Carrel was twenty-nine years old, he was banned from French medicine because he claimed to have witnessed a miracle at Lourdes. Carrel swore that holy water, splashed over a young girl's stomach, had cured her of tuberculosis. French anti-clerical laws forbade physicians from endorsing miracle cures, and so to continue practicing medicine Carrel had to emigrate to the United States.

He worked first at the University of Chicago and then at Rockefeller University. Carrel was the first doctor to develop techniques for end-to-end anastomosis, that is, for sewing together sectioned blood vessels. He claimed to have learned his stitching by imitating his mother, a seamstress. What she did with her embroidery needles, he did when sewing up veins and arteries. For this groundbreaking work, Carrel was awarded the Nobel Prize in 1912, when he was thirty-nine, but this was only the beginning of his career. After World War I, in New York City, he started the first-ever studies in organ transplantation. He sewed a dog's kidney to its shoulder, where the kidney thrived, produced urine, and killed the dog. He took a leg from one dog and successfully sewed it onto another.

Carrel cultured a chicken heart and kept it alive outside a chicken body, claiming the chicken tissue was immortal. In his lab at Rockefeller University, all the walls and furniture were painted black. All the technicians had to dress in black. With Charles Lindbergh, the famous aviator, Carrel began to work on profusion pumps, devices that would deliver oxygen to living organs outside the human body. Lindbergh and Carrel were able to use their profusion pumps to keep cat thyroid glands viable for several weeks outside cat bodies. Lindbergh, whose sister had heart problems, dreamed of a new kind of profusion pump, a heart-lung machine that would keep his sister alive while doctors treated her.

Lindbergh and Carrel both were fascinated by eugenics and race science, and both imagined the racial perfection of humanity. They were two of the leading American fascist sympathizers. In 1935, Carrel published *Man the Unknown*, which was the second-best-selling book in the United States that year, after *Gone with the Wind*. In it Carrel argued, "The democratic principle has contributed to the collapse of civilization in opposing the development of an elite." The introduction to the 1939 edition of *Man the Unknown* worried about "the extinction of the best elements of the race" and proclaimed, "Never have the European races been in such peril as today." Carrel was concerned about the "moral quality of the population" in the United States, where "the number of misfits reaches perhaps thirty or forty million." The German-language edition of his book added new paragraphs that endorsed the idea of using gas to exterminate genetic undesirables.

In 1939, when Carrel was sixty-five years old, he hit mandatory retirement age at Rockefeller University. In 1941, Marshal Henri Philippe Pétain invited him to Vichy France, and there he founded the Carrel Foundation for the Study of Human Problems. It's impossible to assess his personal culpability in what happened there, but the institute was involved in a murky business, propelled by mysticism and barbarity, while the fascist regime brought into action Carrel's eugenic dreams. Just as Carrel had advocated, thousands of people—"misfits" seen as dangers to the "moral quality" of the human race—were killed. After the war, he was widely viewed in France and America as a traitor and a collaborator, though he had his defenders. Dr. Richard Bing, a German Jewish refugee who worked with Carrel at Rockefeller before starting his career at Johns Hopkins, once said, "To me, a young kid, he was wonderful. I have many of his nice, supportive, affectionate letters, and I never saw anything of this 'diabolical' side of his nature."

But there is something in Carrel's life and work that reveals the terrifying business of heart surgery, the cold savagery at the center, the industrial, clinical vivisection and resection of the human body. It's the thing that my mom saw in Jim Malm's eyes, the thing that terrified her.

———

All interventional medicine in the United States now takes place in temperature-controlled sterile rooms. An anesthesiologist administers sophisticated painkillers and narcotics, and expensive electronic equipment monitors the patient's pulse, blood pressure, and oxygenation. In dangerous pediatric surgeries, social workers are on call for both the parents and the child. In 1938, in Lorraine Sweeney's case, all these functions were performed by one woman, Betty Lank, a Canadian nurse who had taken a three-month course in anesthesia.

In the 1930s, all nurse-anesthetists were women, all surgeons were men, and a 1937 speech by Dr. Harold Foss, "The Surgeon and His Anesthetist," describes with cheerful sexism the relationship between the two professionals:

> The surgeon expects, and usually finds in his anesthetist a keenness of mind, an alert intelligence, a loyal, faithful, self-effacing, efficient devotion to the job in hand.... She wants encouragement, helpful and constructive advice and criticism when she is wrong and a word of approbation when she is

persistently doing what she and every one else in the operating room knows to be an especially fine piece of work.

Betty Lank built most of the equipment she used. When there wasn't a blood pressure cuff small enough for her patient, she made one with a piece of surgical tubing. When the masks didn't fit the patients' faces, she soaked them in alcohol to shrink them. She administered her drugs through homemade tubes, clipped from catheters of various sizes. She calmed babies before surgery by giving them bottles filled with ten parts glucose and one-part brandy. She sang them Brahms's "Lullaby" as they went under. She painted stars over their cribs in post-op and described the constellations to them as they recovered.

During surgery, she monitored vital signs by taking her patients' pulse, and counting their breaths, and watching them carefully. In an oral history, Lank remembers the methods of the time as "terrifying" and "awful." For Lorraine Sweeney's operation, she used cyclopropane as an anesthetic. It was highly explosive and had caused a fire in an operating room at nearby Deaconess Hospital. To minimize electrostatic sparks, Dr. Gross's operating room had to be kept above 55 percent humidity. There was no air-conditioning. Betty Lank's surgical notes are stained with sweat and blood.

So, in a hot and humid operating room in summertime Boston, a one-eyed resident and his multitasking nurse—against the explicit direction of the hospital's surgical chief of staff—set out to perform the first-ever corrective surgery on a human heart. Lank administered the cyclopropane through a mask and turned the patient on her side. Gross made his incision between the third and fourth ribs. In his notes, he writes, "As the left lung was allowed to collapse inferiorly, an excellent view was gained of the lateral aspect of the mediastinum," that is, the cavity that holds the heart. He put his finger right on her heart and felt "a very vibrant thrill over the entire organ." His report continues, "When the stethoscope was placed on the pulmonary artery, there was an almost deafening, continuous roar, sounding much like a large volume of steam escaping in a closed room." Using an aneurism needle and a silk thread, Gross pulled the ductus arteriosus shut. Lorraine's blood pressure immediately normalized from 110/35 to 125/90. Gross waited three minutes, watching. The ductus, when he saw it, looked too short to section, so he left it closed. According to his report, "There was only mild discomfort on the afternoon of the day of the operation, and on the following morning the child was allowed to sit up in a chair. By the third day, she was walking around the ward."

He bought his patient a little doll and took a photograph of her slouching in her white frilly dress. Her dark sunken eyes look tired and frightened. Lorraine's mother was not allowed to visit the girl for the extra week that she was held in the hospital "because of the interest in the case." But Lorraine herself was fine. She lived on into her nineties.

———

On the train from Baltimore to Boston, Helen Taussig rehearsed her notes on tetralogy patients as she would present them to Gross. Because of the ventricular septal defect, the venous and arterial blood mixed in the large chambers of the tet patient's heart. Because of the pulmonary stenosis, not enough blood got to the lungs. But with the ductus arteriosus open, some of additional blood went back into the lungs instead of going out into the body. This increased the volume of blood going into the lungs, thus the volume of oxygen going out to the body, and hence improved the health of the child.

So Helen Taussig practiced reciting her theory: one could relieve the symptoms of tetralogy of Fallot by creating an artificial patent ductus. Make a hole, make a shunt between the arteries, and direct more of the blood to the lungs and more oxygen to the body. She got off the train. She went to Longwood Avenue. She found Gross's office. When she explained her idea to him, he laughed at her.

"I think," Taussig remembered later, "he thought it was one of the craziest things he'd heard in a long time."

"Madame," he said, "I close ductuses. I don't create them."

Taussig, a half foot taller than him but begging, asked if he *could*, if it would be possible. She said meekly, "It would be a great help to a cyanotic child."

Gross turned her down.

To be fair to Gross, all his dogs with artificial PDAs had died. Building a shunt between the great arteries is a tricky business— too narrow and not enough blood gets to the lungs; too wide and the lungs are flooded. No one had ever done it before. So Taussig went back to Baltimore.

She decided to try her idea on the newest surgeon hired by the hospital, Dr. Alfred Blalock. He had recently come from Vanderbilt and had a reputation for experimentation. Blalock had made tremendous strides in the treatment of battlefield shock. He was a rising young star in American surgery.

She met him in his lab at Hopkins. He was small, pale, handsome, and intense, with round glasses and dark hair swept back from his forehead, a southern gentleman, directly descended on his mother's side from the president of the Confederacy, Jefferson Davis. On the stool beside Dr. Blalock sat another man, Vivien Thomas. Taller and younger than Blalock, with a longer face and milder manners, he wore a white lab coat, and—this must have been confusing at first for Helen Taussig—he was a black man.

Baltimore was a Jim Crow town. Johns Hopkins had separate entrances and bathrooms marked "colored." Thomas wasn't supposed to drink from the same fountains as Taussig or Blalock. All the other black people working in the hospital held menial positions. None of them wore lab coats. Thomas could have been arrested for eating lunch with Blalock or Taussig. But he sat there, expectant, Dr. Blalock's special assistant, brought with him from Vanderbilt to work in the lab. Taussig made her presentation about tet kids and PDAs.

She might have been nervous, but she had learned from her meeting with Gross. She was not going to tell a surgeon what to do. Taussig withheld her conclusions and simply described the evidence and her observations: the comparison of tet kids with PDAs to tet kids without; the way that tet babies became symptomatic only after their PDAs closed. She presented this as a curiosity, as a puzzle. She wondered aloud if something could be done for these kids "as a plumber changes the pipes around."

Blalock looked at Thomas. Thomas smoked his pipe.

24.

I N THE 1990S, I was a man in denial, hanging perilously onto my health but unwilling to acknowledge the fact. I was a patient way out in the wilds of science. Michael Freed and Marlon Rosenbaum were two brilliant men, both eminent in their field, but together they had no idea what to do with me.

"We have this dilemma all the time," said Dr. Freed, when I had lunch with him in the spring of 2018. We met in Zaftig's Diner in Brookline, Massachusetts, near his home. He had a bagel and lox; I had a cup of borscht and a plate of potato pancakes. I brought him a bottle of Armagnac as a gift for saving my life. He seemed embarrassed by this. I very much enjoyed his company.

Dr. Freed explained that the problem he faced with my heart in the mid-1990s was typical of the history of pediatric cardiology. It really wasn't that different from the problem Welton Gersony and Sylvia Griffiths faced with the hearts of their patients in the late 1950s, when they had to choose between Blalock shunts (safe but temporary) and complete repair (dangerous but potentially curative).

"You've got something that's okay," he said, meaning the Blalock shunt, or my freely leaking heart after tet repair, "and then someone comes up with a new thing," meaning open-heart surgery in the 1950s or valve replacement in the 1990s. "Whenever you try the new thing, there are unknown risks."

In the late 1950s, Blalock shunts left patients with reasonably healthy outcomes. They survived for decades. Corrective open-heart surgeries, initially, were much more dangerous, with high mortality rates. It took time for the lines on the graph to cross: it was several years before the surgically repaired patients began to outlive and outlast the patients with the shunts. In the 1990s, most people like me—repaired tetralogies with big leaks—were doing fine. We were clearly at risk, but valve replacement surgery was similarly risky. There were no data to suggest when, where, and how to intervene on a patient, particularly one like me who seemed reasonably healthy.

Twenty years after my 1971 surgery, it was hard for the doctors to guess who would live and who would die. Surgery had left us all with free pulmonary regurgitation. Blood flowed backward through our pulmonary arteries and into our right ventricles. The ventricles got bigger. Some patients did well for fifty years after tetralogy repair. Some got in trouble after five years. There were no data. We who were living all said that we felt fine. A lot of the patients who died had been lost to care, their cases unsupervised and irrecoverable. Many had died from sudden arrhythmias. In those cases enlarged ventricles were only one of many possible contributing factors; there was no way to correlate those deaths with ventricle dysfunction. For a given patient, outcomes were unknowable. They still are. To this day, the subject remains obscure. It's impossible to know how long a given repair will last.

"We're still trying to get a handle on what the predictive factors are," said Dr. Freed over our lunch in 2018.

In the 1980s, Dr. Freed explained to me over his bagel, imaging technology did not allow doctors to get a clear picture of a heart's decline. When Sylvia Griffiths looked at my heart on an X-ray, she could see that it was enlarged, but the shadowy image didn't let her know which chambers were getting bigger or by how much.

There was no way for Dr. Griffiths to measure right ventricle growth. Only with the echocardiograms could doctors begin to see which ventricle was enlarged in which patient—but even the echo doesn't give a great measure. The pictures depend a lot on the angle of the transducer wand and the skill of the technician, and the data is at best impressionistic. I've seen this in my own more recent echos; Marlon Rosenbaum has shown them to me. Year to year it can be very hard to say in precise millimeters whether a chamber is growing or shrinking or staying the same.

Every spring after 1995, I went up to Boston to Dr. Freed, and he looked at my X-rays and my echos and gave me an exercise test. In trying to plot the course of my heart's decline, he was traveling through a foggy, unexplored territory. He had only the vaguest of maps and no real landmarks. For my part, I knew that my ventricle was collapsing, but I convinced myself that my prognosis was really no different from anyone else's. No one, I told myself, knew how long any heart would last. No heart could last forever. I talked it out with Marcia. I drew her into my insanity. But I refused to let her come with me, ever, to Boston.

Each spring at Children's, I stood in the X-ray room in the pediatric cardiology ward by the pictures of Barney and Minnie and Mickey Mouse, and the technicians raised the cold glass, and I pressed my chest against it, and they gave me the big print in a big brown envelope and told me to walk over to my next stop, the echocardiology lab. The X-ray print in its envelope felt to me like secret evidence that could convict or acquit me. I felt burdened having to carry it, like a man carrying his own death warrant to his executioner.

Please God, I prayed in the echo lab, let it not show that I need heart surgery. As Dr. Freed explained to me, the technology of valve replacement developed alongside imaging technology. In the early 1960s, Giancarlo Rastelli at the Mayo Clinic had demonstrated that it was possible to relieve pulmonary stenosis through the implantation of an external conduit, and by the time I was seeing Dr. Freed in the 1990s, pulmonary valves were beginning to be used in a handful of congenital patients with collapsed or collapsing ventricles. But outcomes were in question. Mike Freed was unsatisfied with the evidence. Valve replacement might resolve my situation—or compound it. I might do worse after heart surgery, even if the surgery was successful. Dr. Freed was unsatisfied, too, with the diagnostic technology. Neither the echocardiogram nor the cardiac catheter offered him hard quantitative measures of my ventricle. My exercise tests showed that I performed somewhat under average, at 85 percent of the predicted rate for my age, but that was meaningless in my case—pretty solid, in fact, for a congenital heart patient. The echos didn't demonstrate conclusively that my ventricle was getting any larger. At what point would the size of my ventricle begin to endanger my health? Would the surgery (dangerous in itself) bring me out of danger from my collapsing heart? Would the surgery leave me with new problems?

In 1997, I moved in with Marcia. I sent out a slim, two-hundred-page, highly polished draft of my novel to literary agents, and I got very kind rejections in reply. Then I gave up on the book ceremoniously. I took all the drafts and notes and versions, which by that time filled two big copy-shop paper boxes, and I put it all on the curb and said good-bye.

In his office, Dr. Freed continued to warn me that the leak in my heart was considerable and that the ventricle was very enlarged. I asked if I needed to take a catheter exam (as if that were the thing to fear and not the collapse of my body). He said we'd talk about it next time. I must have been a double puzzle to him, all my terrors a barrier he had to sail around as he made his way toward treatment of my heart.

Marcia and I were married in August 1997. We danced under a tent on a sunny day in Vermont. A year later, she was pregnant. I got a full-time teaching job, out at the State University of New York at Stony Brook. The commute was a bear from our place in Brooklyn—two and a half hours each way—but I wrote on the train in the morning and graded papers on the way home, and I only had to go out two or three times a week, and I got good health insurance and a retirement account.

What was she thinking, marrying me, a man with a failing heart? What were we doing, having a baby when it was unclear how much longer I would live? The answers come back like vague X-ray shadows. I guess we were thinking what everyone thinks when they make those kinds of commitments. We were in love.

On April 2, 1999, she woke me in the middle of the night to tell me that her water had broken. I was annoyed and said she was imagining things and really we should just go back to sleep. Then we were in the delivery room. Marcia was screaming in pain. She seemed both to want me near her and to want nothing to do with me at all. She was sweating and straining, and then she gave a push, and my daughter Eliza was out.

"A girl!" I cried. "A purple girl!"

I held my baby in my arms. She was so tiny and so frail in her hospital blanket. The whole world shifted on its axis, or my world got a new axis to revolve around, and the axis was Eliza Rose Brownstein.

She was a difficult infant. She screamed all the time. When she wasn't nursing or sleeping, she howled at the top of her lungs. She would wake two, three, four, five times a night. Marcia, sleep deprived and besieged by hormonal shifts, cried in the pediatrician's office and cried when I came home from work. I climbed from the subway station as the sun set in May, and there was my beautiful wife looking shell-shocked and holding my gorgeous daughter, whose face was bright red, whose mouth was set in a perfect, yowling O. We tried everything to calm the baby. Sometimes singing helped. Holding her like a football, with my hand on her chest and her belly on my forearm, seemed to take some pressure off her gassy gut. Someone suggested the sound of a vacuum cleaner might help, so that was the scene in our apartment after work, Marcia running the vacuum, me jogging around the house with the baby on one arm, the two adults singing "This Land Is Your Land," while the baby howled and howled and howled.

25.

WHEN I ASKED Vivien Thomas's nephew, Dr. Koko Eaton, to describe his uncle for me, Dr. Eaton, the orthopedic surgeon for the Tampa Bay Rays Major League Baseball team, offered one word: "humble."

I said I was uncomfortable with the word. All his life, I said, the white world had wanted to humble Vivien Thomas. He had been treated as less than a human being, had lived through segregation and racism, had faced a life of humiliation without once losing his dignity, had accomplished so much when so many had tried to make him feel so small.

Helen Taussig had proposed the surgery, and Alfred Blalock performed it, but Vivien Thomas was the one who—in his lab—invented the procedure, who figured out how to make heart surgery practicable. It was Thomas the lab technician, not Blalock the surgeon or Taussig the cardiologist, who performed the research for the blue baby procedures, built all the instruments, and designed the groundbreaking technique. I said I wanted to use a word other than "humble."

"What can I tell you?" said Dr. Eaton, who spoke to me from his work inside the Rays spring training facility. "That's the word I'd use."

His uncle Vivien had built his own house and all his own furniture. When he hosted family barbecues, he used spatulas he'd made for himself out of surgical clamps. Vivien Thomas's portrait hangs on the wall at Johns Hopkins, but if asked why it was there, Koko Eaton told me, Thomas said only, "I used to work here."

At Hopkins, Thomas was paid janitor's wages. Maids refused to collect his garbage, and higher-ups refused to fill his supply orders. Blalock made him paint the walls of their lab. He was routinely demeaned. In his laboratory workshop, Thomas trained many of the great doctors who would dominate heart surgery for the next decades, but he had to supplement his income by working as a servant for Blalock. At Blalock's parties, Vivien Thomas was the bartender, fixing drinks for his students and colleagues. At Blalock's wedding, Thomas was the chauffeur.

Vivien Thomas hadn't ever wanted to move to Baltimore. He had grown up in Nashville, where he had a large, protective family and community. In Baltimore he was exposed to discrimination in a new way—alone—and he thought the city was dirty. But Thomas had little choice. When his boss, Alfred Blalock, moved from Vanderbilt University to Johns Hopkins, Thomas had to follow him from Nashville to Baltimore: no one else in the world other than Blalock would let Vivien Thomas pursue the work he loved.

When he was young, Thomas had wanted to be a doctor. He was the son of a carpenter, and he had worked ever since he was small. He had saved up money for his education, but when he was nineteen, all of it vanished in the 1929 stock market crash. Carpentry work dried up too. When Thomas first took a job in Alfred Blalock's lab at Vanderbilt, he saw it as "a stop-gap measure to get me through the cold winter months." He thought the economy would pick up, and he could work again, and save again, and make his way through college. But that's not the way it happened.

The work in Blalock's Vanderbilt lab was gruesome at first, and Thomas performed it meticulously. In Nashville in 1929, Blalock was running animal experiments to measure the effect of shock. It was Thomas's job to induce systemic shock in laboratory dogs and measure the effects of grotesque wounds on their bodies. This meant anesthetizing the dogs, whacking them on their hind legs with a hammer, and then seeing how their blood pressure shifted.

"I soon overcame my reluctance to inflict the trauma," Thomas wrote in his memoir.

For a blood pressure gauge, Thomas used a U-shaped tube half filled with mercury. A rubber float lay on one side of the U, attached to an aluminum rod; as the dog's blood pressure changed, the rod moved and etched the changes onto a piece of glazed, smoked paper that rotated around a slowly spinning drum. When it was all over, Thomas carefully amputated the dogs' legs, sewing up the blood vessels and then weighing the legs against each other to see how much fluid had run to the injured leg relative to its mate. He was paid less than he would have been if he were working as a groundskeeper.

Thomas's skills grew and, with them, his responsibilities. He began to design tools and experiments. Vivien Thomas, at twenty years old, was tall and thin and handsome, with very dark skin, long limbs, and long, sensitive fingers. He was famously calm and polite almost to the point of being finicky.

Blalock, by contrast, was a hard-drinking man, with what Thomas called a "reputation for prowess with the ladies and for being a great party man." He kept a case of Coca-Cola in his laboratory fridge and a ten-gallon charred keg of whiskey in his storeroom. As Thomas wrote, "The profanity he used would have made the proverbial sailor proud of him." Thomas warned Blalock not to use such language in front of him if he wanted him to stick around, and Blalock obliged, and so a partnership was formed.

Over the years, the two men's professional lives merged. "It was extremely difficult to tell," recalled Dr. Allen Woods, "if Dr. Blalock had the original idea for a particular technique or if it was Vivien Thomas, they worked so smoothly together." Their work on shock changed the way soldiers were treated on the battlefield. (In his later years, Blalock would say it was his work on shock, not on blue babies, that was the real triumph of his medical career.) When Blalock came to Hopkins, he accepted the job on the condition that he could bring his assistant with him.

Thomas liked Helen Taussig as soon as he met her. "She was tall and slender with a pleasant personality and spoke with a distinct New England accent."

These two reserved professionals, both of them exiled from their colleagues' full respect, seem to have worked very well together. That first day they met in the lab at Johns Hopkins, "she went into great detail about the problems of patients with cyanotic heart disease." According to Thomas, "she was particularly interested in the tetralogy of Fallot."

When Thomas visited Helen Taussig's museum of hearts, he was dumbstruck. He spent days looking over the deformed hearts, the tetralogies. First, he was amazed by the human problem: How could a child live even for a year with a heart like that? And then he was overwhelmed with the technical problems of the surgery Taussig proposed.

Thomas's first problem was to induce the conditions of tetralogy in a lab animal. He did all his work on dogs, just as he had in Nashville, operating on animals as he developed and refined his technique. Of course, he could not punch holes in the centers of the dogs' heart without killing the animals, so he tried several methods of restricting their blood oxygenation: tying ligatures around the pulmonary arteries and excising parts of their lungs. Thomas worked fourteen- and fifteen-hour days, killing dog after dog after dog. Finally, he began to work on the great arteries, trying to redirect oxygenated blood back to the heart, where it would mingle with the venous blood. This worked: it allowed Thomas to build a set of cyanotic lab dogs.

Once he had rejiggered the blood flow in the dogs' great arteries, he experimented with building the artificial ductus. The lab work continued for two years. He invented special instruments for pediatric cardiac surgery. He braided the thread. He cut down needles and sharpened them so they would work on the tiny arteries of a child. He built the special clamps that would thereafter be named for Blalock. As a surgeon, Thomas was a wonder—so precise, nimble, fast, and accurate that the Hopkins doctors assigned him (without paying him any more money) to teach their students how to operate.

Blalock was skeptical that the surgery Thomas had designed would be effective. He thought it would just give the tetralogy patients a small measure of relief. Taussig, meanwhile, had identified a candidate for the operation: Eileen Saxon, fifteen months old, who had been born prematurely and attended to by Taussig since soon after birth.

Eileen had been born in August. Initially, she had been diagnosed with a ventricular septal defect, a hole in the middle of her heart. But her condition had worsened. Taussig suspected that Eileen's relatively good early health corresponded with a PDA, which after a few months had closed.

By March, according to Taussig's report, it had become clear that Eileen had a grave deformity. "After eating she would become deeply cyanotic, roll up her eyes, lose consciousness and appear extremely ill." In June, Eileen was admitted to the Harriet Lane Home. "She was poorly nourished and poorly developed. She had a glassy stare. Her lips were cyanotic. . . . The baby was given oxygen and phenobarbital but remained very irritable and would become intensely cyanotic when taken out of the oxygen tent."

Eileen could not move on her own. She had to be carried everywhere. She failed to gain weight. She could only sleep with her knees drawn up under her chest. "During her recurrent spells," wrote Taussig, "she breathed fast and deep and then suddenly went limp and lost consciousness." By October 17, she was falling into a coma. Without intervention, Eileen was sure to die.

Alfred Blalock had not yet performed the surgery, not on a person and not on a dog. Blalock had watched Thomas work, but he had never done the cutting and sewing. So in November he scheduled a date on which Thomas would teach him how to perform the surgery. On the appointed day, Thomas had everything ready for his boss—the dog on the table, the tools all prepared— but Blalock didn't show. Thomas was getting impatient, when the phone rang. It was Blalock. Eileen Saxon was dying. If they were going to perform the surgery, it would have to be done now, without Blalock ever having performed it in the dog lab.

———

The operation took place on the morning of November 29, 1944. Blalock was so nervous, he didn't trust himself to drive to work and asked his wife to take him to the hospital. Thomas set up the room. "Suture material had been prepared, and supplies included additional bulldog clamps, a seven-inch straight Adson hemostatic forceps (which was useful as a needle holder), a blunt right-angle nerve hook and smooth bayonet-type forceps to pull up the continuous suture." Having arranged it all, Thomas ducked out, too anxious to watch.

Dr. Austin Lamont, head of anesthesia at Hopkins, examined Eileen Saxon and refused to take part in the surgery. She was too small, Lamont thought. If the anesthetic didn't kill her, the surgery would. He thought it would be more humane to let her die on her own. Blalock turned to a junior anesthesiologist, Dr. Merel Harmel, just a year out of medical school, who agreed to help out.

Blalock was assisted by his resident, Denton Cooley, and his chief surgical intern, William Longmire. Cooley would go on to found the Texas Heart Institute and to be the first man to implant an artificial heart in a human being. Longmire was one of the founders of the UCLA School of Medicine and in Los Angeles built one of the foremost heart surgery centers in the world. When Blalock got to the operating room, he didn't look for either of these men. He looked for Vivien Thomas—who had trained both Cooley and Longmire in his dog lab.

"I guess you better go call Vivien," he said. Thomas came to the observation gallery, where he could look down on the surgery below.

"Vivien," Blalock said. "You'd better come down here."

There were seven people in the operating room that day: Blalock, Thomas, Taussig, Cooley, Longmire, Harmel, and a scrub nurse, Charlotte Mitchell. Rain fell against the big windows. The radiator hissed. The room was cold and damp.

"Many of us thought this operation was going to be a big disaster," Cooley remembered.

The patient was wheeled in. Weighing less than nine pounds, she was so small it was difficult to see her under the sterile, surgical drapes. Taussig calmed the patient, held her, and laid her down on the operating table. Harmel, the anesthesiologist, had some difficulty fitting his breathing tube into the little girl's tiny windpipe, but once the oxygenation began, her color improved. Taussig stood by the girl's head. Ether was comingled with the oxygen in Eileen's breathing tube. The patient was so small, according to Thomas, that they didn't take her blood pressure—they couldn't find a cuff small enough.

Blalock asked Thomas to stand where he could see the operation, and so Thomas found a footstool, stepped onto it, and stood looking down over Blalock's shoulder. Photographs of the operation taken from the gallery show six people gathered around the operating table and Thomas, standing tall, just behind the surgeon, in a cap and surgical mask. Denton Cooley, low man on the totem pole, inserted a needle into a small vein in Eileen's ankle, at the ready with fluids and blood for transfusion.

Blalock entered the chest on the left side. He made an incision from the sternum all the way down the side of the chest. Blalock entered the chest cavity through the third interspace between the ribs. The light was inadequate. A common floor lamp had to be brought close to illuminate the cavity. The veins and arteries were so small they looked to Thomas like capillaries. There was more bleeding than expected, which made it difficult to find the great arteries. Blalock found the left pulmonary artery and cut it free of the surrounding tissue.

The artery was "no bigger than a matchstick" to Taussig's eyes. According to Thomas, "The patient's vessels were less than half the size of the vessels of the experimental animals that had been used to develop the procedure." Blalock applied one of the clamps that Thomas had developed to the pulmonary artery and paused to see if the patient tolerated it. Then he applied a second clamp. He asked Thomas if he thought the space was long enough for an incision in the pulmonary artery. Thomas thought it was long enough—in fact, the incision didn't have to be that long.

"Al Blalock's tenacity was remarkable," Longmire remembered. "The cuff of the vessel visible was a fraction of a millimeter, and the incision itself was only four or five inches. I remember watching him open the patient and just thinking it was impossible."

Blalock began to suture the left subclavian artery to the incision he had made in the pulmonary artery, creating a connection that mimicked a patent ductus and diverted more oxygen to the lungs. The sutures had to be less than a millimeter apart from each other and very close to the edge of the vessels. It was a slow, laborious process. As Denton Cooley remembered it, "Dr. Blalock would ask Vivien questions over his shoulder. He would say, 'Vivien, should I do it this way or that way?' Vivien would know the answers."

Thomas watched Blalock sew and corrected him when the stitches went in the wrong direction. "Well, you watch," said Blalock impatiently, "and don't let me put them in wrong." A set of stay sutures went over the initial suture, and then a second set kept it all in place. The clamps were removed. There was practically no bleeding. The vessels were connected.

From a technical point of view, Blalock wrote later, the connection he'd created, an anastomosis, seemed fine. But he was perturbed by the tiny size of the arteries. And he couldn't hear a "thrill," the sound of blood rushing through at adequate pressure.

The anesthesiologist, Merel Harmel, whispered, "The color is improving. Take a look! Take a look!"

Taussig and Longmire looked down at the baby, at the new, cherry-red color of her lips. "You've never seen something so dramatic," Thomas said later. "It was almost like a miracle." Blalock washed the cavity with sulfanilamide and closed it. The procedure took ninety minutes in all.

———

As she lay in the recovery room, no pulse could be felt in little Eileen Saxon's left wrist, and her left arm was much colder than her right. She was alive, but her circulation was poor. Dr. Ruth

Whittemore, Helen Taussig's young fellow, stayed by little Eileen all day and night through the tiny girl's torturous recovery.

"I had to stick needles into both sides of her chest to draw off air that was compressing her lungs," Whittemore remembered. Several times, Eileen's lungs collapsed and had to be aspirated. There was no intensive care unit and no ventilator. No monitor existed to measure the pressure on her lungs, so Whittemore had to invent one. Eileen remained under close watch for two weeks, going in and out of fever. She was given oxygen and penicillin. She didn't leave the hospital for home until two months after she underwent surgery.

Taussig and Blalock published the results of their work in May 1945, and soon doctors from all over—including Robert Gross in Boston—came to see. Hopkins was flooded with patients. Newspapers across America sponsored contests to send cyanotic kids to the hospital. These kids arrived with their own local press contingent. Hallways were crowded with reporters. "Some of the parents did not bother to [consult] their doctors," Thomas remembered. "They came by automobile, train, and plane. Many had not communicated with the hospital, had no appointment in the clinic, and had no hotel reservations; the cardiac clinic was overrun." The children's surgical ward was converted into a ward for heart patients and was nicknamed "the tet ward." There the kids lay in their cribs and beds before surgery, blue lipped, stubby fingered, crouching and squatting to relieve the pressure on their chests, sometimes twenty to a room.

Vivien Thomas's days began at 7 a.m. when he collected blood from postoperative patients. His day ended at 11 p.m., when he called the operating room for the next day's schedule. Blalock demanded that Thomas be at his side for each of the first sixty operations, and if Thomas was missing—picking up or delivering materials to the Harriet Lane Home, which lay two city blocks from the operating room—he was sure to hear himself paged over the intercom. In the summer, the heat in the operating was unbearable. The big, screened windows were flung wide open. The doctors sweated in their scrubs and masks. There was a fan to blow the air around and an enormous spotlight to guide Blalock in his work. The big, hot light stood on a wobbly stand and was forever being jostled by the surgical team or the four or five observing doctors.

Blalock and Taussig toured the world, lecturing and demonstrating their work. Thomas continued to work at Hopkins. It wasn't until the 1970s, after Blalock was dead, that Vivien Thomas was allowed to become a professor of surgery at Johns Hopkins. After his appointment, he made it his mission to train a generation of African American surgeons there.

Alfred Blalock worked with Helen Taussig for years, but it's not clear that he liked her. "If I get to heaven," he once said, "it will be because I could live with Helen Taussig." Other male doctors seemed to have agreed. They called her "the Queen" or "the Mother Hen" because of the way her students, most of them women, followed her.

She trained more than 123 students at Johns Hopkins. The "Knights of Taussig" spread out across the country. In 1947, she published her book, *Congenital Malformations of the Heart*. It was revised in the early 1960s and again in the 1980s and remained the essential textbook of the field for nearly forty years.

Taussig held reunions for her students at her family home in Cotuit, Massachusetts. Her rule for her guests was simple: let her have her mornings for work; she was not their hostess until after lunch. She liked to swim. She liked to sail. She never married. She seemed to have no personal life outside her work. She was the first woman to become president of the American Heart Association, received the Medal of Freedom from Lyndon Johnson, and was made a chevalier of the French Legion d'Honneur. She continued publishing original work into her eighties, when she was studying congenital deformities in bird hearts. She died backing her car out into traffic.

"She was a terrible driver," one of her (male) colleagues remembered.

Many of the patients who got a Blalock shunt lived for decades afterward, and many survived to have successful open-heart surgery and full correction of their heart defects. They were still somewhat blue after their surgeries, but they were active—the shunts allowed long, full lives. There are even some people still living today whose heart defects have never been repaired, who have survived for decades with terrible cardiac deformities, the shunts in their great arteries redirecting their circulation, oxygenating their blood. I got to talk to one such patient.

Belen Altuve Blanton was operated on by Denton Cooley in 1965 in Texas on Christmas Eve. When she was an infant, Cooley put a shunt into the great arteries of her heart. Her parents had flown up from Venezuela for the surgery, and they never allowed her to undergo a second surgery for a repair to her congenital defect.

I first saw Belen in a hotel bar in June 2017, fifty-two years after Cooley implanted the shunt. A petite, stylish woman with a dark mop of hair and a round, pretty, youthful face, she had a big glass of wine and was surrounded by friends. If I had had to guess her age, I would have said mid-thirties. If you'd asked me what was wrong with her, I would have said nothing.

"It's the make-up," she laughed. Then she showed me her hands. She had lovely rings. Her fingers were small, but under each painted nail, they were purple. She had lived her entire life without a functioning right ventricle, the shunt from 1965 compensating for her heart defect.

Throughout most of her life, she had little medical follow-up. In 1972, when she was seven, the family had flown back from Caracas to Houston, where Dr. Cooley had recommended a follow-up operation, but Belen's parents had refused to put her under bypass on a heart-lung machine.

"My parents," she told me, "they were afraid of everything."

Belen grew up sheltered and adored. She was not allowed to swim or to ride a bike. Her parents never taught her how to drive—they would not put her behind the wheel of a car. Her mother said, "You're crazy. With your heart?" She lived well through most of adolescence, but one day when she was seventeen, she woke up with arrhythmia so severe she couldn't move, so tired she could not brush her teeth. At the hospital, they did an EKG and told her she was dying. Belen vomited yellow bile. She passed out and reports that she felt a sense of flying through the dark, deep into a quiet place. A light appeared, as Belen describes it, as if from a doorway. She told me that she saw her godfather, recently deceased, and at that moment, Belen believes, a defibrillator was put to her chest and she was revived. After that, she began to live her life as if she had no heart problems at all.

"I have this thing," Belen told me. "Life is not for drama. I hate drama."

She went to law school, but law was not for her. When she suffered cardiac arrhythmias at parties or in company, she pretended they weren't happening. "I needed to be cool in front of my friends," she said. She left Venezuela for North Carolina. She got married. She had a kid. The child was healthy, but the pregnancy put a terrible pressure on her heart.

Like Bridgette Ratliff, Belen lived for years in heart failure, without ever acknowledging it, without ever seeing an appropriate doctor. When finally she saw an adult congenital cardiologist and was told that she would need a heart-lung transplant, Belen's reaction was furious denial.

"She told me everything, right to my face," Belen said. The doctor described to Belen the pulmonary hypertension she suffered and the damage that her lungs had suffered on account of the lifelong weakness of her heart. "When I got out of her office," Belen told me, "I thought, 'What does this witch know about life?' But you know, she wasn't mean. She was just telling the truth. That's how I started to learn about my condition."

Belen was placed on a list for a heart-lung transplant, and one was scheduled, but then, at the last moment, called off. Belen received the news on the phone, sitting in a restaurant with friends. She had been diagnosed with cardiac cirrhosis—the long-term damage to her lungs and heart had strained and injured her liver, and doctors, fearing complications to those organs, would not perform the transplant.

Belen, when I met her, had no hope for a cure for her condition. But she perseveres. She has met a second husband, John Blanton, who dotes on her. I last saw her at a party, and she was looking fabulous, wearing a spaghetti-strap spangled dress with a giant eyeball design on the front.

In private, she struggles. "I've become terrified of death. I mean terrified." She refuses to go out of her home alone. "I always have this feeling I'm going to pass out, and nobody's going to be there to save me." Still, in public, she insists on being beautiful and strong. She lives as she has always lived, willing herself and imagining herself to be healthier than she actually is.

At the hospital, when she goes under anesthesia, she tells her husband, "Honey, as soon as I wake up, put some lipstick on me." Sometimes she finds herself losing strength. She'll be eating with friends, unable to move, physically incapable of rising from her chair, but by sheer determination she manages.

"My ass will be out of that chair, and I will be walking," she told me. "You can lose anything in this life, but never your glamour."

26.

I N JUNE WE all went to Boston together, the first time I ever let Marcia come with me to the doctor. Eliza was three and a half months old. Her colic was beginning to ease, and all that anxious nursing had made her a fat and gorgeous baby. She was perfectly charming in the waiting room in her green-and-white-striped Zutano onesie. All the other babies in there were heart patients. We were the only parents with a healthy kid, and even in my own fear and doubt and confusion, it seemed crazy how lucky we were to have Eliza.

Dr. Freed didn't prescribe a catheter exam. Instead, he had me get an MRI. I imagined for years afterward that he had done this as a sop to my neurosis—I'd been afraid of the catheter, so he'd figured out another way to get a measure—but when I met with him in 2018, he disabused me of that notion. The MRI was safer than the cardiac catheter, with the patient exposed to less radiation. The numbers it offered were far more precise. In 1995, the cardiology department at Boston Children's had purchased an MRI machine, and it had taken some time for them to master its use. The MRI is generally designed to give pictures of a static part of the body—a brain or a knee—and the heart is always in motion, so it became necessary in cardiology to learn to use the MRI in conjunction with an electrocardiogram, to "gate" the imaging, in cardiologists' terms: to get pictures of the heart at its greatest points of contraction and expansion, in systole and diastole.

So into the capsule of the MRI I went, naked but for a hospital gown. It was like a giant white washing machine, and I was the load of clothes, tossed in on the spin cycle. White whooshing sounds filled my ears. Oh, please, God, let me know, I prayed: Was I going to live or die? The repetitive sound of the machine gave an answer: wha-*HOOOM*, wha-*HOOOM*, wha-*HOOOM*. I listened and listened and prayed and prayed, and the rushing sounds became words: no-*DEATH*, no-*DEATH*, no-*DEATH*. I couldn't figure out if there was a period between the two words "no" and "DEATH": "no. DEATH. no. DEATH. no. DEATH." Was that it? Or was it "no DEATH. no DEATH. no DEATH." If there was a period, I was going to die. If there wasn't, I'd live. Everything depended on punctuation.

I got back to the waiting room. I took warm, funny Eliza in my arms. She was pointing. She was smiling. I caught Mike Freed's eye as he glimpsed us across the waiting room. He looked at the baby and frowned. Something shifted in his aspect, which I understood as follows: It was one thing to play games with my heart as a solitary neurotic twenty-nine-year-old. It was quite another to do so as a thirty-three-year-old family man.

In his office he showed me the pictures and measurements of my heart. The right and left ventricles should be approximately the same size, he explained, but mine weren't. In diastole, when the heart expanded, my left ventricle measurement was a normal 140 milliliters. My right ventricle measured 472 ml. In systole, the left squeezed down to 53 ml. The right hardly squeezed at all; it compacted to 342 ml. My right ventricle's regurgitation fraction—the amount of blood that went backward—was high: 50 percent. Half the blood that should have been going to my lungs was sliding back. Dr. Freed explained to me that these numbers did not signify changes over time. It wasn't clear how much larger my heart was now than it had been when he had first met me. But now we had a definitive measurement.

I objected. I was feeling fine, I said. Didn't it make sense to wait until I had symptoms? Why should I have heart surgery when I was feeling fine?

Dr. Freed rubbed his forehead. He did not say it outright—that I was not feeling fine, that I was fooling myself, just adapting to my lethargy—instead he told me the old story about the frog getting boiled. He had never boiled a frog, he said, so he had no idea if it was true. But I was a little like the frog in the story. The temperature was being raised slowly, and I wasn't noticing what was going on, but by the time I noticed, I might well be cooked.

"You're saying that if I develop symptoms, you won't be able to save me?"

He nodded.

"So I really do need to have heart surgery."

"If you want to see your daughter graduate college, yes."

Later, Dr. Freed gave me his notes. He wrote,

I don't think there are any surprises. Mr. Brownstein is not limited by his heart disease in his everyday activities. Objectively, his maximum 0_2 consumption is somewhat reduced as is his cardiac output at rest. This is undoubtedly due to the free pulmonary regurgitation and dilated right ventricle with a reduced ejection fraction, which compromises his ability to augment cardiac output with exercise. . . . In spite of the fact that I don't think there have been any real changes over the last few years, I think that most pediatric cardiologists and adult cardiologists taking care of adults with congenital heart disease would recommend surgery to replace his pulmonary valve. As we take care of more and more young adults with repaired tetralogy I think the preponderance of evidence is coming down on the side that long term volume overload of the right ventricle is almost certainly going to get him into trouble eventually. . . . I spent some time discussing this with Mr. Brownstein.

I tried to digest what he was telling me. The surgeon would crack my chest and slit my heart open and put a new valve where I didn't have one, and this would arrest the pulmonary regurgitation and allow my right ventricle to recover its pumping power—or at the very least, it would arrest the ventricle's decline and potentially save me from heart failure. We moved toward scheduling a date. My brother was going to be getting married in early August, and I wanted to be there for that. That seemed reasonable to Dr. Freed. And then the semester would begin, I told myself.

"What about December?" I asked. "Would that be crazy?"

"Not *crazy*," Dr. Freed said. "Some people," he said, "like to take care of these things right away."

"I'll schedule for December," I told him.

That summer was brutal. Was I too exhausted? Should I not have been driving? I thought I saw something in my blind spot, and Marcia screamed my name, and then I slammed my foot on the brake, and the car tires skidded over the highway like skates on ice, and we slipped over the embankment, flipping, flipping, over and over again, and came to rest with the airbags in our faces and Eliza hanging upside down in her car seat, beaming and smiling. Thank God Marcia was wearing her seatbelt.

And then, when we were home in Brooklyn and sorting the broken glass from our luggage, we got the news that one of my childhood best friends had died—a beautiful, brilliant man who had lived a troubled life and only recently seemed to have secured himself happiness. He had died on his honeymoon in Martha's Vineyard on account of a sudden, mysterious arrhythmia that affected his heart. It seemed so unjust, so confusing. Eliza came with us to his funeral, the same church where only weeks before, we'd celebrated his marriage. The choir from the Metropolitan Opera had sung when they'd married. His bride had been one of them, a singer in that chorus, and now she was his widow.

In the fall, Marcia went back to work part-time. Eliza was sleeping, growing, thriving, no longer colicky, a perfectly delightful child. She developed interests—for instance, in a soft yellow duck that went into the bath with her. Every morning, I took a walk with her, baby strapped to my chest. I went out to Stony Brook two days a week, and if I managed all my prep and grading on the long train ride back, then my life at home was relaxed and easy. My dad could not get enough of his first granddaughter. He had just retired. He came out to babysit as often as he could. I got a little workspace, almost for free, in a brownstone converted to an after-school tutoring center. It was always empty during the day.

At Stony Brook, I didn't tell anyone about my condition. On the subway stairs, my heart wobbled and jumped. At night I was haunted by anxiety. I had an awful vision: that I'd wake up from the anesthesia in the middle of surgery, and I'd see it, I'd see the saw they used to open my chest. I imagined the spinning steel blade, the teeth blurred and biting, the spitting blood and the skin and the bone, and there I'd be on the operating table, *watching*. I wasn't sure what I was going to do with my life, but I certainly didn't have to decide anything until after surgery.

I worked on my stories. Sometimes at the tutoring center, I browsed the bookshelves and reread stories from my childhood. Back to Narnia. Back to Earthsea. I reread the volumes of classic stories they'd stocked up on for school kids. I had been trying to write stories about my childhood, probably because my old friend had so recently died. I was thinking about his heart and mine, and I began to rewrite my nostalgic stories over the classics all around me. "Wakefield," for example, by Nathaniel Hawthorne: I made Hawthorne's main character live on the seventh floor of my parents' old apartment building. My childhood friends and I spied on him. My narrator fell in love with Wakefield's daughter. I found an old story I'd never read by F. Scott Fitzgerald. I thought I had read everything by Fitzgerald. The story was called "The Curious Case of Benjamin Button"—it wasn't in the big, fat selected stories I'd been assigned in high school; it was in a little volume called *Tales of the Jazz Age* and had an awesome premise but was uncharacteristically bumpy for a Fitzgerald story. The idea was so cool—aging backward, back into the oblivion that came before birth—and the story seemed all about death and memory and writing. I sent the Wakefield story off to literary magazines, thinking, Ha-ha, you've rejected me, you bastards, now go and reject Nathaniel Hawthorne. The Fitzgerald story I rewrote got long and bizarrely convoluted and strange. I wasn't writing it for any point but to mark the hours, to explore my brain, to play with language. I was pleasing myself, if nobody else.

Then it was time to go to Boston. My surgeon, the first time he met me, laid heavy emphasis on the risks I faced, the possibilities of infection, heart failure, and death. ("I think he does that," Mike Freed confided, "because his wife is a lawyer.") A social worker walked me through the steps of the procedure and explained that I would wake up with a breathing tube down my throat.

"What does that feel like?" I asked.

"Well," she said, breaking from her smooth presentation, "it's never happened to me."

The night before surgery, we stayed in a hotel. Eliza woke at midnight, and Marcia went to tend to the baby, but I said, "No. I'll do it." I wasn't sleeping anyway. I had nothing else on the agenda for that night. I got her from the port-a-crib and held her, sitting at the edge of the hotel bed. I thought, if this was the last night of my life, this was how I wanted to spend it, soothing my daughter one last time, letting my wife sleep.

PART THREE

The Open Heart Club, Reprise

27.

M Y MIND CAME back very slowly. Out of a very deep darkness, it returned a little bit at a time. The first thing I was aware of was eighteen words, there in the blackness. I didn't hear the words or remember them. They were like a hallucination.

James James Morrison Morrison Weatherby George Dupree
Took great care of his mother, though he was only three.

The skin of my shaved chest was sutured and bandaged and taped. A tube ran into the left side of my chest, sucking out fluid. My chest bone was bound together by staples. The heart itself was stitched up with a new valve inside, one that had come from a pig. Two wires slipped through the skin, attached on one end to an outlet in the wall, then to a pacemaking machine, and then to my heart. Into my arm went the IV tubes of saline fluid and antibiotics and morphine, and out of my penis came the catheter that went to the bag that held whatever leaked out of me. In my mouth was the breathing tube, filling my lungs with oxygen every ten seconds. But I didn't know any of that. Just the little snatch of Winnie-the-Pooh, that's all, a bit of the A.A. Milne poem my mother must have recited to me thirty years before, the first time I had open-heart surgery, when I was just five years old. That little rhyme was the rope my mind grasped onto as it made its way back.

It was a very long way up, a long time coming to consciousness. The first physical awareness was of the breathing tube, which I imagined as a gun-shaped pipe, maybe two inches wide, shoved all the way down my throat. I felt it pressing into the cartilage of my windpipe. Whenever I tried to inhale, the tube's airflow shut off, and I was strangled back to unconsciousness. Then the tube gave me oxygen, reviving me just enough so that I tried to take a breath. As soon as I tried to do that, I was suffocated. And once I was knocked out again, it gave me oxygen. Again I woke up and tried to breathe. Again, the tube strangled me. This went on for a while, awake, strangled, asleep, awake, strangled, asleep.

I remember a clock on the wall, but I doubt that my eyes were open. I'm not sure I could have opened my eyes if I'd wanted to. But that's what I saw, each time I came to, before the tube strangled me and I passed out again, a black-and-white kitchen wall clock with two hands and twelve numbers, about a foot and a half from the ceiling of an ordinary white wall. It was a couple minutes to midnight. Sometimes the clock moved forward. Sometimes back. Then in the darkness a woman's voice came to me. They were going to roll me on my side, she said, for extubation. There would be some discomfort.

I felt the pressure on my back. I felt the tilt, the turn onto my left side. The split halves of my sternum scraped against each other, like teeth grinding in the middle of my chest. I felt the staples that held together my thorax. There was the shock without the sensation of pain. All my nerves flamed, but they were disconnected from my brain, or from the part of my brain that knew what pain felt like. I understood that there was a rip down in my bones and viscera, but I didn't exactly feel it. I felt very frightened. The tube felt very long. It came out with some gummy mucus, and when it was out, my mouth felt like it had been frozen, dried, and vacuumed, which is more or less what had happened. They lowered me onto my back again, and my body and bones and the tubes and needles all fell back into place. I think I fell asleep.

Out of the dark, my family came close. Marcia was there, and so were my parents. They asked what I wanted. I couldn't talk.

Someone had the bright idea to ask me to write, and I tried scribbling something. I don't remember the pad or pen. My hand was like a flipper. I managed to scrawl the word "drink."

"He's thirsty!" they celebrated.

The nurses said that they couldn't give me water, but they agreed to let me have a spoonful of ice chips, which melted in the desert of my mouth. My heart was still not beating on its own.

28.

OPEN-HEART SURGERY WAS an invention of the 1950s, and like rock-and-roll, another great American invention of the time, it seems like the brainchild less of a single person than of an entire nation.

Heart surgery began with kids like me, and it began in Minnesota. For decades, doctors had been operating around the heart, even on the great arteries above the heart, as in the Blalock procedure, but the breakthrough came when they were able to put their patients on bypass, connect them to a heart-lung machine, and open up the heart itself. This happened first in two places in Minnesota: Minneapolis and Rochester. When in the mid-1950s young physicians like Jim Malm and Sylvia Griffiths wanted to learn what was happening in cardiac medicine, they went to the Mayo Clinic in Rochester to see John Kirklin work or to the University of Minnesota to see Walt Lillehei.

Kirklin and Lillehei were the Beatles and Stones of heart surgery, the Bird and Magic, the Tolstoy and Dostoevsky, competitors and partners, driving each other forward, driving medicine toward its new frontier. Kirklin was more dispassionate and technically minded; his biographer nicknamed him "the Ice Man." Lillehei was impulsive, creative, and wild, a rule breaker. In his memoir, *100,000 Hearts*, Denton Cooley describes a trip he took to Minnesota in 1955, along with a few other young, aspiring heart surgeons. In Rochester, Kirklin was gracious but formal. He had Cooley and company over to his house for dinner, where his wife served them a pleasant meal concluded with a "thimble full" of sherry. Kirklin put everyone to bed before nine, saying there was work to be done early the next day. He met them in the hospital in the morning, and they watched him operate. From Mayo the young doctors went to Minneapolis, where they met Lillehei, blond and blue-eyed, with a chin like a movie star's and a frightening scar on his neck.

For dinner Lillehei took the junior surgeons to what Cooley calls "a little road house on the edge of town," where the bartender said to Lillehei, "Howdy, Doc, gonna have the usual to-night?" The usual for Lillehei meant four double martinis before a steak dinner, and then three more after, and then dancing with the waitresses. Cooley struggled to keep up. He and his friends crawled back to their hotel rooms in the early morning. Headachy and bleary-eyed, they hustled to the hospital the next morning to find that Lillehei had not yet arrived. At 10 a.m., an hour after the surgery's scheduled start, Lillehei wandered in "looking clammy, sweaty, and in need of medical attention himself." The patient was a small child with a hole in his heart. The heart-lung machine was a bubble oxygenator of Lillehei's design. Hungover and maybe still a little drunk, Lillehei was unimpaired. He performed the operation "superbly and successfully," wrote Cooley.

"Every 'original' genius," wrote W. H. Auden, "be he an artist or a scientist, has something a bit shady about him, like a gambler or a madman." Lillehei had a genius unusual in a great heart surgeon—he was prodigiously imaginative, while most heart surgeons are methodical, careful men—and Lillehei was certainly a little bit shady. In the 1950s, he was heart surgery's foremost inventor, teacher, mentor, fund-raiser, and promoter. He was also a party animal who didn't mind working outside the law, and his run at the top of his profession burned out soon after it peaked. Late in his career at the University of Minnesota, he crashed his speedboat, drunk and driving late at night. His wife's pretty face was broken and damaged when it smashed against the dashboard. When the hospital didn't promote him to chief of surgery, Lillehei packed up all his equipment and drove to New York, leaving a single long-stemmed red rose on the floor of his lab. In Manhattan in the late

1960s, while his wife stayed in Minnesota, Lillehei lived the life of a swinging bachelor, got into bar fights, alienated his colleagues, and was convicted of tax fraud. Perhaps the single-most influential heart surgeon in history, he spent his last decades humiliated and unable to practice.

Lillehei was born in 1918 in Edina, a suburb of Minneapolis. His father was a dentist, the child of Scandinavian immigrants, and his mother a pianist. Walt skipped two grades in elementary school but was bored in high school and struggled to pass chemistry. From the start, he was not impressed by authority. "I didn't necessarily believe in signs that said, 'don't do this,' or 'don't do that,'" he said. "If I had a reason to do it, I usually did it."

He remodeled his toy BB gun to shoot .22-caliber bullets. With scrap parts and no manual, he built himself a motorcycle. Walt thought he'd become a dentist like his father, but when he discovered that the entry requirements were the same for medical and dental school, he thought, Why not? And he set out to be a doctor.

At the University of Minnesota, he fell under the spell of Dr. Owen Wagensteen, chair of surgery at the university hospital. Wagensteen was a compelling lecturer and a driven man. He had grown up on a small farm run by his Norwegian father, tending to piglets and hauling manure. When Wagensteen came to the University of Minnesota in the late 1920s, the place was a backwater, but he had a vision. He gathered around him a faculty devoted to surgical research, let them pursue their goals aggressively, and built one of the great surgical departments in history.

As an inventor, Wagensteen is best known for an abdominal suction tube that saved the lives of soldiers with gunshot wounds. (There's an Ogden Nash poem that goes, "May I find my rest in / Owen Wagensteen's intestine.") As a surgeon, he advocated aggressive, radical cancer operations, including the hemicorporectomy, the cutting off of a person's bottom half, and the eviscerectomy, in which the surgeon took out the bladder, gonads, lymph nodes, spleen, rectum, kidneys, and a chunk of the colon. He had a drunken son who was in and out of prison and a wife who hated him. She knew Wagensteen was afraid of snakes, so she often sent them to him, wrapped up as gifts.

In 1938, when Walt Lillehei was twenty, he heard Wagensteen lecture about experiments he had performed on the appendixes of tigers and bears. According to *King of Hearts*, G. Wayne Miller's biography of Lillehei, that was when Walt decided to become a surgeon. He wanted to work with a man who wrangled wild animals. Lillehei finished medical school and, like most doctors of his generation, headed off to war. He crossed the Mediterranean with the US troops and landed in Italy at the Battle of Anzio, where the Allies were pinned down in marshes and Germans shelled them from above.

As a surgeon in a MASH unit, Lillehei saw carnage. "I've certainly seen more of the horrors of modern warfare than I ever anticipated," he wrote home. It was his job to award Purple Hearts to wounded soldiers. "It's a beautiful medal," he wrote, "but not much to give a man in return for his leg, arm, or face."

———

World War II, as much as any single physician, drove the development of cardiac surgery. The US Army built the first surgical ward specifically devoted to wounds to the heart. The military bestowed the grants that led to the development of the cardiac catheter. Ultimately, it was the war effort that led to the great US government investment in medicine. Between 1941 and 1951 the federal budget for medical research grew from no more than $3 million to $76 million. Before the war, penicillin was expensive and difficult to produce, but it was needed on the battlefield. The Federal Committee on Medical Research teamed with Bradley Polytechnic Institute in Peoria, Illinois, and before war's end penicillin was being manufactured cheaply in 15,000-gallon drums.

Harvard doctor Dwight Harken had been experimenting with surgeries to remove infectious growths from the heart (before antibiotics were widely available, these things could develop, vegetations like algae blooms). In the war, he was stationed in England when bombs were falling on London. Soldiers from the European theater were arriving with horrific wounds to their chests, shrapnel lodged in their hearts, and if these wounds didn't kill the soldiers outright, they led to infections of the blood stream, or to blood clots that caused strokes, or, best case, to a life of terror, with soldiers waiting, just waiting, for the metal shard inside to shift from its place and kill them.

As late as 1945, the prejudice against cardiac surgery was so strong that no other doctor wanted to touch patients with these wounds. Harken had to plead his case in order to get permission to operate, and eventually his superiors allowed him to create a unit specifically devoted to thoracic surgery and wounds to the heart. After a struggle, it was built: a set of sheet metal Quonset huts in the countryside by Cirencester, a small town in Gloustershire. These first operating theaters for cardiac surgery had neither insulation nor heating. They were freezing in winter and broiling in summer. But they were equipped with fluoroscopes, EKGs, and (most importantly) penicillin. Patients arrived by the truckloads with hideous wounds to their chests.

Harken failed in his first two attempts to remove shrapnel from the heart of Leroy Rohrbach, an infantry sergeant who had been wounded in a battle near the French town of Saint-Lô. An exploding shell had torn up Rohrbach's chest, and a piece of metal had slipped deep into his heart. Harken was a large, red-haired man with a red face, a screamer and a shouter in the operating room, charming and garrulous outside it. His students later called him "the Great Red Man." On August 15, 1945, Harken grasped the fragment in Rohrbach's chest with his forceps, but it slipped from them and was swallowed up by the beating heart. In November, Harken tried again: again, he clamped the metal in his forceps, and again he lost it. Fluoroscopic images showed the fragment bobbing up and down with each heartbeat. Rohrbach was desperate. He begged the doctors to get it out of him. On February 19, Harken tried again.

He opened the sergeant's chest and retracted the ribs, and this time got a good view of his patient's ventricle. Before touching the metal, Harken placed a circle of sutures around the wound. Then he put a Kocher clamp—a scissor-shaped clamp like a forceps—on the shard. He gave it a pull. "Suddenly with a pop, as if a champagne cork had been drawn, the fragment jumped out of the ventricle, forced by the pressure within the chamber," Harken wrote. "Blood poured out in a torrent." Harken pulled on the sutures around the wound, and they shut tight like the strings of a purse. Still, blood came, and Harken pressed his finger on the opening. "I took large needles swedged with silk and began passing them through the heart muscle wall, under my finger, and out the other side. With four of them in, I slowly removed my fingers, as one after another was tied." But Harken's finger wouldn't budge. His glove was stuck in the threads. "I was sutured to the wall of the heart! We cut the glove and I got loose." Rohrbach's chest was closed up. The patient survived. Eminent English surgeons visited the Quonset huts. Cameramen perched in the rafters above the operating table. Harken operated successfully on 134 chest wounds without a fatality and returned to Boston a hero.

Meanwhile, in Germany, a strange, solitary, driven doctor began entering the heart from a different direction.

———

The story of the cardiac catheter begins with Warner Forssmann, a urologist and card-carrying member of the Nazi Party. As Forssmann describes it in his memoir, *Experiments on Myself*, his childhood loves were technology and the kaiser. As a boy Forssmann saw the Wright brothers fly their plane when they came to Germany, and he was thrilled by military parades, the streets crowded with "cheerful, colorful, flag-waving people." His father died in World War I, and Forssmann's family was left penniless. They scrounged for rutabagas and fermented black bread. For Sunday dinners, his mother roasted crows. By the time he had entered university, Forssmann's intellectual interests had shifted from aeronautics to medicine. He learned about a nineteenth-century French doctor, Jean-Baptiste Auguste Chaveau, who had inserted a catheter through a horse's jugular vein and from there to the heart. Forssmann had a vision: he could slide a catheter into a human heart.

This was in the 1920s. The Weimar Republic disgusted Forss-mann. "The 'Golden Twenties,'" he writes in his memoir, "never were golden except for a small, self-indulgent group." Forssmann fell under the sway of a Dr. Freidel, a pale wraith of a man who wore a dusty, black, and velvet-trimmed gown to work and kept a huge sheepdog in his office. Freidel gave political pamphlets to Forssmann and asked him to distribute them to his fellow students, pamphlets including "The Protocols of the Elders of Zion." Forss-mann admitted, "I'm afraid that here and there some of these ideas just may have caught on."

In 1929, Forssmann got a job as an intern at the Red Cross Hospital in Eberswalde, a small town north of Berlin. He was big and broad shouldered with dark, lank hair and narrow, close-set eyes, a hard-drinking, motorcycle-riding obsessive. He still possessed his mania: he was going to stick a catheter into a human heart.

The chief of staff of the hospital at Eberswalde, Peter Schneider, was a friend of Forssmann's mother, and when Forssmann approached him with his vision of the cardiac catheter, Schneider said, "I cannot possibly let you carry out such an experiment on a patient." Over beers, Forssmann explained his idea to a young colleague, Peter Romeis. Romeis objected. The idea was dangerous, inhumane, and pointless. There was no demonstrable benefit to putting a catheter into someone's heart. Perhaps Forssmann should work on an animal's first. Forssmann did not answer Romeis's objections. He only smiled.

To perform his experiment, he needed access to a phlebotomy kit, a urinary catheter, and an X-ray machine. He also needed an accomplice. He "started to prowl around Nurse Gerda Ditzen like a sweet-toothed cat around the cream jug."

I made a point of dawdling in the canteen after lunch, hoping to meet Nurse Gerda as she left the nurses' dining room. We'd often lent each other books, so it was easy to find something to gossip about; and she'd invite me back to her little office. . . . Gradually, carefully, I steered the conversation round to my hobbyhorse, and found she was interested. . . . So, little by little, I won over my essential disciple. When, about a fortnight after my conversation with Schneider, she said with a laugh, "What a pity we can't do the experiment together!" I decided the time had come.

Forssmann showed Nurse Gerda pictures of Chaveau's experiment and demonstrated how he would enter his patient through the arm and not the neck. They decided to try to sneak off together and do it in the early afternoon. "I knew I'd be able to carry out my black deed only during the afternoon siesta while everyone in the hospital was dozing." Quietly, they went to the procedure room. Nurse Gerda offered up her body to him. She would be Forssmann's patient, Gerda said. He could slide his catheter right into her heart. The doctor asked the nurse to lie on the operating table. "With the speed of light I strapped her down," he wrote in his memoir.

With Nurse Gerda bound hand and foot, Forssmann turned his back on her. He anesthetized himself at his left elbow. Ignoring Nurse Gerda, he made an incision in his own skin and inserted a long aneurysm needle into his vein. Forssmann opened the aneurysm needle and pushed the catheter about a foot into his arm. He packed the incision point with gauze and a sterile split and displayed it to Nurse Gerda while the catheter was deep in his arm. As Gerda watched, he twisted the catheter deeper and deeper. He released her from her bindings and asked her to help him up the stairs, to the top floor of the hospital and the X-ray machine. Forssmann stumbled down the hospital corridor, trailing the catheter. He was climbing the stairs when his drinking buddy Peter Romeis saw him.

"You idiot, what the hell are you doing?" Romeis asked, then tried to grab the catheter and pull it out of Forssmann. As Forssmann describes it, "I had to give him a few kicks in the shin to calm him down." Forssmann reached the X-ray room, Romeis and Nurse Gerda following. "I had a mirror placed so that by looking over the top of the screen I could see in it my thorax and upper arm. As I'd expected, the catheter had reached the head of the humerus. Romeis wanted me to stop at this point and remove it. But I wouldn't hear of it. I pushed the catheter in further, almost to the two-foot mark. Now the mirror showed the catheter inside the heart, with its tip at the right ventricle, just as I'd envisioned it."

In 1929, Forssmann's pictures made newspaper headlines all over Germany. He was able to transfer from his small, provincial Red Cross Hospital to the Cherité Hospital in Berlin, the most prestigious hospital in the country, ruled over by the country's most famous surgeon, Ferdinand Sauerbruch.

At Charité, Forssmann chafed under Sauerbruch's strict hierarchy and conventional command. He disobeyed his superiors and was dismissed. He returned to Eberswalde, where he shot colored dye into his own heart to improve the quality of his X-ray images.

He hoped to develop new ways to deliver medicine directly to the heart, but his ideas did not catch on. This was due partly to his lack of collegiality and partly to his foggy conception of the cardiac catheter's usefulness. Eventually Forssmann gave up on his work with the catheter and trained as a urological surgeon. He joined the Nazi Party in 1931, two years before Hitler came to power. Forssmann worked at Moabit Hospital, where 70 percent of the doctors were Jewish. As his colleagues were disappeared, Forssmann rose in the hierarchy. The hospital was renamed Robert Koch Hospital. The new chair of surgery was Kurt Strauss, a high-ranking SS officer. When all the Jews were gone, Forssmann became Strauss's vice chair of surgery.

It is hard to know exactly what Forssmann did as a Nazi army doctor. In his memoir, he is always the innocent: turning down offers to experiment on prisoners, discovering the slaughters of mental patients only after the fact, and expressing horror. He claims not to share the eugenic zeal of his fellow officers and party members. Throughout, he wants to paint himself as a marginal, ignorant, innocent figure. But Forssmann can't help boasting about his connections. "I put a call through to Goebbels," he writes at one point, and then later he boasts that a colleague "wanted to tell Himmler about my work and introduce me to him." With the German army, Forssmann went into Poland and then into Russia. After the war, he was banned from medical practice for three years because of his Nazi Party membership. In the late 1940s, he returned to work as a urologist. His research into the cardiac catheter never proceeded beyond his early experiments in Eberswalde, but his ideas were picked up by two doctors in the United States, and when they won the Nobel Prize, he won it with them.

———

Andre Cournand and Dickinson Richards were two thirty-seven-year-old military veterans and well-published Columbia professors working in the chest division of Bellevue Hospital. Their motive in experimenting with the cardiac catheter initially had nothing to do with heart surgery: they wanted to measure the effectiveness of their patients' lungs. To do this they had to measure the difference in oxygen content in their patients' arteries and veins. It was easy to get a decent sample of oxygenated blood by puncturing an artery in the arm or groin. The only place where they could get a pure and accurate sample of venous blood was in the right side of the heart. They developed the catheter to get this blood so as to more accurately calculate the effectiveness of a patient's cardiopulmonary system.

Some medical histories claim that while in Paris in 1935, Cournand stumbled across an article describing Forssmann's 1929 work. In Cournand's telling, this is not true. He says that cardiac catheterization came up in a conversation with a former professor who had performed hundreds of pulmonary angiograms, experiments, according to Cournand, that "had been received very critically by the great cardiologists of the time, who told him it was 'monstrous' to do such a thing as introduce a tube into the heart of a patient." When Cournand returned to New York, he and Richards began to use catheters to extract venous blood from the right side of the heart, first in dogs, then in monkeys, and then in human cadavers. Their work was progressing slowly when in 1941 the Japanese bombed Pearl Harbor. Then the US federal government began studying oxygen deprivation in soldiers. Alfred Blalock was put in charge of the "Shock Commission." Cournand went to

Washington and described his work to Blalock, and Blalock said, "You have your grant."

New York offered a steady stream of victims of car crashes, industrial accidents, and violent crime, and Cournand and Richards used their catheters to explore these dying hearts. Cournand measured the pressure and flow. Richards produced exquisite pictures of the heart, representing it in unprecedented detail. After the war, their colleague, pediatric cardiologist Janet Baldwin, one of Helen Taussig's protégées, began using their technology to take pictures of congenitally deformed hearts and to diagnose congenital heart disease more precisely.

All the while, federal investment in medical research continued to increase. The grant-giving budget of the National Institutes of Health (NIH) grew from $180,000 in 1945 to $4 million in 1947. Between 1949 and 1951, more than two-thirds of US medical schools applied for NIH grants to build cardiology research centers and cardiac catheter labs. Federal support was met with charitable contributions and private investments. Between 1941 and 1951 total national medical expenditure grew from an estimated $18 million to $181 million. The American Heart Association, founded in 1924 as a network of doctors interested in the new discipline of cardiology, reorganized itself in 1948 as a volunteer organization, raising money and awareness of heart disease. In Minneapolis, a combination of federal, charitable, and university support led to the construction of Variety Club Heart Hospital, with a forty-bed unit devoted to kids with deformed hearts.

When Walt Lillehei came back from the war, he applied to only one medical residency program, the place where this new hospital devoted to heart surgery would be built. His interview with Owen Wagensteen was brief.

Wagensteen: When can you start?

Lillehei: Today.

Wagensteen: You'll need a white coat.

29.

IEXPERIENCED OPEN-HEART SURGERY as pure blackness. Not death, but a little jaunt to the other side. When I woke up, I was surprised and satisfied to have returned. In bed in the cardiac ICU, I was aware, vaguely, of the nurses' station out the doorway to my right. People bustled out there. I heard beeps and whistles and cries, and there was no appreciable difference between night and day. Anytime I managed to fall asleep, that was the moment someone came to check my vitals, to take my temperature, to make sure of my oxygen flow. There was a button for the morphine, but I was intent on being stoic. I didn't want to take any more of that than I absolutely needed.

That was stupid. "Keep ahead of the pain," my nurse told me.

I was surprised by the look of my chest, which was plucked clean of hair and taped shut and covered with gauze pads, tubes and wires, and stains—the brown ones looked like blood, and the yellow ones (I guessed) might have been antiseptic. My arms had a lot of tape and wires on them. Everything smelled bad.

There was a period of euphoria. Yippee, I wasn't dead! Dr. Freed came by to check on me and told me gravely that my heart wasn't beating on its own. I gave him a goofy, satisfied-customer smile. I told him that was just fine. But soon enough I began to get irritable. They made me stand up, but that only taught me what a mess I was. My whole torso was frail and frightened. I was tangled up in tubes and wires. My legs, my feet, everything was exhausted.

It was impossible to get comfortable with the lousy pillow, and the rigid sheets, and the plastic-wrapped mattress.

Who brought the fucking flowers? I wanted them out. My older brother flew all the way from California. He came in with a pretty jar of marmalade. The sight of marmalade in the ICU just made me want to puke.

"Okay, okay," he tried to mollify me. "But maybe you'll want it in a couple of days. I'll put it here, where you can't see."

"No," I said. "Out!"

Marcia was the only person I wanted to see, the only one who didn't rub my frazzled nerves. She made fun of my catheter and told me stories of baby Eliza's day. She taped a little picture of Eliza by my bed, and that was my icon, my little prayer.

I tried to read. I'd brought along John Le Carré's *Tinker, Tailor, Soldier, Spy*, but I didn't have the focus or really the strength to hold the paperback in front of my face.

"Don't strain yourself," said Dr. Freed, when he caught me. "Just rest."

The pretty night nurse, Brianna, rolled a TV and VCR into my room. She suggested *Big*, starring Tom Hanks. But the colors were glaring—the video light, the way it moved, the oversaturation of the reds, the mugging of the actors—it was intolerable. I had brought along CDs and headphones, but music bugged me, particularly the happy stuff—the Beatles, Mozart, or Marvin Gaye.

The nurses emptied the big collection sack at the end of the catheter. I could not believe that giant bag of urine all came from me or that the tube they held came out of my penis. Where was my penis, under those sheets?

Everything was a chore. The doctors made me stand again. My heart still hadn't started beating on its own. I had those two wires in my chest that kept it beating. My legs didn't really want to support me. Allie Brosch, in the web comic *Hyperbole and a Half*, describes depression as a loss of joy in everything, kind of analogous to growing up, when the life of her toy animals vanished. In her comic, she draws funny pictures of herself at twelve, trying to play with a little toy horse and failing. "Depression feels almost exactly like that," Brosch writes, "except about everything." That's where I was. Music, books, movies, people, my father, my mother, my brothers, standing up, lying down, being awake, being asleep—it had all lost its magic. Throw it all in the garage, send it all to Goodwill.

There were occasional sparks. I didn't want to be left all alone. I made Marcia tell me about Eliza. When Dr. Freed told me that my heart was beating without stimulation from the pacemaker, I was a little mystified. A hope had been confirmed, and yet I hadn't realized all that time that I had been hoping. Out came those two thin wires; they just slid right out of my heart, out of my flesh, into the air, leaving little pinprick wounds. The first music I could listen to was heroin piano jazz, Bill Evans, *Waltz for Debbie*; the sly chords filled the runnels of my mind.

The kindest nurse in the history of the world took the catheter out of my penis, and she was frank and funny about it. I couldn't see her hands at work, but I felt some kind of valve switching, and then out came a tube that went way, way further in there than I could have imagined.

"Get up! Get up!" said Michael Freed.

I began, step by step, to move around my hospital bed. I was weak and dizzy, but once I could do it, I kept doing it. I had the IV pole with me, and I kept going in wider circles, wearing two hospital gowns, one for the front and one to cover my ass. I learned the world around me. My bed was one bed in one alcove out of many patient alcoves around the nurses' station. There were babies in cribs and old men in beds. "Look at him go!" the nurses teased me. "Slow down, buddy!" I ate normal food. I took my first trip to the bathroom to relieve myself. There was a nurse's call button and a cripple's bar, but I balanced myself, and I took a crap. You don't know the pleasures of your body until you lose them.

I tried Le Carré again and became engrossed. I sorted through my CDs. Bach was okay. So was Billie Holiday. Then I put on *New Morning*, not the greatest Bob Dylan album ever but maybe his most cheerful: I've always associated the music with Dylan's recovery from his famous motorcycle crash. The first four chords of the title track are all E minor, just Bob hitting the guitar, one, two, three, four, one chord for every beat. There's something both tentative and assertive about his playing, like he's figuring out his instrument after a time away and taking it out for a first dance. Then the music moves, skips on the half beat to A major. It's wake-up time. The band cuts in. Dylan begins his cockadoodledoo.

"Can't you hear that—rooster crowing?" he sings. He says that he's happy to be alive, and that's how I felt, though I wasn't under Dylan's "sky of blue." I was still there, under the ICU's fluorescents.

30.

"THERE ARE NO more egotistical and more competitive people than surgeons," Charles Bailey once said.

In 1945 and 1946, before the heart-lung machine, Bailey raced the great Dwight Harken to be the first to perform a curative heart surgery in a hospital.

"There is an old saying in India that you never find two tigers on the same hill," said Bailey. "What they really mean is you don't find two *male* tigers on the same hill." That's how he saw it: he and Harken against each other, playing king of the mountain. Bailey—less accomplished, less esteemed, but more aggressive than Harken—did all he could to win.

In the 1940s, before the widespread availability of penicillin, the most common cardiac complaint was rheumatic heart disease. Untreated streptococcus infections spread to the heart and left the valves scarred and stenotic. Bailey believed that, following the procedures Harken had pioneered in the Quonset huts in Cirencester, he could unclog the stuck valves.

Bailey was a small man, irascible, and prematurely bald. He had grown up in New Jersey. His father had been a banker but had lost his job when Charles was young, and the family struggled financially. "He died when I was only twelve," Bailey remembered, "and when I saw him coughing up blood into a basin as my mother tried to soothe him, I just stared at this awful exhibition of how mitral stenosis could terminate a young man's life. He was only forty-two." Bailey was driven to cure the disease that had killed his father.

His mother was a domineering figure, and she had decided early on that her son would be a doctor. "My mother had made up my mind for me before I was five, maybe before I was three." She had wanted him to go into oncology, but the shock of his father's death stuck with him, and Charles became interested in cardiology instead. He saw this as a rebellion against maternal influence. "At that very moment [his father's death] I changed my direction, and [she] was never able to persuade me otherwise."

Bailey went to Rutgers Medical School. "I didn't come from any of the schools that are supposed to produce great people," he said. "Partly because I didn't have enough money to go to these schools. I was a bright boy; I probably could have made Harvard or Johns Hopkins if I had tried, but I would not have been able to pay the tuition." He'd worked his way through college selling ladies' underwear, and he felt that contributed to his skill as a surgeon. "Early on," he said, he was "impressed by the similarity of the mitral valve structure to the old-fashioned feminine girdle." Bailey was famous for his clever hands and cold focus in the operating room.

His plan was straightforward: He would make a circle of purse-string sutures like the ones Harken had made in Cirencester. He wasn't going to pull out a piece of shrapnel from the middle of that circle. Instead he'd punch his finger into the heart and poke the stiff valve open. Then he would pull his finger out—Harken's champagne pop—and pull the circle of sutures shut. Using the same kind of big needles swedged in silk that Harken had used, Bailey would suture up his incision.

He practiced his technique on dogs, and then in November 1945, Bailey opened the chest of Walter Stockman, a thirty-seven-year-old man dying of mitral stenosis. Bailey cut between the third and fourth ribs. He used a rib spreader. Then he cut through the pericardium and achieved a view of the left atrium of the beating heart, right above the closed mitral valve.

He put in a circle of sutures just like Harken's. He cut a hole in the center of the circle. A fountain of blood shot upward. Bailey shoved his index finger into the hole while simultaneously pulling closed the purse strings. Instead of closing up the hole, the threads tore through the muscle, shredding it. "Severe bleeding occurred and a large metal clamp was hastily applied," Bailey wrote in his notes. But the clamp also perforated the muscle, ruining the fabric of the heart. "Massive uncontrollable hemorrhage resulted in immediate fatality."

Bailey was not discouraged. His next patient, six months later, was Wilma Stevens, a twenty-nine-year-old mother of two, dying of heart failure on account of her closed mitral valve. She had fluid in her lungs and difficulty breathing, a puffy abdomen, a swollen, tender liver, and tiny spindly limbs.

Again, Bailey spread her ribs. Again, he cut through the pericardium and made his circle of stitches on her left atrium. On his finger this time, he wore a narrow metal probe shaped like a tube. He pushed the metal probe into the scarred heart valve. The patient turned blue. Bailey had plugged her heart entirely. He used his finger and ripped at her valve. He pulled the finger out, pulled the purse strings shut, and sutured the exterior of her heart. Problem was, he had eliminated Wilma Stevens's mitral valve altogether. With each heartbeat, blood flowed backward into her lungs. She died two days later, and that was when Bailey got his nickname, "Butcher."

Up in Boston, Harken was proceeding with similar operations and was also losing patients. But Harken was a war hero and a successful surgical pioneer. Hahnemann Hospital, where Bailey worked in Philadelphia, lacked Harvard's resources. Bailey's chief, Dr. George Goekler, summoned him to his office and delivered a long lecture. He gave Bailey a piece of paper on which he had typed out and explained the Hippocratic oath.

"[Goekler] ended up telling me that it was his Christian duty to keep me from doing any more of these operations," said Bailey. "I responded with some heat. I told him that I believed in this operation, that I believed I was right . . . and that it was *my* Christian duty to continue."

When Goekler revoked Bailey's operating privileges at Hahnemann, Bailey scheduled another mitral valve surgery, this time at Wilmington Memorial Hospital in Delaware. He drove there to operate. This time the patient was a thirty-eight-year-old man, William Wilson. Bailey got him into the OR, opened his chest, cut into his heart—laying out the circle of sutures first—then pushed into the valve. Again, his metal tubular device got stuck in there. Again, he was forced to rip the device out, tearing the valve with his finger. Once again, he was able to sew up the heart. But again, he left his patient without a mitral valve. William Wilson lived on for five days after the operation. Wilmington Memorial, too, revoked Bailey's right to perform surgery.

He now had operating privileges in only two hospitals in Philadelphia. He was afraid that if he failed at either place, he'd lose the right to operate at both. But instead of giving up, Bailey decided to schedule two operations in one day, one in the morning, one in the afternoon. If he killed his first patient, he could hurry across town and still have the chance to operate on the second.

At 8 a.m. at Philadelphia General, Bailey operated on thirty-year-old Jerome Randall. As soon as Bailey opened his chest, Randall went into arrhythmia and cardiac arrest. Bailey took the heart into his hands and massaged it back into beating. Randall's personal doctor was there in the room and wanted Bailey to continue. Bailey didn't want to; he didn't want another death on his hands. He said he'd only go forward if Randall were first declared dead, and Randall's doctor complied.

Bailey sewed his circle of purse string sutures into the heart. He made an incision in the atrium. He plunged his finger through the clogged mitral valve, opening it. He pulled the purse strings shut and sutured the incision. Minutes later, Randall's heart stopped beating. Bailey took off his scrubs, washed up, put on his sports jacket, got in his car, and drove across Philadelphia to Episcopal Hospital, where he had another appointment to perform the same surgery. He knew he was getting closer, getting better, that despite his failures, his technique could save lives.

"Obviously, I felt there were irrelevant reasons for the loss of the first four patients and that the principle was entirely sound and could be developed but just needed further effort," he said. He parked his car at Episcopal Hospital. He entered the building. He changed into scrubs and met with his team. "The poignancy is so great that I can't really express it," he said in an interview later. "You know that almost all the world is against it; you know that you have a great personal stake and might even lose your medical license. . . . In fact, the thought crosses your mind that maybe you really *are* crazy."

Harken in Boston had by this time killed six patients. Twenty-four-year-old Constance Warner lay anesthetized on the table before Bailey. He made his incision, used his rib spreader, and entered the chest. He put in his sutures; he cut into the heart. On his finger Bailey had a new instrument, a fine cutting blade, designed to separate the valve's leaflets one from the other. He made his incision in the stenotic valve. He removed the cutting tool from his hand, put his finger back in the hole, and widened the space between the leaflets. By touch in the dark chambers of the heart, Bailey separated the leaflets of the valve. He pulled his finger out and pulled the circular suture shut. He sewed up the incision. He repaired the pericardium and closed the chest. Constance Warner recovered.

By the third day after her operation, she was up and walking from her hospital bed to the bathroom, down the hall, and around the ward. She was still in the hospital when the news came in from Boston—Harken too had a patient who had survived. Bailey was nervous. Would Harken claim the prize and be known as the first? The American College of Chest Physicians was having its annual meeting 1,000 miles away in Chicago.

Bailey bundled up Constance Warner, put her on a train, and rode with her to the convention. And there, before a conference of his peers, he presented her, the first patient to survive heart valve surgery.

In Minneapolis, Walt Lillehei was beginning his residency. Ligation of patent ductuses had become the norm. Blalock shunts were being put in all over the country. At Bellevue in New York and at Johns Hopkins in Baltimore, Janet Baldwin and Richard Bing were using cardiac catheters and achieving precise images of the holes in children's hearts. Doctors knew that if they could get into the heart, they could sew these atrial and ventricular defects shut, but it was at the time impossible to enter the heart without killing the patient. If you stopped the heart for four minutes, the patient suffered brain damage. If you stopped the heart for six and a half minutes, the patient died.

Robert Gross in Boston invented a way to conduct cardiac surgery while the heart kept on beating. He called his invention the "atrial well." Gross sewed a plastic funnel into the wall of the atrium of the beating heart of a child. The funnel diverted and controlled the heart's bleeding. Gross used clamps to hold his thread and needle, and he dipped these into the pool of blood in the funnel and down into the heart of the child. Dr. Abraham Rudolph was in the OR, a junior member of the surgery team, the first time Gross attempted the technique, and Rudolph watched in horror as Gross, serenely confident, sewed shut not the atrial septal defect but the child's mitral valve. The atrial well seemed unlikely to yield repeatable success. "Surgical procedures carried out under direct vision," said Walt Lillehei dryly, "are far more likely to be satisfactory than those carried out blindly."

Another way to approach the heart was through induced hypothermia. By cooling their patients, doctors could slow blood movement and give themselves a few more minutes to work inside the heart. During World War II, German and Japanese doctors had experimented on prisoners to determine the effects of extreme cold and had studied the way hypothermia affects the body and the heart. In northern Manchuria, in the small town of Pingfan, Dr. Shirō Ishii had conducted quasi-scientific experiments on prisoners of war whom he called *marutas*, or "logs." (He called them that because his lab, Unit 731, was disguised as a lumber mill.) Ishii electrocuted, vivisected, poisoned, and shot his subjects, seeking to determine the limits of human endurance. He froze his *marutas* to discover the lowest temperature to which a living body could be safely reduced. These tortures were echoed by those conducted by Dr. Claus Schilling at the Dachau concentration camp.

Reverend Leo Miechalowski, a Roman Catholic priest, was a subject of these Nazi experiments and at Nuremberg testified to their brutality. Starving on a work crew at the concentration camp, Father Miechalowski kept fainting and falling down, so in 1942 he volunteered for a new assignment, hoping he would get some bread to eat. Instead, he was brought to the hospital for his new "job," where he was poisoned with malaria. After the Nazis had gotten him sick, nurses gave Father Miechalowski further injections. Some caused headaches; some caused renal pain; some left him unable to speak.

Eventually, the priest was moved to the so-called aviation lab, where he was dressed in an aviator's uniform and fur-lined boots and then submerged in icy water. Wires attached to his back and up his rectum measured his internal and external temperatures. Miechalowski pleaded that he was freezing. The Germans laughed. "Well, this will only last a short time." Periodically, samples of his blood were taken from his ears. His body temperature dropped from 99.7 to 86 degrees Fahrenheit. Finally, Miechalowski passed out. The findings of the torturers' experiments crossed the Atlantic to America.

Dr. Alfred Bigelow, a Canadian surgeon who worked under Alfred Blalock in Baltimore in 1946 and 1947, became interested in the possibilities of hypothermia in the cardiac operating room. Bigelow's inspiration came not from Nazi torture but from observation of small animals. He had grown up in Alberta, where hibernating groundhogs slept in their burrows in the winter, their bodies almost as cold as their frozen nests. Bigelow wondered if one could chill a person similarly and then bring that person back to life. In 1948 and 1949, he tested his theory, operating on 120 dogs. So long as he kept their body temperatures above sixty-eight degrees Fahrenheit, the dogs survived operations to their hearts,

with their brains seemingly undamaged. Bigelow presented his results at a conference in 1950, but the world of cardiology was not
convinced. He never got a patient to undergo his surgery; he got
no volunteers and no referrals.

Charles Bailey, back in Hahnemann in Philadelphia, picked up
on Bigelow's ideas. He purchased a six-foot-long freezer to cool
the dogs in—but the freezer didn't work, or worked too well: it
froze the animals solid as blocks of ice. So Bailey used rubberized
cooling blankets that had been designed by psychiatrists for treating schizophrenics. This seemed to work well enough on dogs to
convince Bailey that Bigelow was right: hypothermia would nearly
double a patient's window of survival, to twelve minutes. Ever re-
sourceful, Bailey found a patient on whom to run his experiment,
a twenty-seven-year-old woman with an atrial septal defect, a hole
between the top chambers of her heart. In August 1952, he rolled
her into the OR. He used his frozen rubber psychiatry blankets
to cool her body. He clamped off her heart. He worked fast—he
cut into her atria, sewed up the hole, and closed the heart, all in
six minutes. But when Bailey unclamped her heart, the patient
went into ventricular fibrillation: her heart started beating uselessly
at more than two hundred beats per minute. Her great arteries
went translucent. He'd let air into her heart accidentally. She died.
Meanwhile, work continued on the heart-lung machine dreamed
up by Alexis Carrel and Charles Lindbergh.

In 1931, while Lindbergh and Carrel were working together
at Rockefeller, Dr. John Gibbon was in training at Massachusetts
General Hospital. As a young doctor, he stayed up all night watching a middle-aged woman die of pulmonary embolism. Just after
dawn, Gibbon's supervisors attempted surgery. They clamped off
the coronary artery, knowing that they had to complete the procedure in less than four minutes. But it took them seven minutes
to get into the lung and get the blood clot out. When the clamps
were released, the patient was dead. Gibbon was crushed. It came
to him with the force of revelation: he would build a heart-lung
machine. For decades after, he devoted himself to this single project, to extend the amount of time surgeons had to operate. Initially,

his work was driven more by the thought of lung surgery, surgery for pulmonary embolism, than for surgery on the heart.

He worked on his heart-lung machine for five years at Mass General. Gibbon married Mary Hopkinson, also a medical student at Harvard, and Mary and John continued their work together at the University of Pennsylvania. In 1941, the Gibbons had built a prototype bypass machine that could keep a cat alive for twenty-six minutes. But their work was interrupted. John was called away to war. He served his tour on a remote South Pacific island.

When Gibbon returned from war, he got back to work in Philadelphia. Mary and John were joined by Thomas Watson of IBM. They weren't the only ones trying to design a heart-lung machine. In Detroit, Dr. F. Dewey Dodrill was collaborating with General Motors on a similar project. In Toronto, Dr. William Mustard was working on his organic heart-lung machines: those blanched monkey lungs hung in big sealed jars. In 1945, after the war, Clarence Dennis, one of Owen Wagensteen's protégés, visited the Gibbons in Philadelphia, and John Gibbon was kind to Dennis and shared his plans for the machine. Even as Walt Lillehei was returning from Italy, Clarence Dennis, on the University of Minnesota campus, was working on a heart-lung machine.

By 1950, Lillehei was Owen Wagensteen's chief resident and rising star, handsome, charismatic, brilliant, and adventurous. The building of Variety Club Heart Hospital was near completion. The work toward open-heart surgery seemed about to begin in earnest, and Lillehei was in the thick of the research. But his colleagues noticed something worrisome—Walt had grown a lump on his neck. Wagensteen had the lump biopsied. It was cancerous, a lymphosarcoma. In 1950, the cure rate for this cancer was 25 percent at five years and less than that at ten. Wagensteen decided to operate.

———

One time, after throwing away the legs of a patient on whom he'd performed a hemicorporectomy, Wagensteen received an anonymous letter: "Now that you've done that," it said, "why don't you cut off your own head?" Some of his residents liked to say,

"Wagensteen hates cancer because it kills more patients than he does."

Walt Lillehei went under Wagensteen's knife. John Lewis, Lillehei's best friend at the hospital, assisted in the surgery. At 7:15 a.m. on June 1, 1950, Lillehei was anesthetized. Wagensteen's team began by working at the throat. David State, who had performed the initial exploratory surgery, cut out the remainder of Lillehei's parotid gland. When that was done, a second surgeon scrubbed in. Richard Varco attacked the rest of Lillehei's neck, taking out all the lymph nodes and glands. It was 11:15 a.m. Four hours had passed. Wagensteen noted that some of the glands by Lillehei's jugular vein were enlarged. The surgeons conferred.

Wagensteen scrubbed in. He split Lillehei's sternum. He went into the chest cavity. He removed lymph nodes, glands, muscle, fat, an entire rib, and Lillehei's thymus. The patient bled profusely. It was 6 p.m. when they sewed him up again. The operation lasted ten hours and thirty-five minutes. Lillehei had needed more than two gallons of blood. When he awakened from anesthesia, Walt was surprised. He had not expected Wagensteen to crack open his chest. He had not agreed to it. After two weeks in the hospital, he went home to his wife, Kaye. The chest wound became infected. When Richard Varco came by to clean it, Walt mixed them both martinis.

More complications: Lillehei's stomach dilated, which meant a trip to the emergency room and another hospitalization. He underwent twelve sessions of radiation treatment on his face. These left him nauseated. He feared he'd go blind. Wagensteen proposed a second surgery, to look around inside and see if there was anything else to take out. Lillehei declined. He was depressed, his body ruined, and his survival uncertain. The odds were good that cancer would come back and kill him.

31.

EVERYONE WAS TELLING me that I was doing great. Mike Freed said, "You look like an advertisement for heart surgery." I was moved from the ICU to a more ordinary hospital room, a private room, which in retrospect I suppose my father had paid for.

An intern came by and said, "I hope I look as good after my heart surgery."

He was young, fit, and Australian, and I couldn't believe that he too was about to have an operation like mine. His father and his grandfather, he explained, had had heart troubles. When he got old, he was most certainly going to need open-heart surgery.

"Dr. Freed maybe let you go longer than you should have," he told me—the first person to say anything like that, that I had waited too long to have heart surgery—but he said that everything was looking good.

The crisis had passed. The new pulmonary valve had stopped the backward flow of blood. The hope was that my swollen ventricle would strengthen and shrink, but that was far from a certainty. No one knew how long the new valve would last. Five years? Ten years? Twenty? The only certainty was that in time it would fail and need to be replaced and that another heart surgery lay in my future.

My dad bought me three plaid shirts. I put one on instead of the hospital gown. I didn't look entirely like myself, but I didn't look like a heart patient either. My old uncle, a distracted mathematical genius, a man I've loved since childhood but who is by nature quite difficult to reach, came creeping down the hall and knocked, a surprise visit. I think he'd expected a dead man and was delighted to find me, and I was delighted to find him, too, smelling of cigarettes and citing Karl Marx. The human world was expanding again for me.

"Take it slowly," said Dr. Freed.

I took a shower. I stood under the water, and for the first time since surgery, my body actually felt pleasure. My skin, used to alcohol wipes, delighted in the prickling warm water. It was so good to be standing—I felt like *me*. I felt strong, and I wanted to wash it all off—not just the dressings but the whole experience.

I toweled myself dry, and there was another one of my dad's shirts. He'd brought the thickest possible flannel, as if, through the volume of fabric, he could express his love. I put it on. I looked in the mirror. Was that me? Then my heart started beating, a frantic, bass-drum beat. I didn't know what to do.

I lay back on the hospital bed. This is okay, I told myself. I am okay.

The beating resolved itself, and my heart felt normal, and I was faced with a question. Should I tell the doctor what had just happened?

I guess I could castigate myself. I could say that my behavior was thoughtless and reflexive: that I was doing what I always do, pretending to be healthy when I'm not. On the other hand, I could claim it was calculated: I wanted to get out of the hospital, I wanted to go home, and I didn't want to undergo any more tests.

But maybe the truth is that the moment when I started pretending that I was okay was the moment that I really became healthy. Maybe that's what *healthy* is, an act we put on when we pretend that we're not dying.

32.

OWEN WAGENSTEEN MADE sure that Walt Lillehei received his salary during his period of convalescence, and in the autumn of 1950, Lillehei went back to work, no longer the easygoing mischievous young man. He had seen war, and he'd been cut open. He was likely to die soon, and after surgery, his head didn't balance right on his scarred and skinny neck.

Now there was a prototype heart-lung machine in the University of Minnesota Hospital, the one Clarence Dennis had built based on John Gibbon's designs. The machine was six feet long and three feet high and had a glass tower arising from its chrome and stainless steel base. Surgery with this device required sixteen professionals: two lead surgeons, two assistant surgeons, two anesthesiologists, two nurses, two technicians, a person in charge of transfusion, someone in charge of blood samples, and four people tending to the machine. Endless moving parts had to be monitored: there were pumps, valves, switches, motors, a flow meter, a magnetized coil of wire, a series of rotating plates, and a reservoir for deoxygenated blood.

In 1951, the team at the University of Minnesota Hospital gave the machine a try. Richard Varco, who had cut the nodes out of Walt Lillehei's throat, was the chief surgeon. Lillehei observed. The patient was Patty Anderson, not yet six years old. She had been hospitalized three times in her short life. She was cross-eyed and weak and had been diagnosed with an atrial septal defect (ASD), a hole between the top chambers of her heart.

The doctors anesthetized Patty at 8 a.m. in surgery's Room II at Variety Club Heart Hospital, a small space with steam radiators, green walls, white tile floors, and windows that the doctors opened on hot days for ventilation. It took Varco four hours to get down to the little girl's heart, which was massively enlarged and beating irregularly. Just past noon, they began to connect Patty to the pump. The process took over an hour, with sixteen people in the operating room making sure all was in place. At 1:22 p.m., Varco gave the order.

"Pump on." And she was on bypass, her heart and lungs being circumvented and her blood being oxygenated by a machine.

He made his incision. The heart bled. The suction was inadequate. The pump was working, but there was so much blood, the surgeons could hardly see. Varco felt around the interior of the heart with his fingers. There were holes in the top and the bottom chambers. The valves were deformed. The diagnosis had been incorrect. Varco sutured shut what he could—eleven stitches closed the worst hole—and then sewed shut the sick heart with its malformed valves. At 2:02 p.m., after forty minutes of surgery, Patty was taken off the machine. At 2:45 p.m. she was pronounced dead.

Elsewhere in the country, surgeons met with similar challenges. In Philadelphia, John Gibbon lost his first bypass patient in the same way Varco had lost his: the pump worked, but the diagnosis was incorrect, and the child died soon after surgery. In May 1953, Gibbon tried again. His patient, Martha Crowley, was an eighteen-year-old freshman at Wilkes-Barre College who had been suffering her whole life with an ASD. When Gibbon sectioned her sternum, connected her to his oxygenator, and opened her heart, he found no surprises, just a hole between the atria about the size of a half dollar. Gibbon kept Martha Crowley on the heart-lung machine for twenty-six minutes as he sewed up the ASD. Satisfied with the closure, he disconnected her from the machine and put her chest back together. Martha Crowley woke up feeling fine. She was cured.

John Gibbon had spent two decades building his heart-lung machine, and he was the first doctor ever to perform a successful bypass surgery. But Gibbon was a quiet man and not inclined to draw attention to himself. It took him a year to publish the results of his successful operation, and when he did so, he put the paper in a tiny journal, *Minnesota Medicine*, where very few of his colleagues would read it. He never announced his success at a medical conference. He operated on two more patients. Both of them died. After those two deaths, he seemed to lose interest. Gibbon never again used his heart-lung machine. As a friend of his observed, "The others were taking the risk and killing babies, and he didn't like that."

To be crowned the king of heart surgery, you had to be more than just inventive and successful. You had to be comfortable playing with life and death. You had to be a daredevil and a showman. Walt Lillehei's head didn't balance right on his neck, but otherwise he was strong. He was ready. He was going to make his bid for the crown.

33.

WE WERE A crowd on the plane from Boston to New York when I was released. Marcia, Eliza, I, my parents. And our friend Hannah, who, along with my sister-in-law Sharon, had come all that way to support Marcia. I was in a wheelchair. On the way to board the plane, there was a little lip in the floor where the mouth of the tunnel met the door of the plane. The flight attendant asked if I could stand, and I almost laughed. Of course, I could stand. Who did she think I was? I didn't really *need* a wheelchair!

I walked down the aisle to my seat, and Hannah said something—I cannot remember her words exactly—about my being not exactly ill. This confused me. I was not *ill*. I had just had heart surgery, that was all. Otherwise I was fine. It wasn't really that big a deal!

Back in Brooklyn, with my clothes on, I looked like a perfectly ordinary citizen, maybe a little stiff, like I'd hurt my back or something. In the mirror in the morning, my chest was different. The hair was all gone, and so was the scar I'd had since I was five. It had been excised. In its place was a thin line that had already superficially healed. It looked like a tracing with a stylus, and that made my shaved chest look like it was made of clay.

I wasn't allowed to pick up a gallon of milk or a pot of boiling pasta on account of the fragility of my still-knitting chest bone. I wasn't allowed to pick up my daughter, which frustrated little Eliza and frustrated me too.

I refused to go back to Dr. Rosenbaum. His diagnosis had proved correct, even prescient. He had saved my life. He was the doctor who had grasped the situation most quickly. But despite that— because of that?—in my head he had transformed into some kind of hobgoblin. All my rage and fear, all my fury about my own weakness and vulnerability, had been transferred over to this doctor who had intervened and told me the truth about my condition and what I had to do about it. He had gone as far toward saving my life as I'd allowed him to, and I could not forgive him for it. I went for my postsurgical checkup to an internist, an old man who was a friend of the family and wished I would see a real specialist in congenital heart disease but agreed to look at me.

I took a cab up to his office on East 39th Street. I got there early and walked around in the January sun. It was my first time out alone in the city after heart surgery, and I felt scared and unsteady. I didn't know if I was feeling okay. But I thought I was feeling okay. I kept checking my pulse, checking my balance. Was I lightheaded? Lethargic? Was that normal after heart surgery?

Dr. Nachtigall's old EKG machine was built into his wall. Its wires attached to the skin with old-fashioned suction cups. It took him a very long time to read the results. He made phone calls to Boston. I was in heart flutter, he said. My atria were beating too rapidly. I needed to go to a cardiologist and have it checked out. So I got on a plane the next day and went back to Boston, where they cardioverted me, which is to say, they put a kind of camera down my throat (that hurt), knocked me out for a minute, and then shocked my heart so it skipped back into its normal rhythm. Then I booked a plane back to New York City.

"This is stupid," said Dr. Freed, about as gently as a person could say such a sentence. But still I didn't go back to Dr. Rosenbaum. I *really* didn't want to see him. My anxiety was all out of proportion with what had actually taken place. Why? All you armchair psychologists in the audience, sing it with me: facing Marlon Rosenbaum meant facing my mortality.

One advantage of having my cardiologist in Boston was that it located all my troubles, psychologically, two hundred miles away.

In New York City, I wasn't a heart patient anymore. But my denial came with its inevitable backlash: I kept wondering if I was in heart flutter. I kept pressing my fingers to my jugular vein, shutting my eyes, trying to figure out if my heart was in a normal rhythm. When I had been in heart flutter, I had thought everything was fine. Now that my heart was beating normally, I worried that it fluttered.

Marcia went back to work before I did. My mom hung out in the apartment with me and baby Eliza. The whole ordeal of my heart surgery was as psychologically painful for my mother as it was for me—maybe more so. She was both anxious and exultant to see me well. She lit a tuna melt on fire in the toaster oven. I grabbed a box of salt and dumped it on the flames. What made her feel terrible made me feel good. Putting out a fire, I was a little bit less of an invalid.

My mom was there when the literary magazines started calling. People wanted to print the stories I'd sent out in the fall. This was new, and this was fun, and my mother was tickled to play my secretary when the *Northwest Review* or the *Hawai'i Review* called. These were journals with tiny circulations—Was that the right word? Did they have "circulations" or just print a bunch of copies?—but it felt nice. My sternum knit itself back together. I was allowed to lift packages again. I went on the happiest grocery shopping trip of my life, delighting in lifting things off the shelf, putting things in the cart. Picking up two bags and carrying them home to the apartment. Holding my daughter in my arms. She ran to me. Up, up, up! I put her down, and she wanted me to pick her up again. Marcia and I were very ginger rekindling romance. There were weird tricks and hitches in my chest, like someone was plucking guitar strings in there. I called Michael Freed about it, and he said the symptoms I described didn't sound like a real worry. So much had been cut and sewn and moved around in there, it could be anything.

Still wondering if I was in heart flutter, I went for a run. I think it was my second or third time jogging after surgery, a rainy April day. I didn't go very far. Maybe a slow, gentle mile, maybe less.

My heartbeat accelerated, and that felt good. But then, when I stopped running, my heart didn't slow. I walked back toward our building in the drizzle. I rested, but the fast heartbeat didn't stop. I went up the stairs—we lived on the third floor of a row house—and I paused at each landing. But my heart was still going like I was running.

I came home. Marcia said, "Lie down for a minute." I did and the heartbeat normalized, but when I stood to get a glass of water, my heart sped up again. I lay down again. It slowed. Marcia made me call Dr. Freed. He took my call. He went through it all with me very carefully, the jog, the heart rate, and how I felt. Any dizziness? How long had it taken to resolve itself? How was I feeling now?

He paused and mulled it over. "If it happens again, call me."

It did happen again, toward the end of summer. I was in the hall of our building, looking down the central stairs. I had Eliza in my arms. On the floor below was our neighbor's babysitter, and she was talking to me, innocuously, about the babies growing and about the weather.

I was smiling and pretending to enjoy our conversation, but really I wanted to get back into our home. She talked to me about the little toy poodle she took care of along with the little girl and how the poodle thought that it was her main job, as if it were the baby and the baby were the dog. As she chattered, my heart started going BANG BANG BANG BANG BANG.

I said, "All right," hoping it meant, simultaneously, "Enough of this" and "Good-bye," but the woman downstairs wanted to tell me more about the toy poodle's eating habits and how the little poodle liked to play.

Eliza was fussing. My heart kept going BANG BANG BANG BANG BANG BANG. I said, "Got to go!" I went into the apartment, put Eliza down, and lay on the couch and waited for the banging to pass. When it did, I reached toward the phone, but I didn't pick it up or dial. I knew I was supposed to call Dr. Freed. But I didn't.

Instead, I read to Eliza, *Where the Wild Things Are*. In Max's room, a forest grew.

34.

ROBERT GROSS HAD some success with the atrial well. Doctors were also able to repair some atrial septal defects with hypothermia alone. But to get deeper into the heart, they needed to perform bypass surgery—to oxygenate the blood with a machine while they operated on the heart.

Between 1951 and 1955, by Walt Lillehei's count, there had been eighteen attempts at cardiac bypass surgery at four different hospital centers. Only one patient had survived, John Gibbon's. The mechanical oxygenators, to Lillehei's mind, had too many moving parts, too many possibilities for disaster. He thought about babies in the womb, the way a fetus survived when dependent on its mother's cardiovascular system. He wondered, What if another person took the place of the heart-lung machine? What if the blood of the child went into its mother to be oxygenated, and then the mother's oxygenated blood went back into the child as it lay upon the operating table? Could a child survive surgery dependent on a parent's body? Lillehei called his idea "cross-circulation."

Before approaching a human subject, he tried his technique out on dogs in the lab. His machinery was store-bought: beer-keg tubing and a $500 dairy pump called a Sigmamotor T-6S that could move multiple streams of liquid in several directions. Lillehei anesthetized two animals and laid them out on separate tables. Then he connected the donor dog's femoral arteries and veins to the subject dog's aorta and vena cava. He tied off the subject dog's heart. He operated. During the surgery, one heart beat for two animals.

With cross-circulation, Lillehei was able to perform bypass operations inside his dog subjects' hearts. The results were consistent over months of experimentation, and he proposed using his new procedure on children.

Dr. Cecil Watson, chairman of the Department of Medicine at the University of Minnesota, was appalled. With two patients instead of one, the risks of infection were doubled, as were the risks of brain damage. There were so many possible complications: The difference in size between the two bodies raised all kinds of questions of blood-flow rates and quantities of anesthetic. What would knock out the parent would kill the child. They could both die. "A two-hundred percent mortality rate!" said Watson.

Lillehei had studied his animals thoroughly, during and after cross-circulation, then had euthanized them and autopsied the bodies. His team had checked for changes in the dogs' carbon dioxide and hemoglobin levels, blood pressure, and pulse. Postoperatively, they'd microscopically studied samples of the animals' livers, kidneys, hearts, lungs, and brains. The results were overwhelming. Cross-circulation, if carried out correctly, would do no damage at all to either parent or child. Owen Wagensteen looked over the data and supported Lillehei in his fight against Watson.

The first patient was a one-year-old boy, Gregory Gliddens, the eleventh child of Lyman and Frances Gliddens from Hibbing, Minnesota. Lyman worked in the Masabi Range iron mines. The Gliddens had lost a previous child to congenital heart disease, and Lyman was willing to serve as his tiny son's artificial heart.

The surgery was slated for March 26, 1954. Lillehei's first case of the day was a routine hernia operation. Then he turned his attention to cross-circulation. Two beds were squeezed into Room II of the Variety Club Heart Hospital, the room in which Richard Varco had tried to perform his bypass surgery. The anesthesiologist used cyclopropane, the same explosive gas Robert Gross and Betty Lank had used in Boston in 1938. A mask attached to a black bag was put over Gregory's mouth, and then the doctor squeezed the bag, measuring out the dose. Lillehei sectioned the boy's chest, and when the doctors had a clear view of the heart, the boy's father,

Lyman Gliddens, wobbly with drugs, groin shaved, was brought into the operating room.

The doctors put Lyman under. They didn't want him moving or panicking during the surgery. Lillehei attached canulae to the major arteries and veins in Lyman Gliddens's groin. Then he attached them to his clean beer-keg tubing. Similar tubes connected to the dairy pump, and these went into little Gregory's heart.

"Pump on," said Lillehei.

The Sigmamotor T-6S began to churn. The rate of flow had to be carefully calibrated. Too slow, and Gregory would die. Too fast, and the blood would flood Gregory's tissue.

Lillehei found the ASD and sewed it up. He made sure there were no leaks and no other holes. He removed Lyman and Gregory from the pump and closed the chest cavity. Everything seemed perfect until little Gregory, in the recovery ward, developed an infection in his chest. No doses of antibiotics, no suctioning of the lungs, no massaging of the heart seemed enough to save the child. Days after surgery, Gregory died.

Lillehei was undaunted. He was sure that cross-circulation worked, and he found another patient: Pamela Schmidt, a four-year-old with a ventricular septal defect (VSD), a hole between the big bottom chambers of the heart. Pamela was sickly, weak, short of breath, and coughing up blood. On account of the hole in her septum, she had suffered chronic infections and been hospitalized four times for pneumonia.

The operation was scheduled, but then delayed when Pamela suffered yet another attack of pneumonia. There were other difficulties. Pamela's mother's blood type did not match the girl's. And Pamela's father, a factory worker, had too low a hemoglobin count. He was anemic. The hospital's hematologists recommended against his being used as a blood donor. The Schmidts were anxious; they knew about Gregory Gliddens's death. But Lillehei promised them that his was the only way that their daughter would survive.

Walt drove a big, shiny Buick convertible. He wore gold jewelry. He cruised the pretty nurses. He had seen martial slaughter in Italy. He had been eviscerated on the operating table and had come back to life. He was on a mission. He was not going to be put off by a hospital administrator, a case of pneumonia, or a previous failure. When Pamela Schmidt recovered from her lung infection, the operation was scheduled to proceed, and Pamela's father, Ronald Schmidt, was to act as donor. He was five times the size of his little girl.

Again, two beds were set up in Room II. Again, the patient's chest was sectioned, and the father was anesthetized. The doctors used the same dairy pump and fresh beer-keg tubing. Lillehei wore no surgical magnification glasses (those hadn't been invented yet), and he borrowed a headlamp from an otolaryngologist.

With a stiletto-bladed knife, he punctured the patients' arteries. Soon two sets of tubing ran between the beds. Little Pamela's blood ran from her vena cava into the Sigmamotor T-6S and then through a transparent tube into her father's leg. Blood from her father's lungs ran through the pump and right into Pamela's aorta, into her brain.

Examining the trabeculated wall of little Pamela's septum, Lillehei found the VSD. He sutured and knotted and sewed the hole shut. There were no other leaks. All was going well, but when he began to close the incision he'd made into the ventricles, Pamela's heart slowed. The ventricles and atria beat out of time. The coordination of her heartbeat collapsed. Pamela's heart spasmed out of control, bloodless and sputtering. Then—ninety seconds after it had gone wrong—the heart righted itself and beat normally. The arrhythmia passed as mysteriously as it had appeared. Lillehei made the call.

"Release the tourniquets!"

Blood filled the little girl's heart. Pamela's heart kept a healthy rhythm. The father and daughter were disconnected from the tubes and the dairy pump. Everything was stable.

In 1954, professional ethics forbade physicians from advertising themselves to the public. Charles Bailey, when he took his patient on a long train ride to a medical conference in Chicago, had been showboating. John Gibbon, after his quiet victory, had been perhaps overly modest, but he was scrupulously correct.

Quiet and modest wasn't Walt Lillehei's style. The University of Minnesota's publicity team put together a four-page news release, complete with photos purporting to show Lillehei operating on Pamela. (In fact, the photos were staged, the doctors posing in an autopsy room.) Lillehei called a press conference in the theater of the Variety Club Heart Hospital. He took the stage, commanding and glamorous. He told the sad and difficult story of Pamela's life before surgery. He showed slides of the pictures from the press release. He showed diagrams of a heart with a VSD.

He discussed his dog-heart experiments. "We have long felt that there must be some simple way of working inside the heart. When elaborate machines designed as a substitute for the heart and lungs proved unsatisfactory we tried using the animal's own lungs and substituted the simple mechanical pump for the heart." He reviewed the failures of his peers and compared his technique to theirs. "Our method," he said, "is widely applicable by surgeons experienced in heart surgery."

The press release was distributed. Little Pamela Schmidt was pushed into the room by her beaming, crying parents. She had ribbons in her dress, big brown eyes, and freshly combed curls. The family posed for pictures with Lillehei. "She's a little fighter," Schmidt said of his daughter. "She'll never give up."

The news made the front page in Minneapolis and echoed all over the world. "Impossible Surgery Now Done" was the headline in the *New York Times*. London's *Daily Mirror* called it "an operation as extravagant and fantastic as any ever written in a shilling science 'thriller.'" The Minnesota chapter of the American Heart Association (AHA) named Pamela Schmidt "the Queen of Hearts" and in its publicity materials showed pictures of her riding on a tricycle. Senator Hubert Humphrey sent Pamela a birthday card.

During the spring and summer of 1954, Walt Lillehei was the only person in the world performing cardiac bypass surgery. Through the summer, his success rate was strong. Six out of eight patients survived the surgery and thrived. He was the most famous heart surgeon in America at the time, and desperate parents drove their children to Minneapolis, hoping he would save their kids. Money rolled in from private sources like the Variety Club, from public charities like the AHA, from the Minnesota state government through the university, and from the federal government, where Walt's new buddy Hubert Humphrey worked. Lillehei became more and more ambitious. In late August, he moved beyond ASDs and VSDs and attempted a full correction of a tetralogy of Fallot—the first attempt ever at a complex congenital heart defect.

The patient was Mike Shaw, a ten-year-old whose divorced mother worked in a Minnesota poultry-processing plant, cutting the wings and legs off chickens. Mike was so cyanotic that he could barely walk. His mother couldn't afford a car, and so she pulled her boy around in a red wagon. Doctors had scheduled Mike for a blue baby operation at University Hospital; they could safely put in a Blalock shunt and potentially give the boy new energy and years of life. But Lillehei intervened. He offered to cure the boy entirely, but he said it had to be one or the other: if they chose the blue baby operation, then, Lillehei said, he would not be able to justify signing the boy up for a cross-circulation.

Mrs. Shaw decided to go for the promised total cure.

Unfortunately, her blood type didn't match Mike's, and neither did Mike's father's. Mike was AB negative—only one in a hundred people would match him—but with the help of the hospital, the AHA, and the Blue Cross, Lillehei found a potential donor, Howard Holtz, a twenty-nine-year-old highway worker and father of three boys.

Lillehei told Holtz that the surgery was the only chance to save the boy's life. Holtz agreed to participate. "I just wanted to do what I hope someone would do if my child were a blue baby." And he lay down on the bed in the hospital room next to little Mike Shaw—Mike with his chest sawed open and Holtz drugged and stripped and shaved. The tubes were attached. The dairy pump started churning. "The following day," wrote Mrs. Shaw in her journal, "we noticed the color returning to [Mike's] lips and fingernails and ears. He was turning a nice rosy pink."

Lillehei scheduled a report of his success for December at the next gathering of the American College of Surgeons in Atlantic City. He was going to show that cross-circulation was a solution for even complex deformities. But then, Lillehei's luck turned. On September 7, just a week after the tetralogy of Fallot operation, he lost a patient. A seven-month-old girl died of heart block on his operating table. The following week, he lost another. Then another. Over a period of nine weeks, Lillehei performed eight operations, with six fatalities.

On October 5, he lost his first blood donor. Geraldine Thompson had taken her daughter to see heart specialists in Boston and Colorado and Texas before she settled on Lillehei. She'd met with Denton Cooley and Robert Gross. Her eight-year-old daughter Leslie had a VSD and had undergone any number of X-rays, catheterizations, and examinations. On October 5, 1954, Geraldine and Leslie were lying side by side in the operating room, connected to the Sigmamotor T-6S. Something went wrong. The anesthetist hadn't connected the pump and tube correctly. A technician noticed air bubbles heading into Geraldine Thompson's thigh. At the sight of the air bubbles, Lillehei cancelled the surgery, closed the patient's chest, and detached the mother from the device. But it was too late. Geraldine Thompson's heart was beating, but the air bubbles had met her brain, and she would never wake up again. Her mind was wiped clean and empty.

That December, Lillehei took the stage at Atlantic City to report his tetralogy of Fallot triumph. On stage, he was his usual charismatic, assured, and enthusiastic self. But the audience knew. Lillehei was heckled.

"Admit that you have a vegetable in the hospital!" someone screamed.

Helen Taussig, told that Lillehei had succeeded with a tetralogy patient, said, "Too bad, now, he'll continue."

Lillehei did continue. All his patients were not treated equally. Calvin Richmond was a black sharecropper's son in Little Rock, Arkansas, whose parents could not afford to send him to Minneapolis. A local charity drive run by newspaper and TV raised

$3,000 and sent him to Lillehei. The Arkansas Air Guard flew the thirteen-year-old boy to Minnesota. "I wonder if he recognizes what preparations have already been made for him ahead," wrote a reporter.

Unfortunately, Calvin's blood type didn't match his mother's, and no one else would act as a donor for the boy. The team at Minnesota looked to the local prison for volunteers, but no white person would allow their blood to mix with a black child's. No black donor seems to have been approached. As a result, Lillehei's team used a dog lung for Calvin—something closely resembling the apparatus William Mustard had set up with monkey lungs in Canada. The *Washington Post* trumpeted the news: "Heart Mended as Lung of Dog Aerates Blood." The boy survived. It was one of the last cross-circulation operations to get national attention.

———

John Kirklin wore his hair in an odd Caesar-style cut, with abrupt bangs high on his forehead. A tall, thin, pale man with a narrow face, large glasses, and a small, flat mouth, he was decorous and precise. At the Mayo Clinic, an hour-and-a-half drive from Minneapolis, he viewed what was happening at Variety Club Heart Hospital with some skepticism. Later he said, "I think the medical world . . . intuitively knew that the cross-circulation technique was not going to be widely accepted and/or used. Against that background there was no other alternative but to go with the heart-lung machine." Kirklin visited Philadelphia to see what Gibbon was doing. He went to Toronto to see Mustard. He visited Dewey Dodrill in Detroit. "Dewey Dodrill's machine was built for him by General Motors, and it looked like it—it looked like a car engine," Kirklin said. "Dr. Gibbon's machine had been built by IBM, and it looked like it—it looked like a computer." Kirklin built a machine of his own.

In March 1955, he began lining up patients. His first bypass surgery was successful. His second was not. Kirklin performed eight open-heart surgeries on patients with holes in their septa. He had a 50 percent mortality rate and published the results in the *Mayo*

Clinic Proceedings. Almost simultaneously, Lillehei's assistant, Richard DeWall, developed a simpler oxygenator.

The story, probably apocryphal, is that DeWall and Lillehei came up with the idea of a bubble oxygenator in a bar, looking down at a glass of beer. Why not just fill the blood with oxygen, DeWall asked, just aerate the blood with bubbles and then let the bubbles filter out? He built the device with the same Sigmamotor T-6S dairy pump plus some stuff he'd found in the lab and $15 of odds and ends: a cork, a coil of beer-keg tubing, some narrower tubing he scavenged from a mayonnaise factory, a reservoir, two needles, and two filters. The blood was filled with bubbles of oxygen, then sent through an antifoaming agent and down a long, helix-shaped coil of hose. The extraneous oxygen floated to the top, and the bubbles burst. The oxygenated blood then ran into a reservoir and then into a tube that went into the patient's aorta. The device, the DeWall Oxygenator, was a success, and by August 1955 Lillehei had stopped using cross-circulation entirely.

More and better machines came to market. In 1957, Denton Cooley finished his own prototype, a three-chambered device that looked like a percolator and was dubbed "Cooley's Coffee Pot." In the first four months after its completion, Cooley in Texas did thirty-nine bypass operations. By the end of the year, he and his Texas colleagues had performed 137 open-heart operations, the most anywhere in the country. That same year, Kirklin published his textbook, *Cardiac Surgery*. The age of heart surgery had begun.

35.

IT WAS SEPTEMBER 2000. George W. Bush had not yet been elected president. I was out in front of the library on the paved concrete campus of the State University of New York at Stony Brook. I was eating an ice cream sandwich. My friend Astrid sat with me, drinking a cup of tea. We were enjoying the sun.

I was a man returned from the dead. I was jogging a few times each week. I was practicing yoga. I told a joke that no one else thought was funny: I'm in training for my next open-heart surgery. (Rim shot. Silence.) Eliza had grown curly hair and chubby cheeks and walked around on little, spindly legs. My stories appeared in little magazines. Literary agents wrote me. I was putting together a manuscript. The value of our Brooklyn apartment tripled, and we were looking to sell. We were browsing houses a dozen blocks away, where the neighborhood got a little less ritzy. We decided to have a second child. I said to my friend Jeff on the phone, "If this is it, if there is no more success at all, I'm okay with it."

Astrid laughed. I checked my watch. The trains back to Brooklyn left every few hours. If I missed the 4:40, I wouldn't get home until nearly midnight. But we still had a few minutes. Astrid, a stylish and fit older woman with trim gray hair, started telling me about her daughter's life. Her family all seemed to me charmed and successful and brilliant and gorgeous, but she explained that her daughter's boyfriend had a grave health problem. She was describing this illness to me, and I was leaning in to listen, when all of a sudden I found that I couldn't follow her words at all.

Something in my body had shifted, like a reversal in the poles of my electricity. My skin buzzed. I was lightheaded. There was a strange ferrous taste in my mouth, like the charge of a small battery.

"What is it?" Astrid said.

"Nothing," I told her, but the change must have registered on my face.

I said, "Don't worry."

My heart was slamming against my ribs. I stood up, experimentally, to check my balance. Standing felt okay. I told Astrid what was happening. She told me to sit back down.

Astrid is a poet and a translator and a potter and a physical therapist, the wife of a prominent biologist, a mother of two young adults. She is a woman twenty years older than me, a woman to trust in a moment of crisis, but I dismissed her concerns. I checked the time. It was a long way from the library to the station. I had to catch my train. I said good-bye. I started on my way. She insisted on accompanying me.

We went down the stairs of the library, across one of the narrow roads that bisected the campus, and down a second narrow set of stairs toward the path that led to the playing fields and baseball diamonds. The kicker on the football team was practicing. Footballs spun end over end against the polarized sky, then down through the uprights. My heart was trying to break out of my chest.

I felt no pain, and I tried to deny my panic, but the symptoms of my arrhythmia were the same as the symptoms of panic: the heart racing, the lightheadedness, and the stupidity. As my heart went wild, my brain went white. Mind and body ran in opposite directions, leaving the rest of me in the existential lurch. It was like a twinge in the knee, I told myself. It would pass.

But it didn't pass. We got to the train platform, a piece of raised concrete by a two-lane blacktop in the part of Long Island where the air smells like the salty bay. There was a convenience store across the street and a pay phone by the little steps of the platform. Astrid urged me to sit, to rest, and not to board the train.

"Call Marcia," she said.

"Okay, okay," I said, as though she were the one acting hysterical.

With Astrid by my elbow and nervously watching, I picked up the pay phone, dialed home, and admitted to Marcia that my heart was pounding. Astrid thought I shouldn't get on the train, I said, but really everything was fine. It had happened before, I admitted. No big deal. It had always gone away. Everything would be okay. I didn't want to miss my train. There it was, headlight in the distance, horn sounding as it got closer.

I told Marcia that I felt fine.

"You're probably right," she said. "It's probably nothing. But if it keeps going, get the conductor."

The train whistled and braked, metal wheels screeching. I hung up the phone. Astrid said I shouldn't get on, no matter what Marcia had told me.

"Don't be reckless," she said. "Be safe."

But apart from the panic in my head and the pounding in my chest—both of which I was doing my best to ignore—I felt perfectly fine. The train doors opened. I got on board, leaving Astrid disconsolate on the platform.

I found a bench of three unoccupied seats. Stony Brook is the second-to-last stop on the ride the whole length of Long Island to New York City. I carried a portable CD player, headphones, and a wallet of music. The conductor punched my ticket. I lay across the length of the bench, put on some string quartets, laid the CD player on my savage breast, and watched it bounce to the crazy rhythm of my tachycardia.

The stations went past. St. James. Smithtown. In those days all the posters were for new internet businesses. Wines.com. Pets.com. The whole world was floating in imaginary money. Kings Park. Northport. The landscape shifted from rural to industrial. The conductor walked by my seat. I promised myself that if the attack didn't stop soon, if my heart didn't slow by the next time he passed, I'd stop him and tell him I wasn't feeling well.

We passed Huntington and the station for Cold Spring Harbor. The world outside was suburban. The guy in front of me had a phone, and he talked loudly enough that I could hear him over the oboe in my headphones.

"Fucking three o'clock," he was saying, "and the guy says to me, 'The exhaust pipe's rusted out.' He says, 'The brake pads are worn.' Then he gives me the estimate. Hundreds of dollars. Fucking hundreds. I go, 'All's I came here for was a battery.' He says, 'What can I tell you? This is what I see with your car.' I say to him, 'Did I ask what you see?' And we're standing there, and by now it's fucking three-fifteen."

Through the headrests of the seat in front of me I could see the man's hairy hand and his ear. I had the idea to tap his shoulder, to ask him to dial 911 for me, but the thought was like a dream. Everything was becoming abstracted. Syosset passed and Hicksville. His oration continued.

"I can pay for it. That's not the problem. You know I can pay. I got my Visa, Discover, fucking American Express. I'll get miles and points. That's not the problem here. You know what the problem is. And by now it's like fucking three-twenty-five or something." The man got off at Mineola.

The thumping in my chest didn't slow. The conductor came through, collecting tickets, saying next stop was the last one, Jamaica Queens. I got up, surprised that my body was still functioning. I put on my backpack. I lined up at the door with everyone else. The door opened, and I crossed the platform for the train to Brooklyn, and I stood there, looking down the track for my train, as if my heart were not going BOOM BOOM BOOM.

What was I thinking? I wasn't thinking. Two hours since my heart had started its pounding, and it still wasn't hard to stand. It wasn't hard to walk. I found a seat and handed my ticket to the next conductor, who punched it and handed it back to me, and we rode over East New York, the hospital, the high school, the housing projects, and cheap fast food, Kennedy Fried Chicken, halal butchers, and flat-fix joints. At Atlantic Avenue, I got off the train again and was afraid to climb up the stairs, but it worked, my body went up step after step.

From the Long Island Rail Road, I changed to a crowded subway train, two stops from Atlantic to Grand Army Plaza. I had to stand, and the train rocked under foot. BAM BAM BAM went my heart, which made me feel so alone, so isolated in the crowded train. In my backpack were files of papers and paperback books and Tupperware from lunch and my CDs. I felt a pain not in my chest but in my back, and in my left shoulder, and rising up the left side of my neck. My vision was narrowing. Out of the train at Grand Army Plaza, up the stairs through the turnstiles, past the ticket booth, and up another set of stairs.

Time had now developed a thin quality. I was hoping it would all stop—the tachycardia, my heart, everything. Death seemed like rest, like a relief, like a long warm bath. Hysteria turned to resignation. I doubt enough blood was getting to my brain, had been getting to my brain for hours.

The pain spread more intensely and dug more acutely into my left shoulder blade. I went up the subway stairs and into the twilight with everyone else who was coming home from work. I was in my familiar neighborhood. My house was just a few blocks away. Our apartment was on the third floor. Up the stairs I went, with the wild whacking of my heart, when each step might have been my last. Marcia was home. So was Eliza. And my dad. He had been babysitting, and he had stuck around to see me.

When I was little, my dad had protected me from the world by not letting anyone know I was ill. My father acted to shield me from the world's pity and to extend the illusion of my safety and immortality. Now I didn't let him hug me.

I didn't want him to feel my chest—he would panic; he would go crazy about it. I gave him the brush-off. His anxiety was the last thing I could deal with now. I told him I was tired and snuck past him and to bed. My neck and shoulder ached as I lay down. BANG BANG BANG went my heart. I heard my father leave, heard Marcia lock the door behind him, and only then did I pick up the telephone and call Boston. I explained what was happening to the nurse on the phone.

"Hang up," she said. "Call 911."

I said, "Really?"

Marcia stood in the door with our child in her arms. "They want me to call 911," I said to her. "What do you think I should do?"

36.

A S SOON AS surgeons began cutting into the myocardium, they began to disturb the conduction systems of their patients' hearts. John Gibbon, Charles Bailey, Dwight Harken, Walt Lillehei, and John Kirklin all lost patients whose hearts would not beat after surgery.

Paul Zoll, a colleague of Harken's in the Quonset hut hospital in the British town of Cirencester, worked with Harken again after the war at Harvard. Zoll was a small man, with a thin face and enormous ears. Colleagues were struck by the odd combination of Zoll's elfin looks and his dour disposition. He saw dozens of patients die of heart block on the operating table, both in war and after, patients with their heart muscles stitched up but unable to beat. He became obsessed with the problem.

In the early 1950s, Zoll found a way to keep these patients alive. His wartime experience had taught him, as he put it, "how easily excitable the myocardium is. You just touch it, and it gives you a run of extra beats—so why should the heart, that is so sensitive to any kind of manipulation, die because there's nothing there to stimulate the chest? It wasn't sensible." Though Zoll said he had a "poor background in electronics," he knew that electrical stimulation was the likeliest solution to the problem.

Zoll used a device called a Grass Physiological Stimulator, designed to deliver regular pulses of electricity in laboratory experiments. He attached two electrical leads from the Grass Stimulator to the skin of a blocked patient's chest, strapping the leads down with a leather belt. The stimulator gave off sixty shocks a minute. With each shock of Zoll's device, the patient's entire upper torso convulsed. All the chest muscles clenched, sixty times a minute. Under the leads, the patient's skin developed burns and ulcers. The heart beat, and the patient survived, but the pain was unendurable. "The problem with the original external pacemaker," said Zoll, "was that it hurt too much."

Zoll's first patient, an adult after valve surgery, was attached to the stimulator for more than forty-eight hours, his skin scorched, his pectoral muscles and diaphragm convulsing. The second, also an adult, stayed alive for three days. "His heart did not pick up on its own," Zoll recalled. It was unclear how or when the doctors could get the man off the machine, unclear if Zoll had built a life-saving or torture device. "Even my cardiac fellow said, 'Maybe we shouldn't be doing this.'" Seymour Furman, one of Zoll's interns, remembered, "We had a patient that I recall, a patient when I was an intern, who had been on a Zoll pacemaker for a long period of time, and finally committed suicide by turning off the switch, just after a pep talk which the house staff, myself included, had given him about the wonders of the future to come, which we didn't believe in, and he equally didn't believe."

Eventually, Zoll was able to devise an interior lead that went down the patient's esophagus and more directly attacked the heart. No longer did the skin burn; no longer did the chest muscles convulse with each shock. But the machines were unwieldy, and they weren't portable. So long as patients were on Zoll's pacemakers, they were confined to their hospital beds.

In Minnesota, Walt Lillehei was bedeviled by the same problem as Harken and Zoll. Every time he sutured the septum of a small child, he risked interfering with the conduction system of the heart. It was a terrible problem: after surgery, one in every ten of Lillehei's patients suffered heart block. Following Zoll's lead, Lillehei took a Grass Stimulator from a lab in his hospital and hooked it up to his patients' chests. But he found that using a Zoll pacemaker on a child was impossible.

"Getting a shock like that fifty, sixty times a minute is torture," said Lillehei. "With some infants we were able to restrain them so they wouldn't tear [the chest electrodes] off, but they would develop blisters and ulcers in four or five days. So that was totally inadequate."

Lillehei began attaching electrodes directly to the hearts of his blocked patients—connecting the wires to the heart muscle before he sutured them up. Experiments on dogs showed that direct connection to the heart required far less electricity than did external stimulation. A thousandth of an amp "drove the heart beautifully," said Lillehei, and the charge at that low level was imperceptible to the patient.

This became protocol at Variety Club Heart Hospital. In 1957, eighteen children were confined to their beds after surgery, electric stimulators attached to their hearts. In seventeen cases, the children survived. The doctors found that once the heart started beating on its own, they could gently pull the wire, and it would emerge out of the heart muscle and out of the chest without the need to ever reopen a suture. But having the children tethered to a pacemaker and to an electric outlet was untenable.

"Many of these [patients] were kids," said Lillehei. "They wanted to wander around and get active. Well, they *were* active." They wanted to get out of their beds, but "they couldn't get any further than the cord. We had to string wires down the hall," said Lillehei. "And then, if they needed an X-ray or something that couldn't be done in the room, you couldn't get on an elevator, so you had to string them down the stairwells. It seemed that almost everything you wanted was on a different floor."

A power failure on October 31, 1957, frightened the staff. The hospital had auxiliary power—none of the kids on pacemakers died—but Lillehei saw the risk, and he worried about the opposite of a power failure, a sudden power surge that might overwhelm the pacemaker kids. He dreamed of getting these patients out of their beds, getting them to move about the hospital, attaching them to some kind of portable device. He talked the problem over with

Earl Bakken, a graduate student working as a part-time electrical technician in the hospital labs. Outside the hospital, Bakken ran an electronics repair shop out of his garage. His partner was his brother-in-law, Palmer Hermundlie, who had a day job in the lumber business. Bakken, a short man with big glasses and a sharp nose, wasn't an electrical engineer but a tinkerer. He fixed EKG machines in the hospital and radios and toasters in his business from home. When Lillehei described the problem to him, Bakken's first idea was to use a car battery, but then he happened to read an article in *Popular Mechanics* titled "Five New Jobs for Transistor Batteries." The article showed the circuit designs for a metronome.

In his garage workshop, Bakken cribbed the designs for the metronome and, using mercury batteries, built a little machine that set off a charge once every sixty seconds, regulated as surely as a musical beat. The machine was about the size of a paperback book. It could hang on a cord around the neck. Bakken showed it to Lillehei. Lillehei was impressed.

Ten days later, a young patient lay on the operating table, chest open, heart sutured but refusing to beat. Lillehei applied his electrodes directly to the child's heart, and before stapling together the breastbone and sewing up the skin, he attached the wires to the metronome pacemaker Bakken had built in his garage. Bakken came into the recovery room the next day and was surprised to see his machine hanging around a little boy's neck, the wires running from the machine to the boy's heart, keeping the boy alive. This was the first implanted electronic medical device ever.

In 1958, Bakken built the Medtronic Model 5800 pacemaker. The device was housed in layered, carvable Bakelite housing, the words "Medtronic Pacemaker" in stylish white letters against the black. It had two handles and a strap to connect it to the chest, as well as a blinking red light to assure patients that it was working. It became a device not just for postoperative children but for older patients who needed long-term stimulation of their hearts.

Soon after Bakken's breakthrough, two Swedish doctors, Rune Elmqvist and Åke Senning, introduced the first implantable pacemaker, one small enough to sew into the flesh. Bakken and Medtronic followed suit. According to Kirk Jeffrey, author of *Machines in Our Hearts*, the development of the implantable pacemaker coincided in the United States with the establishment of Medicare. The federal government soon was helping elderly patients purchase these lifesaving devices, and pacemakers became a profitable business. Medtronic sold 1,200 pacemakers in 1962, 7,400 in 1966 and 1967, and 25,000 in 1969 and 1970. The company suffered a net income loss of $16,093 in 1968, but by 1972 it made an annual profit of almost $4 million. Pacemakers became a common piece of medical equipment.

Hospitals needed doctors to monitor the patients with difficulties in their hearts' electrical conduction systems, and so electrophysiology became a growing medical field. As Jeffrey wrote, "The very existence of the technology prompted researchers to intensify their investigations" into other arrhythmias and electrical disorders of the heart, including potentially lethal conditions like mine.

A pacemaker could get a stalled heart beating, but what to do when the heart started on a rampage, beating wildly, beating too fast?

37.

THE EMS GUYS littered our apartment with paper—Band-Aids and syringe wrappers. They hooked me up to a portable EKG. They gave me shots. They slid a needle into the crook of my elbow and set up an IV. They told me to strain, like I was trying to take a shit. (Apparently, in some cases, this can stop an attack of arrhythmia.) But nothing—not drugs, not exercises—could slow the crazy rhythm of my heart.

I remember lying in a curtained-off section of the emergency room with Marcia by my side and my heart beating ferociously. She held my hand. She teased me. "Brownstein, you really know how to bring the excitement." I gave my history to the attending physician. I asked if I was going to die. The doctors gave me more injections. Grimly, they told me they were going to have to shock me out of it. They were going to have to do it while I was awake. They took out the big electric paddles, rubbed them together, and said, "Clear!"—just like in the hospital TV shows. They applied them to my chest, and my whole body jumped and jolted. After that, my heart beat at its normal rate. I was exhausted, but I was calm.

My sense, internally, was of a ravaged quiet—like a street swept clean after a hurricane. The skin of my chest was seared, as if badly sunburnt. Marcia's face showed sweet relief. The doctors wouldn't let me go home. I needed to have surgery, they said. They would not release me from the hospital until I got an implanted cardioverter defibrillator (ICD) sewn into my chest. It wasn't safe for me to walk around the world without one. The next arrhythmia attack might kill me, so I needed a machine inside me, one that would shock my heart when it started beating too fast.

I really should have gone back to Marlon Rosenbaum. A mystic aura of terror had grown around him in my mind, an aura separate from the man himself. He had come to represent something for me, something I could not face. Was I ashamed that I had run from him, and that he had been right about my condition, and that I had been wrong? Perhaps vanity was involved as well as denial. At any rate, I made arrangements to go to Mount Sinai Hospital, where Dr. Steven Fishberger, a former student of Mike Freed's, was practicing pediatric cardiology. Dr. Fishberger worked closely with an eminent electrophysiologist, Dr. Davendra Mehta. Dr. Mehta would implant my ICD.

I rode an ambulance across the East River. I was awake for most of the procedure but loopy on anesthetics. A cloth border was hung in front of my face. The doctors tugged on the skin of my chest, and I felt their cuts like scissor snips and the cold baths of antibiotics washing out the pocket of the wound. Dr. Mehta guided wires down through my subclavian artery and screwed the leads into the muscle of my heart. I remember Dr. Mehta in scrubs coming by my head and speaking to me softly. "We have to check the device." They were going to put me to sleep; they were going to induce arrhythmia; they were going to make sure that the ICD could do its job to shock my heart with forty joules of electricity and knock it back from tachycardia to its normal beating. I woke up in the recovery room. Dr. Fishberger, the kindest of men, came to check on me. He brought some cookies.

"Lorna Doones," he said. "The choice of cardiologists."

There were bandages below my collarbone and a strange new bulge in my chest. The skin under the bandages was swollen and tender. I could feel the device, a little palm-sized piece of metal, squirming about in a wash of painful pus. When I stood, I felt its weight pulling downward. There was an illusion that I was wearing a necklace with a heavy medallion, like a police badge, but the medallion was the ICD, and the necklace was my skin. I put my clothes on. The ICD slid around, adjusting itself. Marcia and I met Dr. Mehta in his office.

Davendra Mehta is among the most elegant physicians I have ever met, a man with the kind of self-possession that flatters his interlocutors. Out of his scrubs, in a jacket and tie and sitting behind his desk, Dr. Mehta explained the device to me as if he and I were peers—as if it were only natural to be as smart, as stylish and good-looking, and as knowledgeable as he.

In a healthy heart, Dr. Mehta explained, the heartbeat is governed by the sinus node, that small bundle of electricity-generating cells that sits above the right atrium. The electricity from the sinus node travels in a complex pattern through the beating muscle cells of the top of the heart. The two small top chambers of the heart convulse, and then the charge gathers itself once again in the atrio-ventricular node, which governs the second firing of the heart, the contraction of the ventricles. Down goes the charge, through the septum, the central wall of the heart, through conduits known as the bundle of His and the bundle branches. At the base of the septum, the charge flares out through to the Purkinje fibers, which rise up to the exterior walls of the ventricles and run through the muscle like spreading rills at the end of a river delta—these fibers control the ventricles' beating.

A normal fast heartbeat, said Dr. Mehta, is called "sinus tachycardia," that is, a rapid heartbeat under the governance of the sinus node. That's what happens when you run up stairs. The arrhythmia I had suffered on the train ride was "ventricular tachycardia"; that is to say, my ventricles were beating on their own. When I was sitting in the sun with Astrid, the bottom half of my heart acted like I was running, while the top half acted like I was sitting still. As a lifelong heart patient and a surgery survivor, I was susceptible to these things.

Any damage to the muscle of the heart, Dr. Mehta explained, risks damage to the heart's conduction system. In my 1999 surgery, something had been severed or disturbed in the circuit of the heartbeat, and so my heart would not beat on its own. This is known as heart block. After approximately forty-eight hours of electrical stimulation in the cardiac ICU in Boston, my heart had recovered from its block, and the sinus node reasserted control. But damage had been done; my heart was continually reconstituting its conduction system, and there were some glitches where the heart had been cut. Sometime after I came back to Brooklyn, a new electrical conduction circuit had asserted itself—the stressed-out pattern of atrial flutter. Electricity ran in a loop around a scar, and the top chambers of my heart added some frivolous beats to their usual march-time dance. Back in Boston, through cardioversion, the electrical shock had eliminated that problem, but then, in the months after, the heart—adapting and readapting to the damage and scarring and recovery of the myocardium—had developed a new circuit yet again, a circular charge running around the bottom of my heart, a new electrical pattern that resulted in my ventricular tachycardia, or V-tach, my new arrhythmia.

The scar on the skin of my chest, so narrow and stylus fine after surgery, had thickened too. It was now a quarter of an inch wide, and I imagined, as the doctor talked, that similar changes had happened inside me.

Dr. Mehta explained everything smoothly and suavely, and I listened like an eager student. The V-tach in itself would not necessarily kill me, he said. I had tolerated it well. But V-tach can easily flip to ventricular fibrillation, or V-fib, the rhythm of death, where the big bottom chambers of the heart flap fast as a humming bird's wings, as fast as three hundred beats per minute (bpm), so fast that the chambers become useless and no longer move the blood at all. That was invariably fatal. My machine, said Dr. Mehta, would monitor every beat of my heart. If my heart rate became accelerated, the device would give me treatment.

"You mean I'll get a shock?" I said.

"Not necessarily."

The ICD had three modes, Dr. Mehta continued, and the modes were determined by the speed of my heart in beats per minute: there was a first threshold at which the device simply recorded the heartbeat; a second threshold at which it delivered antitachycardia pacing (ATP), little gentle pulses akin to a pacemaker's; and a top threshold at which the machine would fire, delivering forty joules of energy into the muscle of the heart. If the device sensed an accelerated heartbeat (first threshold), it would begin recording. If that heartbeat exceeded a preprogrammed rate (second threshold), the device would give me ATP. The ATP pulses would be mild enough that I would not feel them—the hope was that the pacing beats would trick the heart out of arrhythmia. But if the ATP didn't work (third threshold), I would get the shock. The shock would be quite painful.

"What does it feel like?" I asked.

"I've never experienced it," he reminded me, "but they say it's like getting kicked in the chest by a horse."

I should be careful when I exerted myself, he warned. "The machine," said Dr. Mehta, "is an idiot."

The ICD did not always recognize the difference between sinus tachycardia and ventricular tachycardia. It could distinguish between fast and slow beats but not between healthy and sick ones. My device gauged its thresholds based on the speed of the heart. It would react the same way if I was racing up a hill or if I was in V-tach. Because my V-tach ran at 150 bpm, said Dr. Mehta, the threshold for firing was relatively low. I would have to be careful when working out. I would get a shock anytime the machine sensed a sustained heart rate over 150 bpm. This was the disadvantage of the device.

The advantage was that my arrhythmia would not kill me. So long as I had the device in my chest, I was safe.

"A hundred percent safe?"

Dr. Mehta smiled. Nothing was 100 percent, but genuinely safe. I was not going to die of arrhythmia when I had the ICD inside me.

Marcia and I left the hospital, and we went home. The phone rang in the morning. It was Astrid. I thanked her for trying so hard to save my life. I apologized for not listening to her. She was relieved. She was happy, she said, so happy to hear my voice again.

We went to the Brooklyn Botanical Gardens, Marcia, Eliza, and I. The last roses were in bloom, and the trees were changing color. As I lay back on the lawn, with my baby daughter crawling around and my wife beside me and the fat white clouds moving across the sky, I felt the terrible luck of my life, the stupid happenstance by which I was there at all, despite all my idiocy, my seeming attempts to destroy myself. The green of the grass, the blue of the sky, the wet smell of earth—I felt it all so keenly, the miracle of everything.

I still can't believe it: that I was born where Jim Malm was practicing, right after he mastered the art of tetralogy repair; that my heart held on just long enough, while the blood leaked backward and my ventricle expanded, for imaging technology and medical consensus to form around surgical intervention in 1999; and that I survived that crazy train ride somehow and was met in the hospital by newfangled technology that would guarantee my life. Had these arrhythmias come in the 1980s, when I was wearing my Holter monitor to high school and being tested for them, the doctors would have had no way to contain the threat to my life. But now they did.

Baby Eliza put her face over mine, huge and smiling. Then she climbed up on top of me, her little foot and chubby weight right on the incision, and her poor father yowled in laughter and pain.

38.

THE FIRST IMPLANTED defibrillator was placed in a human chest in 1980 at Johns Hopkins. The machine was a half-pound brick, five inches long. Dr. Levi Watkins Jr. performed the operation. Watkins was the first African American surgeon on staff at Hopkins and a protégé of Vivien Thomas, who was still working at the hospital, now as a professor. Thomas himself helped Watkins design the surgery and prepare for it, running experiments in his dog lab. The patient was a desperate case: a fifty-seven-year-old woman who had had a heart attack and bypass surgery and whose frequent spells of arrhythmia were causing her to faint and putting her life at risk. She needed more than a pacemaker. She needed something that would reset her heart when the sinus node lost control of its beating. The doctors cracked her chest, laid the big device into her abdomen, and attached it via patches to the exterior of her heart.

In the operating room, watching the procedure, was Michel Mirowski. A short, thickset, balding, and bespectacled research scientist in his mid-fifties, Mirowski wasn't used to wearing scrubs. He was a researcher, not a surgeon. He had conceived of the implanted defibrillator in 1966 and had spent his career wandering—from Israel to Mexico to Baltimore, then back to Israel, then back to Baltimore again—obsessively working on the problem. Mirowski had received virtually no grant money in his quest to build the machine and minimal corporate support. He and his partner, Dr. Morton Mower, had been obliged to finance their work on their own, even purchasing their own lab dogs at $1 apiece.

In the early 1970s, the implanted defibrillator was seen as an unwieldy, unnecessary, even sadistic device, enormous, uncomfortable, and as likely to go off unnecessarily as to save a patient. An early critic called it "an imperfect solution in search of a plausible and practical application." Others described it as a bomb sewn into the human body. Some compared its use to Nazi experiments on prisoners, a particularly cruel comparison, given Mirowski's history.

He was born in Warsaw in 1924. As a boy, his name had been Mordechai Frydman. He'd changed it when he was fleeing the Nazis. His early childhood had been happy—he was the bookish son of a man who ran a profitable delicatessen. "I had a liberal view of the world which was in conflict with the Jewish reality in Poland," he remembered. "I thought I was, first of all, Polish—obviously a mistaken impression." He was an assimilated, middle-class child. But with the rise of fascism in Poland, his placid early life vanished. "Even the police were sympathetic to the right-wing trends," he remembered. "They stood aside when fascistic toughs beat and even killed Jews, and this was before the Nazis arrived."

In September 1938, German planes dropped bombs on Warsaw. Mirowski walked streets where the sides of buildings were torn open and the rooms exposed like dollhouses. In November, his mother died of heart failure—probably as a result of scars from childhood rheumatic fever. On December 1, all the Jews in Warsaw were ordered to wear yellow stars. "The schools were closed, and the persecution began. I remember German officers cutting off the payess," the long sidelocks worn by Hassidic Jews, "to humiliate them. I told my father that I wouldn't wear that yellow star and that it seemed foolish to stay in Warsaw."

Mirowski's father made him take a new name so he could pass among the German invaders. And he gave his son two final pieces of advice before they parted. "Be a physician," he said, and "be a Jew." On December 5, the boy left the city. With a friend, he headed east, walking through woods and fields, hitching rides in the backs of trucks, sleeping in railroad stations, suffering asthma attacks. The boys traveled two hundred miles, down the Vistula river, past the suburbs and the resorts where bourgeois Jews had once spent their summers, through the German territories, to Lvov, which was held by the Soviets.

He tried to enlist in the Russian army but was too young, so he ran further eastward, across Ukraine to Kiev, sleeping in parks. The Nazis entered Kiev in September 1941, and Mirowski and his friends fled ahead of their advance, riding on the tops of trains, eating whatever they could scavenge. They headed north, into Russia. In Rostov, the boy found work on a building crew, before he had to run again, 1,000 miles southward, to Krasnodar, where he hustled, rolling loose tobacco into papers and selling cigarettes. From Krasnodar, Mirowski went further east, ahead of the advancing Germans, all the way to Baku, the great oil-rich city on the Caspian Sea. In the Uzbek city of Andijan, he worked up to eleven hours a day at an airplane factory.

He was now 2,500 miles from home, fighting off tropical fever, going to the library every day to study. He found work with a traveling group of singers, storytellers, and musicians, hanging signs and posters, a job that gave him coupons for bread. In 1944, finally, he enlisted in the Polish army and so survived to the end of the war and returned to Poland with the liberators. Everything he had known was gone, his family dead, his neighborhood rubble.

"I saw the camp near Gdansk where the Germans had converted human corpses into soap, and there was a lot of it still available," he remembered. "As far as Poland was concerned, it had become a cemetery for me."

Mirowski arranged with some fellow refugees to flee illegally to Palestine and arrived in 1947 only to find there were no medical schools there. He ended up studying medicine in France. "I knew I wouldn't be staying," Mirowski remembered. "Only in Israel or in the US could someone like me be a first-class citizen."

In 1954, he traveled back to Palestine. He found a job in Tel Aviv, in Tel HaShomer Hospital, working under Dr. Harry Heller, whose erudition and professionalism engendered a kind of worship in Mirowski. In Heller, Mirowski encountered the kind of doctor and mentor that he might have studied with had the war never happened, had he remained Mordechai Frydman, the clever deli man's son, and had he gone off to Berlin for school.

"A typical German professor," Mirowski said of Heller. "Every day that we made rounds together was a holiday for me." But Heller was suffering from bouts of tachycardia. "My wife asked me why I was so concerned," Mirowski remembered. "'Because he will die from it,' I told her. And he did, two weeks later, at dinner with his family."

Mirowski had seen so much death—but here at last was one cause he could combat. He devoted the rest of his life to building a device that could save a person from sudden cardiac death due to arrhythmia. In the early 1970s, external electric defibrillators existed—Paul Zoll had built the first, and then another Boston doctor, Bernard Lown, had adapted the machine to alternating current—but defibrillators were large and unwieldy, weighing thirty to forty pounds, and the idea of putting one in a person's chest seemed absurd. In Baltimore, Mirowski worked with Helen Taussig and met his partner, Morton Mower. Despite the lack of grant money and the widespread doubt that their idea was plausible, Mirowski and Mower persisted, and by 1980 they had built their big, bulky, but initially successful device.

The principle of Mirowski and Mower's machine is the same as the principle of the device that was put in my chest: when the heart beats too fast, it gets recalibrated with a shock. But my ICD is something quite different from the big, heavy brick Mirowski and Mower invented. My ICD weighs just a few ounces, and its sensors and memory are computerized; it varies treatment according to symptoms and can be adjusted to respond to the conditions of different hearts. ICD technology continues to improve: now patients don't get wires put in their hearts. The latest models are smaller and nestle on the side of the patient's chest, monitoring and treating arrhythmias. I'll get one of those someday or maybe something even more futuristic.

But for now, I am satisfied. Like so much else in cardiology, my ICD seems to have emerged through a haze of chaos and impossible history, just in time to rescue me.

39.

LET'S PAUSE IN this discussion of progress to remember the patients who did not survive. Not everyone has been as lucky as I have been.

I met Doron Weber on a spring day in New York at a diner on the Upper East Side of Manhattan. A bald, gregarious man—a New York intellectual type quite familiar to me—Doron is the author of one of the few great books about congenital heart disease, *Immortal Bird*. It's a memoir of the death of his son Damon.

A decade had passed since the book's publication, but I felt I could still see the grief over his lost boy on the man's body. On a sunny spring day, he looked worn, like he'd walked to the diner through a storm. We chatted over breakfast. I got a bagel and a fruit cup. He ordered eggs, bacon, home fries, and toast. We did a little writerly shoptalk: books we liked, agents we'd worked with, editors we knew. When I say my heart went out to Doron, I hate the cliché, but that was the feeling, an ache in my chest moving toward him.

The title of Weber's book comes from Keats's "Ode to a Nightingale": "Thou wast not born for death, immortal Bird!" And that's how I feel about my daughters, Lucy and Eliza. Everyone is born to die, but not them. For Doron in his memoir, his son Damon is a powerful spirit fastened to a dying animal. Damon's defective heart is not, for Doron, *Damon*. And Doron's ambivalence about doctors and hospitals is evident right from the start, when Damon is diagnosed and taken to the neonatal ICU:

> Three-day-old Damon lays inside a clean bubble, separated from us by modern technology, a pint-sized astronaut marooned in his own world. We slip our hands through the little portholes to touch him but this only brings home how distant and sealed-off he is . . . a captive of the medical profession.

The Webers need the physicians to save their child, but ultimately they want to free their son from the prison of the hospital.

Though he is born with just one ventricle, though he undergoes several surgeries, including a Fontan operation, which reroutes the blood around the failed parts of his heart, for thirteen years Damon is successful. He hikes up mountains. If he's ever winded or having trouble, he hides it. The Webers' life is eerily similar to my family's. They live in the same neighborhood we do. Damon goes to Brooklyn Technical High School, where my daughter goes to school. He's a patient at New York–Presbyterian, just like me. Mike Freed makes an appearance, consulting from Boston. Damon does well at Brooklyn Tech. He makes friends. He stars in plays. But life is not easy. A decade after his childhood surgeries, and though his heart seems to be pumping adequately, his blood begins leaking protein.

> "Yeah, just give me a minute." Damon retrieves from the closet a big box with all his "fixings." First, he disinfects the injection site with alcohol swabs. Then he applies a yellowish smear of anesthetic cream to his abdomen and covers the cream with a thin patch of cellophane, which he fastens with a makeshift belt. . . . We watch together until the cream has done its work. Then Damon unwraps a fresh syringe and needle and inserts the needle into a small ampoule of heparin. He retracts the plunger and fills the syringe with the clear, straw-colored liquid to just the right level, flicking it to ensure there are no bubbles or floating particles.

Then, with a determined sigh, Damon jabs himself.

His condition is a mystery. Protein-losing enteropathy (PLE), it's called, and no one knows how or why it occurs in post-Fontan kids. About half the children who get PLE die, but again, the numbers are small, and the diagnosis is imprecise, so the statistics are difficult to parse. In his first year of high school, even though his liver is so swollen he looks pregnant, Damon wins a part in *The Importance of Being Earnest*. The moment he steps on stage with his slicked-back pompadour, twinkling eyes, and pompous thumbs hooked into his Victorian lapels, Damon commands attention." But he also looks small and frail at curtain:

> My son bends at the waist with panache, draping his belly with one deft arm, while his red locks tumble forward. Temporarily buoyed by the energy on that stage, he's the picture of actorly decorum, yet he's barely holding it together. I know from his friends he's been falling asleep during rehearsals, and even now, I can see him husbanding his meager resources to stand there and look normal.

Damon loses energy. His skin turns swollen and pasty, distorting his once beautiful face. The doctors are confused. The great surgeon Jan Quaegebeur says to Doron, "I think you're overreacting and things may not be as bad as you're making them." But things are awful. Eventually, Damon needs a heart transplant, the aftermath of which is a horror show. Doctors are absent when they ought to be present.

"What have they done to my son?" Doron cries. At the very end, when all the mistakes have been made, when all attempts have failed and the doctors have given up their struggle, Doron rushes to Damon's bedside in the ICU.

> "D-man, listen to me!" I lift my voice and appeal to him as if we're fellow soldiers fighting in the trenches and we could still win this war. "I want you to forget all these goddamn machines and this whole ridiculous setup here! Forget this silly hospital

and these silly doctors. Just go deep *inside*. I know you have the strength—it's time to use it. Okay?" I pump my fists, as I have so often for him, and urge Damon on with every fiber of my fraught being. "Come on, D-man, let's bust out of this joint and just go *home!*"

Does love obscure Doron's vision or enchant it? In the cardiac ICU and the neonatal ICU, he sees so much more than what's actually there.

The essential prayer of the long-term heart patient is silent and unspoken, and always it is implicit in the prayer Doron recited as Damon died, the desire to flee from the world of medicine. *Let's bust out of this joint and go home.*

40.

TIMOFEY PNIN, RUSSIAN émigré, sits in a park in a small town in upstate New York and feels a shift inside him, an alteration in the substance of his body. "He felt porous and pregnable," Pnin's author, Vladimir Nabokov, writes. "He was sweating. He was terrified." *Pnin* was written in 1957, before the advent of electrocardiology, so Nabokov—who has a word for everything—has no language to describe precisely what is happening to his hero's heart. "Was his seizure a heart attack?" Nabokov asks. "I doubt it."

When doctors examine Pnin closely, "the cardiograph outlined fabulous mountain ranges." Pnin gets no diagnosis for his condition. He regards his heart "with a nervous repulsion, a sick hate, as if it were some strong slimy untouchable monster that one had to be parasite with, alas." In the moment when he is sitting on the park bench, he feels that monster has betrayed him, as if "the repulsive automaton he lodged had developed a consciousness of its own and not only was grossly alive, but was causing him pain and panic."

Arrhythmia makes the self other and the other out of the self. One's heart is not one's own. An implanted cardioverter defibrillator compounds this unnerving experience. In the patient's chest there are now two competing alien intelligences, not only the arrhythmic heart but also the ICD, with its chilly robot brain, ready and willing to blow the crap out of the body.

An ICD battery lasts about five years, and when the battery runs out, the whole thing has to be excised from the chest, and a new one has to be attached to the electric leads that screw into the heart, and the skin has to be sutured up above the device. On a chilly first day after it's been implanted, a new ICD can get cold before the rest of the body, like a bunch of icy coins in your pants pocket, but in this case the pocket is your skin.

The first time my ICD gave me a shock, I was on an elliptical trainer at the local YMCA, listening to Talking Heads, feeling strong and recovered and going as fast as I could. "We are vain and we are blind," said David Byrne. And then—David Byrne went silent. Everything went dark. Something tore through my chest, like a brick was ripping through my thorax, and my first thought was that a bomb had gone off behind me. But then the lights went back on. "I hate people when they're not polite," said David Byrne. Everyone else was exercising, as if nothing at all had happened. My heart was no longer thumping with exercise. It was steady and quiet. I stepped off the machine. I put a towel to my face.

One of the weirdest things about a defibrillator shock is that when it hits, the pain is total and self-obliterating, but when it's gone, it's gone. There's no residual tenderness or swelling or mark. I walked home. I called a doctor.

The second time, I was teaching my daughter how to ride a bike. I ran hard, pushed Eliza up a gentle slope, and then—I was doubled over, and she was pedaling. The third time I was running through deep snow, trying to catch a bus. You learn, somehow, to integrate these things into your life, though they are traumatic.

After her childhood heart surgery, Meg Balke had been an athlete, a competitive swimmer in high school and a professional trainer as an adult. But the birth of her second child taxed her heart, and Meg developed life-threatening arrhythmias. After an ICD was implanted in her chest, she continued to operate her business—a Strollercize franchise in Florida. One day in the park, with her baby in its jogging stroller and several new moms in exercise clothing pushing strollers behind her, Meg (tall, thin, redheaded, and fit) jogged up a hill, and her ICD fired. She didn't fall. She didn't falter. She just slowed down and had her troop walk the last fifty yards of the routine.

I met a patient named Jenny who was working as an events coordinator when one day, in a stairway in her office complex, her ICD shocked her ninety-eight times in the course of thirty minutes. Jenny is a youthful, attractive woman with long, blond hair and a wide-open midwestern face, and her harrowing decline in health led to a heart transplant. She showed me the scar on her chest where the defibrillator had been—with a new heart, she didn't need the device anymore. But still, the trauma lingered. She could not enter a stairway anymore. She always took the elevator. And she still suffered phantom shocks from her missing ICD, moments when she tensed and seized, imagining that her defibrillator was blowing her away. I get these too, these imaginary shocks. They hit me often when I'm on the cusp of sleep.

I have learned to be careful, to always take my medicine, and to wear a heart monitor when I ride a bike or climb a mountain. I have also learned to be grateful. For each badly timed explosion, there have been a dozen times when my ICD has saved my life, usually without my knowing it. My heart runs whacky for just a few seconds. The defibrillator sends out its gentle antitachycardia pacing, and the ATP beats dissolve the arrhythmia before I know it's even happened. I might be commuting home, cooking dinner, or having a cocktail with a friend—these ATP-cured arrhythmias are nothing to me. I only learn about them in the doctor's office, when the device is interrogated and reveals its history.

"Remember where you were on November 19 at 5:10?" the nurse will ask. And I'll have no idea, and no memory of the episode of V-tach.

Soon after my ICD was implanted, Marcia got pregnant again. We moved into our new house. My daughter Lucy was born, and my ICD was there in my chest, counting beats in the delivery room. Just a month after Lucy's birth, I was on the Long Island Rail Road, and the conductor announced, "If you look out your window, you'll see the World Trade Center just got hit by a plane."

My first book came out. My ICD was with me as I crossed the stage and won an award. I got a tenure-track job, published a second book, and then spent years writing an experimental novel about black-face comedy—one that was never published. My ICD was in my chest as I read the rejection letters.

The device didn't cure my arrhythmia; it just made sure my V-tach didn't kill me. I published some stories. I got tenure. I started a new book, about three marriages in one family. It wasn't clear how much longer the pig valve in my heart would last—the lifespan of those things can go from one year to twenty, so every six months I'd get an echocardiogram to see how well it was holding up.

As I got older, the pace of my arrhythmias slowed. I started experiencing attacks at rates below the threshold at which my device was set—my heart would be pounding at 140 beats per minute, and there was nothing to do but to wait for those attacks to pass.

I was riding my bike around town, I was teaching and writing and raising my kids, but soon the attacks became more frequent, and I no longer had the ability, or the will, to pretend I was healthy. The ICD was there under my skin. The pig valve was in my heart, wearing out, a little bit, every day. I left Steve Fishberger's practice and was treated by Deborah Gersony (thank you, Deborah!), an adult congenital heart disease doctor and the daughter of Welton Gersony. She was the first trained adult congenital heart disease doctor in New York City. (Marlon Rosenbaum became a doctor before such training existed.) But Deborah Gersony left medicine, and eventually I had to go back, tail between my legs, to Marlon Rosenbaum, who was the doctor in New York best qualified to treat me.

Like so many long-anticipated meetings, my reunion with Marlon was anticlimactic. I was anxious in the waiting room, but Marlon could not have been more professional and decent. There he was, a soft-spoken, unprepossessing man, hurried and distracted, rumpled even though his shirt was clean and pressed.

"This is Gabriel," he said to Nada Farhat, the brilliant and kind RN who works closely with Marlon. "Gabriel, whom I've known for a long, long time." There he was—an actual man, uncoupled from the black hole of my imagination.

I tried to make up for past confusions. I apologized for running away from him. I went on about it, but he stopped me. He tilted his head to one side. He squinted slightly. He remembered the exchange with Dr. Freed. He admired Mike Freed. He said they were friends, really. He said that a lot of people hadn't believed him in 1995 when he was arguing for replacement of pulmonary valves in patients like me. He didn't seem surprised that I had chosen the path of nonintervention.

I told him that I had been really, really afraid of heart surgery. He raised his palms slightly, as if to say, *Who isn't?* I told him that he had been right and that I should have listened to him.

"Sure," he said. And he put a stethoscope to my chest and then to my back. "Breathe," he said. I have put myself in his hands ever since.

Often, when I see Dr. Rosenbaum, there's a fellow in his office training to work in adult congenital cardiology, and often he'll tell his fellows the story of my case and of the different ways that he and Dr. Freed saw it.

"It just goes to show," I've heard him say.

"You have to go with the data?" I've asked.

But that's not the moral of the story. There wasn't any data. There's still no real data, he's explained to me. All the doctors know is what they see. "If you replace the valve in an adult tetralogy patient," Dr. Rosenbaum told me, "you'll see that a year later the right ventricle has shrunk 30 percent." But that doesn't address outcomes. Doctors have only an eighteen-year follow-up on a handful of patients and no control group, so there's no real proof that with intervention there's less tachycardia, heart failure, and death.

The moral, it seems, is the difficulty in imagining new ways of treating patients and the difficulty of getting the medical establishment to change its practice as new ways emerge. Marlon Rosenbaum, trained as an adult cardiologist, came to congenital heart disease with fresh eyes, and what he saw seemed obvious to him: people in general do better with pulmonary valves. A leak in an enlarged heart could not be tolerated indefinitely. But since Jim Malm's time, this had been how pediatric cardiologists had cured people like me. It was part of the algorithm Malm and his peers developed—the heart was repaired without a pulmonary valve. This practice, over thirty years, had been incredibly successful. A whole generation was living long, happy, healthy lives. We were doing great. I was doing great. In the 1990s, the risks of surgery and heart valve implantation were real, while the benefits were entirely hypothetical.

I've often wondered, What if I'd had my valve replaced in 1995? Would I have an ICD in my chest now? Would I be plagued by the arrhythmias? When I ask these questions of Marlon, he winces as if he's been pinched. He does not want me to blame myself for my condition.

"Any time you cut into the heart," he's explained, "you run the risk of disturbing the conduction system." And the V-tach doesn't necessarily correspond to the enlargement of the ventricle. "It's multifactorial," he has said to me.

Besides, it's not clear anyone would have replaced my heart valve in 1995. The difference between Dr. Freed and Dr. Rosenbaum wasn't nearly so large as I had imagined. Marlon Rosenbaum did not have a patient undergo valve replacement until 1999, the same year I had my surgery in Boston. He presented that case to his colleagues, and the night before the operation was scheduled, an eminent visiting doctor from London argued vehemently against intervention.

"He thought I was crazy," Marlon said.

In 1995, adult congenital cardiology was not an established field. Kids whose hearts had been repaired in the 1970s and 1980s were mostly seeing their pediatric cardiologists, if they were seeing cardiologists at all. Diagnostic technology changed too. It was the MRI of my heart, a test unavailable when I left Marlon's practice, that presented the hard data about my ventricle. And even in 1999, when I had my surgery, adult congenital cardiology was in its infancy. It wasn't until 2010 that doctors could train in established adult congenital cardiology fellowships. There was no board-certifying exam in adult congenital cardiology until 2015.

"When I started," Marlon Rosenbaum told me, "people would say, Why do you want to do *that?*"

As recently as the 1990s, he was the only doctor in New York City devoting himself to adult congenital cardiology patients. There are now four other congenital heart disease (CHD) centers in the city. Dr. Rosenbaum has a practice with thousands of adult patients and two CHD doctors working under him.

Current medical practice dictates that patients make the final choices about their health. In *The Heart Healers*, James S. Forrester, former chief of cardiology at Cedars-Sinai Medical Center, writes, "From our first days in medical school we are admonished never to order, only to advise." "This has to be your choice," Forrester tells his patients. But a choice made in ignorance isn't a choice at all.

I've been back in Marlon Rosenbaum's practice for about a decade, and in that time I've had continuing troubles with my heart. The valve has weakened, and I've suffered new and difficult arrhythmias. But I've learned to listen to him and to be ruled by his recommendations. I ask him questions, and if I ever didn't understand his advice, I wouldn't hesitate to get a second opinion. But I've learned that to make good decisions I can't be ruled by fear. Educated patients want to view their decisions critically, to hear their doctors' recommendations with some skepticism, but skepticism without knowledge isn't thinking. It's just a reaction driven by vanity and fear.

41.

"E VERYONE WHO IS born holds dual citizenship," wrote Susan Sontag, famously, "in the kingdom of the well and in the kingdom of the sick. Although we all prefer to use only the good passport, sooner or later, each of us is obliged, at least for a spell, to identify ourselves as citizens of that other place."

For most of my life, I've behaved like a spy or a refugee, a citizen of the kingdom of the sick traveling under false papers in the kingdom of the well. But as I have grown older, the borderline between Sontag's two kingdoms has gotten blurry, and so has my sense of citizenship. On a given day, I no longer know which territory I belong to—the kingdom of the healthy or the kingdom of the sick—and I no longer know which passport I'm supposed to carry. Sontag wrote those famous words in 1977, and maybe her geography is a little out-of-date. More and more of us live like me, in a territory unimaginable fifty years ago, a strange border country ruled by medicine.

I've been teaching in the same English department, at St. John's University, for more than twelve years, and by now I know which of my colleagues has survived a stroke and which an infection that crossed the blood-brain barrier. Some have confided in me about their antidepressants and their high-cholesterol and hypertension drugs and their cardiac arrhythmias. The estimate is that by 2025, 164 million people in the United States will be living with chronic illness, and that number doesn't count the ones who were spared long-term disability because of pins in their ankles and their hips after skiing or football injuries, or the ones who don't have rheumatically scarred heart valves because they took penicillin when they were kids with strep throat, or the ones who never got measles because they and their neighbors were vaccinated, or the ones who never got cholera because their drinking water was clean—in other words, we all should count ourselves among the saved, living in the kingdom of the well by the grace of doctors and public health measures. Medicine penetrates our lives so deeply that it's invisible. We forget that we have been rescued. I am not the only one whose insides have been changed. Hemoglobin structures differ among those in the developed world and those in less prosperous countries, largely because the former have been shielded from diseases.

Like everyone with great privilege, we take our privilege for granted. When I was a kid, even when I was thirty, I felt singled out by my heart. But now I feel less like an outlier and more like a trenchant example. We're all in the Open Heart Club now.

———

I was on my bicycle, going around the perimeter of Brooklyn to Queens, from my house to the Rockaways, sweaty but happy, and then heading home on a narrow path by the side of the Belt Parkway. My heart, which had been steady around 115 bpm, leapt on my wristwatch monitor, all the way to 148 bpm. I stopped biking, waiting for the shock, but nothing happened. The rapid heartbeat continued. I saw the monitor's number go down to 144 and back up to 147. Again I tensed, gripping the handlebars, feeling the panic rise. The shock never came. The arrhythmia resolved itself on its own, down to one hundred, then to sixty. Hesitantly at first, but eventually with some confidence, I biked my way home.

It started happening more often. The palpitations hit me at rest. I'd be eating out, and I'd hand the menu to the waitress and feel the V-tach begin in my chest. I went to Dr. Rosenbaum's office. He raised his finger in the air and recommended a radio ablation. They would put me under some sedation, guide a catheter into my heart, and with the electric wire of that catheter attempt to burn the arrhythmia right out of the muscle of my heart. It seemed a frightening proposition, but this time I didn't ask too many questions. I took Dr. Rosenbaum's advice.

I was rolled on a gurney into a chilly OR. Doctors shaved my groin and gave me a shot of local anesthetic down there. They ran a catheter up my thigh, through the abdominal aorta and down into my heart. They induced the arrhythmia, and my body began to shake. Dr. Danforth Zhee (I'll call him), my young electrophysiologist, stared at a computer screen. Dr. Zhee called out sectors of my heart by letter and number. I felt a buzz each time the catheter burned the interior of my heart muscle.

The ablation seemed to work, for a little while. I went biking. I went hiking. I was back in the kingdom of the healthy. But in the fall of 2015, the V-tach started to hit me more frequently, started to hit me at night. BOOM, BOOM, BOOM. The bed shook with the crazy pulse of my ventricles. My doctors prescribed new drugs, Sotalol instead of Atenolol, but no medicine seemed to work. Every night, I was up pacing the kitchen, staring at the monitor on my wrist, 147, 148, 149.

For Christmas vacation, we went to visit my older brother, Daniel, in California, and he set us up in his neighbors' place, a big, stucco, ranch-style house in the pretty border between Oakland and Berkeley. I don't know if jetlag exacerbated the symptoms of my arrhythmia, but in that week my V-tach was awful. I was up three and four times a night with my heart pounding. My brother's neighbors' house had a big, squared-off staircase between its first and second floors, and all through the night, I found myself going up and down, up and down, hoping and praying that the whacking in my chest would stop.

"This is torture," said Marcia, about getting awakened three times a night. "This is how they drove Oscar Wilde out of his mind."

In February, I had another ablation: again my chest was shaved, again the cold adhesives were applied to my skin, and again I was rolled into the catheter lab. The cold, clean room, the massive banks of instruments, the big screens and big white plastic cameras, and the technicians at their monitors behind the window. Nurses put on their sterile gear and set up the IV and the instruments. They played soft 1970s rock from someone's iPod, Billy Joel, Elton John, Carole King. The Vercid numbed my brain. The catheter slid into my thigh. The equipment beeped each time my heart beat. Dr. Zhee and his assistant stood anxiously by their computers, calling out numbers and watching the screen, their crazy game of Battleship.

I really like Dr. Dan Zhee. He reminds me of my smartest friends from the Bronx High School of Science. His hair is always neatly parted, his shirt is always pressed, and his white doctor's coat is always clean, but somehow he manages to look casual. He slumps a little. He never moves fast. Early on, Dan gave me his cell phone number and encouraged me to call him by his first name. A Harvard grad with a degree in public health as well as medicine, he seemed to me like the kind of super-bright guy who had ruled the foosball table at college, who would only talk about something if he were an expert, who always competed to win. But in the OR that day in February 2016, Dan could not get through the first step of the ablation. He could not stimulate my arrhythmia.

It was absurd. I was going into V-tach three times a night, two times a day, every day, but somehow, while I lay there on the operating table, given every kind of electrophysiological lure, my heart wouldn't budge. Dan Zhee kept trying, again and again, to get my heart to do its whacky dance. Again and again, my heart refrained. My sinus node, so willing every other day of the year to cede control, now stayed jealously at the helm: steady at sixty beats per minute she went. Dan Zhee knew my heart well from the first ablation, and following what he knew, he burned the hell out of its insides, working the spots where the pattern had been last charted. I began to feel his frustration. I began to feel the burning in my chest.

"Sorry," said Dan, and I was given more Versed.

This went on for a couple hours, until finally he gave up and rolled me into the recovery room, where, promptly and unbidden, my heart went into its familiar arrhythmia.

I asked Dan if he could roll me back into the OR once more and give it another whirl. He told me that was impossible. These things were tricky and complex, he told me. I shouldn't lose hope.

"Sometimes, there's a settling in period," he said.

Dan, with all his brilliance, confidence, expertise, and degrees, all his drugs, computers, monitors, cameras, radio waves, and catheters, suddenly seemed like a building superintendent with a monkey wrench taking a few whacks at a boiler and hoping the heat would rise to a third-floor apartment.

At work, I stared at ceilings and waited for meetings to end. I dragged myself through my classes. Still I had not experienced any defibrillator shocks. Still I was driving to Queens. But I could feel that an end was coming, that I would be incompetent soon enough. The drugs prescribed were more powerfully tranquilizing, but the symptoms persisted. I had the slow pounding attacks every night. I was up in the kitchen at 2 a.m., hopping up and down and hoping my heart would beat right, sometimes even hoping for a shock to put the arrhythmia to an end. In the day, my attacks were more acute. I got up from the couch, watching TV with my family, and listed suddenly to the right and had to lean against a wall. My knees buckled, but I didn't fall. The next morning, I sat down in the driver's seat, pulled the belt across my chest, and imagined the jolt to the heart, the sliding car, the crash, the dead pedestrian.

At dinner one night, Lucy said, "So we're not going hiking this summer, right, Dad?" And I said I didn't know. I said the doctors might be able to fix my heart.

"They're not going to be able to fix it, Dad," she said, thirteen years old and wise to me.

I had fooled myself into thinking she didn't know what was going on, that she was unaware of my weakness, that she didn't know that I was up every night, that she had believed me when I said my hospitalizations were no big deal. But she maybe had a better grasp of it all than I did. I gripped her hand. She looked at me, big eyed and soulful.

"Let's try to be optimistic," Dan told me the day he adjusted my device and scheduled my third ablation. But I wasn't optimistic anymore. I was sure my run of good luck had finally ended.

I left Dan's office, got to the street outside the hospital, and checked my phone. There was an email from my literary agent, David McCormick. I had never mentioned my heart problems to David—or to anyone in the publishing world—and had only told my closest friends in my department. David had been sending around my novel about three marriages in one family, and a fifth editor had rejected it. David had been very enthusiastic about the book at first but now thought that I should consider revising it. I knew he was right. The book needed revision. But I also knew no matter what happened, I could not rework it. I wasn't the person I had been when I'd started the book.

A dozen years before, mine had been named the best first book of fiction by an American writer, but the award had always seemed somewhat fluky to me. As I stood in the street outside the hospital, my career as a writer now seemed done. Was I a has-been or a never-was? The Buster Douglas of the literary world, I figured, a palooka who one time got lucky and knocked out the champ.

Who had I been kidding anyway?

———

All I had to read on the way home from the hospital was Toni Morrison's *Beloved*, which I was supposed to teach the following week in my contemporary novel class. But I couldn't read it. The train got more crowded as we moved through Manhattan, and all of it seemed so depressing to me. There was a pretty nurse riding home from the hospital across from me, and I watched a man try to flirt with her. He had aviator glasses, and his thick tawny hair was combed back 1970s style. His eyebrows rose on his expressive face, and his hands made broad gestures. She nodded demurely. She looked away. Both of them had hearts, and both their hearts were going to fail, and they were both busy pretending that this was not inevitable. I climbed back up the steps of the subway as the sun was setting in Brooklyn.

I decided to buy salmon for dinner. Then I went to the friendly fruit and vegetable market and bought my daughters the kind of mandarin oranges they love. At the wine shop, I got a bottle of vino verde, then another. I bought cut flowers, something I never do. I thought of a friend and neighbor, Tom, who had died earlier that year. He was a handsome man with a sympathetic face. He had two boys and a beautiful wife, and the family owned a shaggy dog. Throat cancer ate at him for a long time, through onset, treatment, remission, and then a wicked demise. I had seen Tom through his illness climbing up the subway steps, headed home after work, at the end of his day as an art director in Midtown, and I'd always felt sorry for him, and he'd always smiled. We exchanged pleasantries, and sometimes, "How are you?" came out of my mouth, and he would always say, "Fine," even when his throat didn't work anymore. His voice turned to a croak, then a high-pitched whisper, and then it was gone. As I made my way home with my flowers and fish and wine and oranges, I thought I understood a little better what his smile had meant, how much maybe he enjoyed those last months of life, savoring a stupid, ordinary thing like coming home from work.

Marcia was on her way back from a job in New Jersey. I made dinner—that was my happiness—I got to make dinner while my children did their homework and joked and complained. But after dinner my sense of happiness was gone. I had at the time an old rocking chair in my office, an orange-pleather faux-modernist thing that once belonged to my in-laws, and I was sitting in the rocking chair with my feet up, going through Facebook, clicking "Like" every time a picture of a baby appeared, when I drifted off, and I was neither awake nor asleep when suddenly the ICD fired. The computer flew up and down on my lap. I must have screamed.

"Are you all right?" called Marcia from the kitchen.

"I'm fine, I'm fine," I said, partly because that's what I always say and partly to hide my terror from my kids.

I went to the bedroom. Nothing like that had ever happened in all the time I had had my ICD—the shock out of nowhere. I lay down on my bed to clear my mind and think things out.

My heartbeat slowed. I felt it in my chest, like a tickle, like a seed planted there, the beginnings of arrhythmia. I tried to stand. I knew my heart was about to speed up. I had the idea that if I got up and moved, I'd stop the V-tach from happening. I put one foot on the ground and had the other one in the air when the shock came again. This time it sent me sprawling. I lay on the floor. I pounded the carpet.

"What do I do?" I asked Marcia.

"You call your doctor," she said.

Dan Zhee was quick to call back when I paged him. He knew right away what was wrong. He had reset the device so it would respond to arrhythmias slower than 150 bpm, but in doing so he'd somehow shrunk the time between the ICD sensing my arrhythmia and the machine giving me a shock. When the V-tach started, there wouldn't be any gentle pacing beats tonight. Right away, as soon as the V-tach commenced, the thing would slam me. And the V-tach seemed to happen every time I relaxed.

He recommended against a visit to an emergency room. It was past 9 p.m. I'd be there all night, he said. I'd never get any sleep. If I went to the ER, they'd probably admit me to the hospital. He knew that I would be more comfortable at home and asked what drugs I had in my medicine cabinet. I told him. He prescribed more than twice the dose of beta blockers I'd ever taken—both kinds that I had in the cabinet, Atenolol and Sotalol; we added a one-milligram pill of Ativan, and I'd already had three glasses of wine.

"That should do it," he said. "Get some sleep." He told me to meet him in his office first thing in the morning, and he would reprogram the device.

"You're not in any danger," he assured me.

I took the pills and went for a walk, figuring that it would take some time for the drugs to take effect. When I came home, the kids were in bed. I talked to Marcia. We tried to reassure each other that the night would go okay. I decided, as kind of test, to slow my heartbeat gradually. I sat on the living room floor and tried to meditate. It's something I normally don't do, but I am a reader of Buddhist self-help books, and I borrowed a mantra from Thich Nhat Hanh:

"present moment," on the in breath, "beautiful moment," on the out. I said that three times, then the device shocked me.

I got up. I went to the kitchen. When the shock hit, the pain was total; when the shock was gone, it left no trace. I felt like I was being tortured, but there were no torturers, just our cat in the dark kitchen with me.

I went to the bedroom. Marcia told me to just follow the doctor's advice. I was in no danger, he had said. I should try to get some rest. I changed into my pajamas. I flossed my teeth and brushed them. I lay down, and the sheets were cool, and Marcia's body was warm, and I picked up my book and turned on my reading lamp, but I couldn't read.

The memory of pain exists more in the body than it does in the mind. Even if there's no bruise, no mark, or no tenderness, the flesh seems to hold the ghost of the feeling. We had this idea, Marcia and I—the kind of idea people invent when their hopefulness makes them stupid—that I could lie back and relax, that even if I got shocked once more, maybe if I stayed quiet, maybe then I'd be able to sleep. Maybe after one shock, the V-tach might leave me alone.

But lying in bed that night, I flinched each time I felt my heart slow. I kept sitting up, lying down, and then sitting up again. I left the bedroom. It was not yet midnight. I looked at the couch. I thought maybe I could lie down there, relax, have tachycardia, get shocked, and then stay still, and then maybe I could sleep. But when the shock came, I was on my feet again, pacing the kitchen. I took out a sponge and some spray bottles, and I began to clean.

I sprayed down and wiped up the countertops, the table, and the cabinets. I swept the floor. I straightened up the living room, putting all of Lucy's schoolwork in one pile and Eliza's in another. I looked at the couch again. I was so tired. I decided to try it one more time: to lie down and see if I could get some sleep. As I lay there, I tried to unclench my muscles. I tried deep breathing. My mind would not be tricked into sleepiness, but my body got warm and heavy.

I felt waves of cold and warmth, pins and needles, the accumulated exhaustion of a winter without sleep. Don't move, I told myself. Don't move when the shock comes. And it was the repetition of those words, "don't move, don't move," and the fantasy that I would relax, that I would get shocked and somehow get quiet and sleep—it was the fantasy of sleep that set my mind adrift, and as soon as it did, as my mind departed consciousness, I felt the thunderclap in my chest, and it bounced me off the couch, onto my feet.

The philosopher Elaine Scarry writes, "Physical pain—unlike any other state of consciousness—has no referential content." Pain belongs only to the sufferer; it can't be communicated. As Scarry puts it, "To have great pain is to have certainty; to hear that another person has pain is to have doubt." Another person's pain exists beyond the human senses—something like ultraviolet light or high-frequency sound or dark matter, something you simply cannot perceive—and pain also exists beyond words. As Scarry has it, we can describe a "burning" pain, a "hammering" pain, a "stabbing" pain—we can use metaphors for the instruments that cause pain, but to express the actual pain itself, the best we can do are curses, screams, and ululation.

I made myself a cup of tea. I tried writing in my journal. I began to try to recount the whole day, the minutia of the day before I had seen the doctor, working at my desk in the morning, washing dishes, and listening to A Tribe Called Quest. Each time I finished a paragraph, I looked up at the clock. Each time I looked at the clock, the minute hand crawled. I regarded the couch the way a whipped dog looks at an electric cattle prod.

I'm telling this story as carefully as I can. I've tried to get it right—the times of night and each instance of shock. I wrote it all down in my journal the day after it happened. But I only wrote down six shocks, not the nine that my ICD recorded. These three missing shocks are maybe more eloquent than all my high-flown references or language. When the shocks hit, I was not myself.

I sipped my tea. I picked up my teacup and walked circles around the table. By 2 a.m. it felt hard to stand. I imagined myself in a puddle on the floor, getting shocked and shocked and shocked again, too whipped by the ICD even to be able to scream and wake up Marcia. I made a second cup of tea. I stood out on the stoop in bare feet and let the cold air wake me. I went back inside, and with nothing better to do, I tried to get some work done, which in this case meant reading *Beloved*. I sat up straight, pencil in hand for underlining. In my focus and my posture and fidgety note taking, I kept my pulse above sixty beats per minute.

In the book, Sethe had been raped and whipped, and the white rapists had sucked the milk from her breasts. She was making her way from slavery and the plantation through the Kentucky grass to the Ohio River, where freedom lay. Her feet were so swollen she could not walk, and her back was flayed and bleeding. The book didn't exactly cheer me up or distract me, but it did remind me where a balky defibrillator lay in the hierarchy of life's miseries.

I made a third cup of tea. Again, I stood outside on the stoop in the cold. I had the idea that I would get dressed and walk from home in Brooklyn to the hospital. If I took my time, I'd get there at 6 or 7 a.m. I'd pass through Times Square. I could stop in the East Village for coffee and breakfast. I could get to Washington Heights for another meal, and then wait for the ICD clinic to open. But what if I got V-tach as I walked, I worried, and the device started to shock me? I'd be lying on a deserted corner screaming, alone, in pain. How quickly my mind invented its pictures—strong me crossing the Brooklyn Bridge at night, vulnerable me on the sidewalk, shocked and spastic—like there was a fluttering switch in the back of the brain, running from fear to denial and back again.

I had an idea that maybe after 2 a.m. the V-tach wouldn't come anymore. The night before I had slept peacefully from about 2 to 6 a.m. I thought it was maybe worth trying again, lying on the couch one more time to see if I could get rest. I started sorting through papers, moving old magazines and homework and envelopes into the recycling. Each time I dropped the papers into the trash, I'd plan on finally going to the couch to lie down, to rest. But each time I looked at the couch, I'd start going through the cubbies and drawers and shelves of the living room, looking for more garbage. Soon enough the place was clean, and it was just me and the couch.

I lay down, terrified. My brain chirped hopefully that the period of arrhythmia was past. My body tensed and shuddered, waiting for the shock. I did something I've never done before: I sang myself lullabies. I thought the singing would keep my heart rate up, keep me from going into arrhythmia, and what came to my mind were the old songs I had sung for my daughters when they were infants. Pete Seeger does a version of "Froggy Went a Courting" with a sweet little refrain, and when all of Pete Seeger's words were gone, I started making up my own:

It would be great to get some rest, *ding-dang-dong go the wedding bells.*

With no ICD exploding in my chest, *ding-dang-dong go the wedding bells.*

After that, I tried the "Hobo's Lullaby," and when "Hobo's Lullaby" was done, I lay there in delicious sleep for I don't know how many minutes until the alarm clock in my chest blew me to smithereens.

It was by then nearly 5 a.m. I made myself coffee. At 5:30 a.m., the newspaper delivery banged on the front door. At 6 a.m. Marcia's alarm went off, and soon the kids were in the kitchen eating breakfast. I went down to take a shower and get dressed, trying my best around my daughters to pretend I was okay.

Elaine Scarry writes,

> It is the intense pain that destroys a person's self and world, a destruction experienced spatially as either the contraction of the universe down to the immediate vicinity of the body, or as the body swelling to fill the entire universe. Intense pain is also language-destroying: as the content of one's world disintegrates so the content of one's language disintegrates, so that which would express and project the self is robbed of its source and subject.

Pain, for Scarry, is an erasure of the individual. Nabokov writes something similar about Pnin's arrhythmia:

I do not know if it has ever been noted before that one of the main characteristics of life is discreteness. Unless a film of flesh envelops us, we die. Man exists only insofar as he is separated from his surroundings. The cranium is a space-traveler's helmet. Stay inside or you perish. Death is divestment, death is communion. It may be wonderful to mix with the landscape, but to do so is the end of the tender ego. The sensation poor Pnin experienced was something very like that divestment, that communion.

This is life on the borderland between the kingdoms Sontag describes: the constant threat of dissolution of the self, the constant attempt to assert that the self is somehow intact still.

Each experience of the ICD shock was obliterating, but as I showered, in the comfort of my own home, using my favorite tea-tree oil conditioner and the skin softening soap, as I flossed my teeth and brushed with baking soda toothpaste, as I looked in the bathroom mirror and saw the same face I always see, I filled that erasure with a story, the story I like to tell myself so often, that everything was fine, that everything was normal. I tried to rebuild the space suit of my ego and my space traveler's helmet. I put on a pair of jeans, a nice T-shirt, a new sweater I had bought at J.Crew. And with a cup of coffee and a shave, I at least appeared to be my everyday self.

The kids left for school. Marcia drove me to the hospital. I wasn't comfortable beside her. I sat up so my back didn't touch the seat. I shook my hands. I tapped my feet. I insisted that we stop for gas, and I got out to pump it. I was afraid of being still, afraid my heart would settle, afraid of V-tach and the shock. At the hospital, she dropped me off and went to park, and I made my way to the security desk—same place I had been before, not twenty-four hours earlier, when I had gone to visit Dr. Zhee's office. I showed my driver's license to the same guard who had been on duty yesterday. I told him where I had to go. I took the same elevator. I wore my long winter coat and good shoes.

I went to the electrophysiology clinic on the fourth floor. There's a familiar desk, and a waiting room, and an enormous TV. Usually, the seats are full of patients and their families, and because it's a city hospital, people can get loud and pushy, and while the nurses are kind and smiling, the secretaries develop a kind of bureaucratic hard shell. But there was no one there when I arrived. The television was on. Marcia came and sat down in the plastic chairs and began to do the crossword puzzle. I paced up and down the hall, afraid to rest. It wasn't long before Dan Zhee came, and when he saw me, he smiled.

"You're all right!" he said.

"I'm fine," I told him.

"YOU ARE NOT!" said Marcia. And she told him how many times I'd been shocked.

Dan rushed me to an examining room. I refused to sit on the examining table—I was afraid if I sat my heart would slow.

He interrogated the device using his big suitcase-sized laptop and the magnifying-glass-shaped wand that rested over the lump in my chest. He could not have been more honest or more apologetic. He corrected the programming on the device, and I looked at the computer screen as if I could help.

"Are you sure you fixed it?" I asked.

He was sure, he said. He bumped up the schedule for my ablation. He walked me to the waiting room, apologizing all the way.

As we said good-bye, I said, "I accept your apology."

He looked at me seriously. "I'm really, really sorry," he said.

The next time I saw Dan Zhee, he zapped the hell out of my arrhythmia, and my heartbeat has held steady ever since.

42.

THAT WAS WHEN I started to write this book. I joined the Adult Congenital Heart Association and flew to Orlando to the ACHA convention, where I met people with conditions similar to my own. And simultaneously, I learned that my pulmonary valve, the one implanted in 1999, had worn out and that I was in need of a replacement. It was my year of reckoning.

Amid the wreckage of another failed novel, I still got up every morning to work. I was writing more and more about my heart, writing scraps and memories and journal entries. I became obsessed with Nicolaus Steno. As I read and reread the biographies, Steno's life seemed to me a fable with a moral I could not fathom, something about how to face and how not to face mortality—something about the intersection of ontology and death. Steno was willing to see what no one else could see, to do what no one else would do, but despite his brilliance and unconventionality and genius, he was constantly thrown up against the limits of the comprehensible, the borders of the flesh and the mind, and these limits undid him.

It was the spring after Donald Trump's election that I flew south to Orlando to meet the other members of the Adult Congenital Heart Association. By that time, I already knew my heart valve had to be replaced, and I wasn't sure when I was feeling or imagining my symptoms of weakness and exhaustion. I still looked and acted more or less healthy. Dr. Rosenbaum said I was in no immediate danger. The procedure for replacement had been scheduled. But I couldn't tell if I was well or sick or somewhere in between.

I was looking around for a cabstand in the Orlando airport, when I leaned on the podium marked "Information" and somehow lost my balance. I thought something had shifted inside me again, an arrhythmia, an embolism. But then I realized that the podium was on wheels. It had slid out from underneath me.

Everyone was wearing a sweatshirt in the frosty air conditioning. Outside it was so hot and humid that I could hardly stand. The shuttle to the conference hotel drove past glittering buildings, highway dividers, and swamps, a landscape that brought to mind Norman Mailer's 1968 description of Miami Beach: "Over hundreds, then thousands of acres, white sidewalks and white buildings covered the earth where the jungle had been. Is it so dissimilar from covering your poor pubic hair with adhesive tape for fifty years?" Fifty more years had passed, more adhesive tape had been applied, and all Florida went on pretending that it was perfectly comfortable. President Trump had pulled out of the Paris Climate Accords. My body, the scenery, the nation to which I belonged, all of us were powered by scientific technology, and all of us pretended busily that the scientific facts were unreal.

Then I was in the big anonymous hotel ballroom, facing it, several hundred patients with identification tags hanging around their necks. I was approached by a short, friendly man in an NPR T-shirt.

"Chris Halverson," he said, reaching out his hand. "Six open-heart surgeries. Pulmonary atresia with VSD."

"Gabe Brownstein," I replied. "Tetralogy of Fallot. Two open-heart surgeries, an ICD, a valve replacement scheduled for the summer."

We formed into little groups, everyone naming their defect and surgeries. We transitioned easily into recitations and comparisons: about our doctors and our symptoms and our fears and our devices. People laughed, describing times they'd collapsed in movie theaters or been rushed into operating rooms with their aortas rupturing.

Danny Spandau and I spent hours together, in the bar, over meals, at the pool. People began to ask if we were brothers, two Jewish guys, ten years apart, both living with repaired tetralogy of Fallot. He introduced me to Meg Balke and Melissa Hartman, two Florida ACHA members who had helped him and supported him emotionally while he went through his valve replacement surgery. In the bar I met Belen Altuve Blanton, who showed me her blue fingers and made jokes about her cyanosis.

I met people whose lives have been profoundly affected by their heart defects. There was a young woman from Grand Rapids, Michigan, a beauty with tiny, childish features and hypnotic gray eyes. But the quality of her gaze betrayed her disability. She had been born at home, without a doctor's care, and her septal defect had led to an embolism, which led to a stroke that damaged her brain. She could not read or write or drive. She was such a small-town girl—she spoke of the two heart hospitals in Grand Rapids as if I would be familiar with both. She was rooming in the hotel with a woman about her age, and her roommate had been born with Shone's disease, a defect of the aorta. At the conference they were a pair of giggling young beauties who seemed to have known each other all their lives. Both had spent their summers at camps for children with heart disease. They both said it was wonderful for kids with scars on their chests to be around other kids with scars on their chests, especially when they were swimming, to have their conditions normalized.

One day over lunch I met a woman named Amanda who was born with a rare genetic disorder, chromosome 18p deletion, which occurs in only 1 in 6,000 live births, and of those babies, only 9 percent suffer from a heart defect. Amanda was short, her big glasses perched on her little nose. She had problems with her eyes, with her hearing. She had scoliosis and a repaired harelip. She had been through so, so much: four heart surgeries in a single year, recently, and then a bloodstream infection that required cutting out part of her lung and kept her hospitalized for weeks.

"Oh, man, that was terrible," said Amanda, shaking her head, and shaking off her cruddy luck. Her style was casual, her attitude adorable, and her husband followed her like a faithful hound.

Amanda's cardiologist, Karen Stout, hugged her in the bar. "I love her," they said to me, almost simultaneously. I saw Marlon Rosenbaum get a little tipsy, and met Dr. Doug Moodie, a big man with a big voice, a senior cardiologist from Texas, who talked to me for a long time about Denton Cooley, whom he'd known well.

I met bereaved parents. There was a couple whose son didn't know he had a heart defect until he collapsed running his third marathon—he'd survived, but it had left them all shaken. There was a woman who, when I told her my surgeon was Jim Malm, gasped, and tears filled her eyes.

"I usually say I have just one daughter with a heart defect," she said, but the truth was she had had two. One was alive, the other was gone, and the child she had lost had been operated on by Jim Malm. Her daughter had survived the surgery—she had lived to her early twenties—but one weekend in the Hamptons, she overdid it: too much sun, too much drink, too many drugs, and she collapsed. I couldn't ask what part her daughter's heart defect played in her death. I could only say how sorry I was.

I took a nap every afternoon, and I wondered, as I always do, how much my naps were due to my decreasing heart function and how much they were due to the demands of travel and conventioneering. In the mornings I did laps in the swimming pool, and tired quickly, and got anxious about my heart rate and my ICD, and I was glad I didn't get shocked in the water.

A panel led by Dr. Curt Daniels of Ohio State University discussed the certification of adult congenital heart centers, a process Daniels was overseeing whereby hospitals could demonstrate their capacity to appropriately treat adults with congenital heart defects—that the hospital had the necessary staff, equipment, and expertise. The certification would allow patients to know where to go to get the proper care.

One of the doctors' big concerns was collection of data over time and lack of information about patients. The United States had once been the world's leader in the development of heart surgery and cardiological care but was now falling behind. In Canada, in Germany, and in the United Kingdom, national health-care systems allowed for organized data collection, whereas in the United States data collection was ad hoc, center by center. Huge numbers of adult congenital heart patients in the United States—about 90 percent of us, according to the ACHA—were lost to care. Without knowing the course of their patients' lives, doctors could not figure out how to treat them.

Mark Roeder, the president and CEO of the Adult Congenital Heart Association, welcomed us all. Before coming to ACHA, he had worked for the National Multiple Sclerosis Society and the Susan G. Komen Breast Cancer Foundation. His mission, as he saw it, was to make the condition—adult congenital heart defects—known to the world and to spur research and data collection.

"We are the number one birth defect," he told the assembly. His goal was to achieve a national profile, to establish a brand. There were now approximately 2.5 million of us in the country. More and more of us were surviving heart surgery and living to middle and old age. We were a new kind of people, and we wanted to be recognized and taken care of. The phrase "adult congenital heart disease" should not be so obscure. Patients should be able to say it, Mark Roeder said, and be understood. Later, privately, he explained how dire the situation was—how poorly the United States tracked its congenital heart disease patients, how the statistics were all estimates, good data and ratios from Canada projected onto the vast US population, where data collection wasn't as systematic. And it was so hard to publicize: "'Congenital' is such a misunderstood word," Roeder said.

At the end of the weekend, there was a big dance. Danny Spandau had a white jacket and confident, restrained moves. Big Doug Moodie wore a double-breasted suit and, though he was in his mid-seventies, got down to J. Cole. I was sitting with Jenny—the woman who had had recent heart transplant surgery, whose defibrillator had once shocked her ninety-eight times in a single half hour. She looked at Dr. Moodie and mentioned that when she was an infant, her father had taken her to Texas, and there Dr. Moodie had said it might be right to give up hope, that it was unlikely Jenny would survive that much longer. She told this story without a trace of bitterness. The music changed. It was "Uptown Funk" by Bruno Mars. She wanted to get on the dance floor. I went with her. Jenny was wearing a hippie skirt, and she threw her blonde hair around like a freak flag.

Oh, yeah, she told me, she'd always been a good dancer.

43.

ON THE PLANE back from Orlando, I watched *Logan*, the Hugh Jackman X-Men movie—a contemporary retelling of the Frankenstein story, with fewer epistolary digressions and more violent chase scenes than in Mary Shelley's nineteenth-century novel. I loved it. The Frankenstein doctor is Zander Rice, played by the British actor Richard E. Grant. He works for a company called Transgen, which is breeding superpowered mutant children in test tubes and raising them to be deadly weapons. The children are chased by tanks, and there are flashbacks to the prison-like hospital in which they were raised. A thuggish henchman with a cyborg arm uses a file folder to blow out candles on a birthday cake. Toward the end of the movie, I got so excited, my left elbow kept spazzing out and hitting the armrest of the seat of the guy sitting next to me—a big guy whom I'd seen screaming into his cellphone when we were getting ready to board the plane. But he was very understanding.

"That's a good movie," he said.

For me, the appeal was visceral. Coming back from the conference, I could see how the movie played into my fantasies. The children in the hospital weren't sick. They were superpowered mutants. The doctors were evil and scary, sticking the kids with needles and keeping track of them on charts. The big and faceless hospital was a jail. And then the hero daddy appeared in the person of handsome and dissolute Hugh Jackman, and he broke the kids out of the hospital, and freed them from their captors, and took them to a paradise mountain refuge where they could live without doctors and just be themselves. It was like the filmmakers had heard Doron Weber's urgent ICU prayer—"D-man, let's bust out of this joint and go home!"—and they had spun from it an action adventure cartoon.

The plane landed. Back in New York, President Trump was on the radio, on TV, in the newspapers, inveighing against Obamacare. He promised a new kind of health-care system that would be "great" and "tremendous." Briefly, he admitted his willful incomprehension—"Who knew health care could be so complicated?"—and the national conversation revealed the extent of our American terror and denial. It's not just me. We all live in the borderland between health and sickness, and we all don't want to talk about it. We all depend on our doctors, but we all want to pretend we're fine and free.

A few months after I came back from Orlando, I had brunch in Brooklyn with five old friends. In a sunny row house backyard, we gossiped, recommended movies, and bitched about politics. Two little boys bounced balls. Two girls played with electronic devices. One of my friends, in town from California, had just been through breast cancer treatments. After chemo and a double mastectomy, she'd had silicone implants put in, and her hair had grown back glossy and brown. She looked fantastic. She was working again, producing films and traveling. A second friend, a financial editor, was living with multiple sclerosis, and he had to take a shot of Avonex each week, but he was still studying martial arts and going to the gym daily and was planning a backpacking trip for the fall. A third, a lawyer, had just gone through complex surgery on her sinuses, while her husband, an architect, had recently realized why he was a foot shorter than his brothers and why he'd spent his life farting. An endoscopy revealed the state of his duodenum, and he'd been diagnosed with celiac disease. After a change of diet, his energy levels were up, and his skin had never looked better. The fifth friend, whose medical history I knew least, was an actor and had recently auditioned for a Cialis ad in which he had to chop a log and bring it to his ladylove by the fire.

"You don't have to do much with this one," the director told him. "It kind of sells itself."

None of us mentioned our health or medications except in the most vague and conventional ways: "How you doing?" and "You look great!" Our conditions were invisible and unmentionable, as was our children's dependence on medicine.

My daughter, strong and suntanned after spending her summer vacation as a volunteer clearing hiking trails on mountains, told us all the silly jokes that she had learned in the woods. She was beautiful and brilliant, and I was bursting with pride. But Lucy was born prematurely and spent the first days of her life in a neonatal intensive care unit. (The birth was traumatic; I made the mistake of peeking into a room and seeing an orderly mopping up my wife's blood.) In her early years, Lucy was plagued with severe ear infections. As a toddler, she had to have an operation to take the pressure off her eardrums so she wouldn't lose her hearing. Before she went to grade school, she had a second outpatient surgery to repair a hernia in her thigh. In elementary school she got strep throat seven times and once, in the countryside, contracted a MRSA infection. Summer was ending, we had made sure her vaccinations were up to date, and she was getting ready to go back to school, an A student, a competitive debater studying robotics. If you'd asked me, was she healthy, I'd say absolutely. I'd say that she had never contracted a serious illness in her life.

Maybe what Ali Zaidi said of congenital heart patients is true of all of us. We no longer know what "healthy" means—we no longer know health as a state separate from medicine. If the folks in that Brooklyn backyard party had lived their lives in the arcadia imagined at the end of *Logan*, a place in the mountains away from all doctors and their interfering ways, we wouldn't have done very well.

No one wants to be a patient. Historically speaking, people began denying the value of scientific medicine at about the same moment that scientific medicine began saving lives. When Joseph Lister came to the United States, he faced tremendous resistance among physicians who did not want to believe his ideas about germ theory, antiseptics, and sepsis. His patients, too, liked to believe they didn't depend on him, even after he cured them. Perhaps Lister's most famous patient, William Earnest Hemley, wrote the poem "Invictus" right after Lister saved his life in a series of grueling and daring surgeries. After the operations were over, Hemley burst forth with his famous work, words quoted variously by Nelson Mandela and Timothy McVeigh: "I am the master of my fate / I am the captain of my soul."

We like to think we're in control. We like to believe that we are independent. That's how we tell stories of medicine, how John McCain "lost his battle" against cancer or how Jonas Salk "triumphed over" polio, as if our fates were captained by our own capable hands. But that's not true. We don't go it alone. We depend on each other, we depend on doctors, and this interdependence makes our lives possible and good. At the ACHA conference and elsewhere, I've heard heart patients described as "heart heroes" and "heart warriors," but my informal conversations indicate that most adult congenital heart patients dislike those terms. Experience has taught us. We are ordinary people with extraordinary luck, beneficiaries of splendid technology.

No one person, no one group bequeathed us this technology. If you consider all the women and men who made modern cardiology possible, the doctors and patients, the nurses and technicians, the people who volunteered and donated to charitable causes, the ones who paid taxes, the politicians and government bureaucrats who allocated funds, the device and pharmaceutical manufacturers, and the brave families of the kids who underwent early heart surgeries, you get a mass movement that includes the widest range of citizens. Pediatric cardiology is something that our parents' and grandparents' generation bestowed on us and something that their parents and grandparents could not have imagined. We should accept this and be grateful for it.

When my mother was a kid, she got scarlet fever. It was the 1940s. Antibiotics were not available. The strep infection in my mom's throat spread to her chest. Her parents were terrified that she would grow up crippled or worse. This kind of terror was

ordinary life, but then the US government teamed with the Bradley Polytechnic Institute in Peoria to mass-produce penicillin, and
now ordinary life is antibiotics. Each year in elementary school,
my kids got strep. They got their throats swabbed, they went to
the doctor, and they got better. The rest of the kids in school got
the same treatment, and no one thought about it much—that
they were all being treated, prophylactically, for pediatric heart
disease.

We're all in the Open Heart Club now. We all depend on our
doctors. My dependence on medicine may seem extreme, but really
it's exemplary. When my dad was in med school in the early 1960s,
congenital heart disease was one of the top ten causes of death in
this country. Now 85 percent of children with heart defects survive.
We thrive. We're all over the place. Whether or not you choose
to believe it, you are the beneficiary of the same technology that
saved us. Every time a pregnant woman gets a sonogram, the doctors check for signs of possible heart defects. In every hospital in
every industrialized country, there are protocols in place for every
birth, operating rooms set aside, ambulance drivers at the ready,
and surgeons waiting to be paged. Were you or your child born in
a hospital in the industrialized world in the last half century? Well,
then, all of this was there, waiting for you. Welcome to the club.

I know. If invitations were sent out, very few people would
RSVP. No one likes to see your children being stuck by needles.
People freak out at the thought of pills and vaccines, let alone
scalpels and heart-lung machines. I understand. I have lived my life
in a similar state of denial. It's how most of the people around me
live. Well-insured, lucky, and cushioned from sickness, we do our
jobs and dance at weddings and make love to our spouses and yell
at our children as if the next trip to the hospital isn't just around
the corner. But we're kidding ourselves, and our state of denial is
evident in the way we talk.

"Health care" is a fudge word. The combo of "health" and
"care" seems designed by marketers so that we never have to say
the words "sickness" or "medicine." "Health care" blurs the distinc-
tion between the care we give ourselves—like exercise and diet—

and the necessary care we get from doctors. The phrase "health insurance," too, is self-deceiving. The only thing we can be sure of regarding our health is that it won't last. Our political language is a language of denial, constructed so we never have to speak the words that scare us.

For my parents' and grandparents' generations, the battle against disease was a national cause. When, on April 12, 1955, Jonas Salk's polio vaccine was proven to be successful, the whole country celebrated: "More than a scientific achievement, the vaccine was a folk victory," wrote Salk's biographer, Richard Carter. "People observed moments of silence, rang bells, honked horns, blew factory whistles, fired salutes, kept their traffic lights red in brief periods of tribute, took the rest of the day off, closed their schools or convoked fervid assemblies therein, drank toasts, hugged children, attended church, smiled at strangers, forgave enemies." We have lost that sense of urgency.

I live a charmed life, as do my friends with their Brooklyn row houses and my tenured colleagues at work, but just outside this circle live my neighbors less fortunate than I, slipping from the borderlands into the kingdom of the sick. There's an absence in my book, a blank spot. Though Danny Spandau and Bridgette Ratliff and Belen Altuve Blanton and Alan Sabal all fell out of care for years or decades, they were all brought back under the umbrella of medicine. For every patient whose story I've told, there are nine others out there who are not under the care of the appropriate doctor, people who don't have insurance or money, people who live too far from an adult congenital heart center, and people who don't believe they're sick. Some of them are doing fine. Others have leaky valves and swelling ventricles. Some ignore their terrifying arrhythmias. Others are in heart failure, just wishing it away. I spoke to an Israeli cardiologist who said that the divide in New York City wasn't that different from the divide in her home country. There are people with full citizenship in the medical world, well-insured people like me, with healthy heart muscle, and then there are people whose citizenship in the world of health is less secure, whose hearts are falling apart.

"Our patients are the underdog," said Mark Roeder, president of the ACHA. "American medicine is complicated. The average citizen is really challenged to negotiate the process on their own. There are a lot of well-intentioned and very smart people trying to work to change the machine that's in place—but," he held his breath for a bit—"it's a long, *long* process."

The moral problem isn't complicated. We have inherited the magic medicine that gives us the power to rescue children from death, and we have inherited the wealth to pay for it, greater wealth and more effective medicine than ever known in the history of the world. If we choose not to share our magic medicine with our neighbors, if we leave them on their own and make them mortgage their homes to pay for their children's surgeries (as many parents in the United States are forced to do), then we are doing evil. We might begin to repair this evil by being honest with ourselves, by accepting the fact of our good fortune.

In *Logan*, physicians and government officials are portrayed as dark figures engaged in a frightening conspiracy to strip us of our humanity, and I've seen a lot of movies and TV shows that run with that same idea, evil doctors in scary, faceless conspiracies to experiment mercilessly on innocent human lives, stripping people of their individuality. Doctors are spooky, doctors are powerful, and—maybe because we're so dependent on them—we continue to view them with suspicion. But if doctors and government officials have been engaged in any faceless conspiracy, it's been one in which, over decades, they have worked together ceaselessly, and with tremendous effect, to make our lives longer, healthier, and more productive. Abbott, Taussig, Thomas, Blalock, Malm, Swift, Griffiths, Freed, Rosenbaum, Zaidi, Zhee, and Farhat: all of them are a small part of a massive, complex universe of healers who have made all our lives possible.

The enemies of these healers are many. There are terrible diseases and craven greedy supervillains yearning to make money off our suffering. But one important adversary that doctors face is simple denial, the desire to pretend that it is because of our own intrinsic good qualities that we are healthy, to pretend that we do not depend on medicine, that our neighbors are not vulnerable, and that we cannot help our fellow citizens.

Medicine, like climate change, is a difficult subject narratively and politically for Americans because the solutions lie less in individual struggles and rights and more in collective obligations and responsibilities. When it comes to medicine, we cannot rely on our gut feelings, our good habits, our individual strength, and our hopes and prayers. We need to rely on what the experts tell us— experts, in this case, being our doctors. We are not alone. We must love one another or die.

44.

JULY CAME, AND so did my valve replacement. I woke up early and anxious. The bedroom was dark. I crept out of bed as quietly as I could, but I woke Marcia before I reached the bedroom door.

"Big day," she said, from under the sheets.

"Excited for it?" I asked her.

"Oh, yeah."

I showered while she was up in the kitchen, having breakfast. I put on a new linen shirt and a pair of cotton pants. Some people show up for their surgeries in fanny packs, sweatpants, and flip-flops, but not me. Hospitals are not resorts; the patient is not a guest. If you don't assert yourself in the hospital, you can get treated like a piece of meat. So I dressed for success, and I lay on the bed until Marcia knocked on the bedroom door.

"Come on, buddy," she said. "Time to go."

It was ninety degrees out. Check-in was at 8 a.m. The app on her phone predicted a thirty-seven-minute drive to the hospital. I gathered my stuff: noise-cancelling headphones, phone for music, and a novel by Elmore Leonard. I took the necessary cards from my wallet, and then I scribbled my prescribed doses of medicine on an index card. I folded the index card around my health insurance ID, my Amex card, and the ID for my implanted defibrillator. I wrapped the whole thing in a rubber band.

Outside it was Brooklyn on a summer morning, people heading to work, carrying iced coffees and sweating, others heading back home from the park with their dogs and babies. Marcia pulled up in front with the car. Here is one of the many small sticking points in our marriage: she likes to use the Waze app and avoid traffic, while I would rather risk a traffic jam than listen to that computerized voice. The rule is, the driver gets to choose, but I was hungry and hadn't had coffee, and I was very, very, very grouchy. I complained. I didn't want to hear that fucking Waze lady voice. Marcia futzed with her phone and ignored me.

"Just drive," I said.

"Just wait," said Marcia. She programmed in the hospital address.

The night before we had gone out to dinner, to a new place we'd discovered, Dawa, in Woodside, Queens. It was clean and pretty, a forty-minute drive from our house. The owners were father and daughter. He made Mongolian food; she made contemporary farm-to-table. The restaurant felt like some dream of New York City that managed to gentrify without violating a neighborhood, and the meat pies were amazing, and so was the squash stew with buckwheat pancakes. We were going to head back, we told each other, and in the car we talked about which friends we'd bring.

The robot lady told Marcia to turn left on 9th Street and routed us through the Battery Tunnel and around the south end of Manhattan up toward the FDR Drive. We turned on the radio expecting headlines about Trump, the Charlottesville Nazi march, and congressional dysfunction, but that morning's news was a transit breakdown at Penn Station. Reporters described crowds packed into the subways. As we cruised the highway, I thought how happy I was not to be in those tunnels underground. Then I remembered where I was headed. We pulled up to the hospital. Marcia wanted to drop me off in the little roundabout they have for patients. I insisted on getting off in the street.

"Whatever," she sighed.

I hopped into the middle of traffic—a New Yorker never feels healthier than when stepping in front of an on-coming van—and marched to the hospital's front door. The guard at the desk asked if I knew my way. I nodded. The only wrong turn you can make is labeled in big letters: HEART TRANSPLANT.

In 1999, to put in a new pulmonary valve, they had to crack my chest and carve into my heart. In 2017, the new valve would slide in via catheter, without any cutting into my thorax or myocardium. The valve would travel in through my thigh, through a puncture wound wide as a ballpoint pen. The catheter would travel up through my abdominal pulmonary vein, right into my heart.

In *The Heart Healers*, published in 2015, James Forrester of Cedars-Sinai calls watching a valve replacement via catheter "the single most jaw-dropping, mind-boggling event in my career in cardiology." The first ever was performed on the aortic valve in London in 2000. The first aortic valve replacement in the United States had happened in 2007. Pulmonary valve replacement via catheter was more complicated, not experimental but not commonplace. At the ACHA conference, a month before the procedure, I went to a physicians' panel in which experts explained the operation to cardiologists and surgeons unfamiliar with the job. "This is a hard thing," said Dr. C. Huie Lin, director of the Houston Methodist Adult Congenital Heart Program. "Probably everyone shouldn't jump into it right away." Dr. Jamil Aboulhosn of UCLA warned attendees that "taking it to the pulmonary position is really demanding." He described pushing and pulling the catheter through the passages of the heart, with the heart resisting and going into arrhythmia.

Again, I had been lucky. My pig valve had lasted longer than expected, which turned out to be just long enough that now doctors could save me without open-heart surgery.

Marlon Rosenbaum had told me that my heart valve was failing in the fall, after I had gone hiking in the White Mountains, wondering as I climbed if my lethargy was a result of aging or something more serious. I had met my new surgeon, Dr. Alejandro Torres, in October, in his office in the old Babies Hospital building, the same building where my parents had met Jim Malm in 1966. Dr. Torres was about my age, very thin and very friendly, wearing an orange pullover. He had a charming Argentine accent and sunken eyes, and he smiled often as he described the valves and catheter delivery systems that were available.

There was one brand, the Melody Valve, that might not be large enough for the opening of my valve. There was another, Edwards Sapien II, whose delivery system might be too stiff to maneuver through the thicket of my scarred heart. Dr. Torres didn't seem particularly satisfied with either.

I said, "But if it doesn't work, we just try again, right?"

Dr. Torres smiles a lot, but he didn't smile when he said, "No." If it didn't work, that would mean open-heart surgery.

I do not think I can express to you how much I wanted to avoid undergoing open-heart surgery again. Beyond the physical and emotional trauma of having my body split in half, there was the danger: heart muscle can take only so much cutting and recutting. Each successive operation is significantly riskier. I braced myself for the procedure, hopeful and frightened, and we scheduled a date for January. Then, in December, Dr. Torres called me.

Edwards Pharmaceuticals had announced that its new valve, the Edwards Sapien III, would undergo an FDA trial for catheter valve replacement in the pulmonary position. Dr. Torres thought this product would be perfect in my case and better than any on the market—a big-enough valve, a flexible-enough delivery system—and so I agreed to join the trial. We got ready to set a date as soon as we heard back from Edwards. But the trial never started. Month after month, Dr. Torres and I waited. All through the winter and spring, as I finished my classes, as I wrote the proposal for this book, as I went to the ACHA conference, he and I were exchanging frustrated emails.

More and more, I worried about arrhythmias coming back, and more and more, I felt myself getting tired. In the mornings I wrote and read about heart surgery and about Nicolaus Steno, and in the daytime I tried to hold it all together, to pretend I was okay. In March, one day, I could take it no more and confessed to my brother Ezra that I was terribly frightened. He said, "Of course you are, Gabe, it's heart surgery. It's scary." I explained to him that it wasn't the procedure that frightened me; it was the waiting.

He was a little flummoxed by this. "So now you want to have heart surgery?"

Yes. My fear wasn't the doctors anymore. Now it was my heart.

Then in May, I got a call from Dr. Torres. Edwards Pharmaceuticals was not going to run a trial for the Sapien III valve replacement in the pulmonary position. The valve Dr. Torres wanted to use was not going to be FDA approved for my heart. Still, he had no doubt: this was the valve and delivery system he wanted. This was the one most likely to save me from having to undergo open-heart surgery. So subtly at first that I didn't understand his drift, Dr. Torres floated the possibility of off-label use of the Sapien III and its Commander delivery system.

The biggest risk of going forward, he said when I finally understood him, was that I would get stuck with the costs. That could mean the price of the valve, about $30,000, or the price of the whole procedure—the cath lab, anesthesiologist, nurses, the whole shebang, about half a million dollars total. I talked it over with Marlon Rosenbaum. In the end it didn't seem much of a choice. If the insurance company refused coverage, I'd have a good argument, Marlon said: catheter replacement was much cheaper and much safer than open-heart surgery, and I was only following my doctor's advice. If I didn't use the right valve, it seemed clear, I'd be putting myself at unnecessary risk.

———

In the waiting room of the cath lab, curved, frosted windows looked out over Riverside Park and the Hudson River. Flat-screen TVs played CNN. The receptionist sat at a big, round desk in the front, banked by a couple of computers. My sharp dressing did me no good. She didn't even say hello.

"You been here before?"

I told her yes.

"So the address and insurance haven't changed?"

I offered her the insurance card, but she didn't need it. She raised her chin and looked through her glasses at the computer screen. She squinted. She sighed, raised her eyebrows, and marked something down on a piece of paper. She swiveled in her chair and flourished her paperwork, this whole ballet of irritation performed without a glance or a word my way. There were forms for me to sign, first on paper, then on a tablet computer.

"No," she said, "you gotta touch with the tip of the pen or else it don't notice. Not like that! Press hard and you're gonna break my pen. You wanna read it or just sign it?"

I finished my business and handed the tablet back.

A form came out of her printer. "Give me your wrist," she said.

"Left or right?"

"It don't matter."

She might have been forty; she might have been sixty. Her hair was dyed black. Her blouse had a big collar. Her necklaces were gold. Was she Hispanic or Italian or Jewish or Greek, from the Bronx or Queens or Westchester? She was the troll at the bridge. From her printout she peeled off a sticker, and she wrapped the sticker around my wrist, and the sticker turned into a bracelet. With a wand, she scanned my new barcode, and *alakazam*, I was a patient again.

"You could wait over there."

Marcia snuck up behind me and caressed my neck. I jumped like I'd been bit. She laughed and apologized. She offered me a section of the *Times*, but I couldn't stand to read it. I couldn't keep up conversation either. I couldn't tolerate the wait. I was itching, itching for them to call out my name, but when the young woman with the clipboard finally said, "Gabriel Brownstein," I wished she hadn't.

I kissed Marcia. I walked through the swinging door, past a secretarial desk. There was Dr. Torres in a checked Brooks Brothers shirt.

"Good to finally see you," we said simultaneously—then we laughed, and I was led away.

The cath lab at New York–Presbyterian is a hive of snaking, circular hallways, with dozens of alcoves for patients. Each patient alcove has the standard equipment: hospital bed, heart monitor, blood pressure cuff, television screen, gloves dispenser, waste disposal, and defibrillator paddles, all in shades of beige.

"Have you been with us before?" my hostess asked.

"Oh, yes," I said. "Frequent flier."

I took off my clothes and changed into the hospital gown. I slipped under the sheets. The nurses began attaching me to all my familiar wires and monitors. Marcia showed up and tried to distract me. She talked about Lucy, whom I had dropped off just a few days before in the Berkshire Mountains in Massachusetts. She talked about Eliza at my parents' house. She told funny stories about the people she worked with, and she reminded me that I was easily the hottest patient in the cath lab. A stylish woman passed on her way to visit a loved one.

Marcia said, "You think I could pull off a maxi-dress?"

We got to know the people who worked on the floor. There was the sullen, self-involved nurse who complained about her plantar fasciitis as she hooked me up to the heart monitor's wires. There was a young guy, transferring over from ER to cardiology, curly haired and muscular, macho and sweet. He kept screwing up and had to take my blood samples twice because he'd mislabeled the first vials.

"You're braver than I am." He shook his head. "I could never do what you're doing."

I didn't know how to respond. I wasn't *doing* anything.

The nurse with the mustache was a comedian. He shook his finger at Marcia, "I hear there's a troublemaker here!" But he was the one who fixed the heart monitor when it was beeping annoyingly, and he showed the trainee from ER how to turn off my ICD and how to wrap the icy defibrillator patches around my shaven sides.

A young physician's assistant read cautiously to me from a script. "Okay, Mr. Brownstein, I want to make sure you understand?" She wore lip gloss and spoke in questions. "The risks include bleeding and infection and the risks of any surgical procedure, okay, Mr. Brownstein? And there's a risk of serious injury?" She squinched her face. "Also death?"

Dr. Torres stopped by in his scrubs.

"You got the right valve." I tried to joke with him. "So, it's all going to go perfectly, right?"

His short hair was on end. His narrow face didn't smile. His sunken eyes were dead serious. "It's the best technology we have," he said. He put his hand on my shoulder, and he left.

"Shit." I turned to Marcia. "He didn't say it was going to work."

"Gabriel," she said, "no doctor is going to promise you that."

We held hands. She started to thumb wrestle me. She won. I said she'd cheated. "No," said the trainee nurse from ER, "her moves are totally legit." Then it was time.

There's something very cinematic about the view from the rolling bed through the hospital corridors, like your eyes are the camera and the gurney a dolly. All the wires from your monitors have been connected to a telemetry box—a kind of Star Trek tricorder—and it rides along with you, and as they push you down the corridor, the nurses stop teasing and cracking wise.

In the cold cath lab, I refused assistance as always as I slid from my bed to the operating table, trying not to seem too awkward and vulnerable in my hospital gown and with all my wires and stickers trailing off me. The nurses took the wires from my telemetry box and connected them to the monitors all around. Fluoroscopy cameras and big black-and-white flat-screens hung above to capture and display the catheter's progress into my heart.

"How much do you weigh?" asked the hipster anesthesiologist, scribbling down numbers in a Moleskine notebook.

The nurse in training said, "I'm going to shave your groin."

I heard the buzz. The hospital gown was less than a fig leaf now, just a puddle of cloth on my abdomen. I felt my oncoming death, just for a second—the grip of fear, the release of prayer—and as I lay there, my prayers shifted from myself to my children. I had had fifty good years. If I died now, it would be no great tragedy. Marcia was strong. She would be okay. I counted money: the value of the house, and my retirement account, and the life insurance from work, and her parents would help with college tuition. I asked God to bless my daughters as another nurse put in a new needle, this one into my right wrist. Then I was gone.

———

My heartbeat was displayed on electronic monitors, my groin was shaved, and the anesthetic had shut down my brain. The nurse put a pillow under my head. An intern used a stainless steel blade to pry open my mouth. He levered open my jaw, and when he got a clear view of my larynx, he slid in the oxygen tube. I would no longer be breathing on my own.

Dr. Torres and his team made an incision on the left side of my groin, slicing into the flesh and then cutting down the femoral artery. They slid the guide wire in. Over this wire, they slide their first catheter, all the way up the abdominal aorta, over the aortic arch, alongside the leads of my disabled implanted defibrillator, against the flow of blood, through the aortic valve and into my left ventricle. This catheter would stay there throughout the procedure to monitor internal blood pressure, with particular attention paid to the coronary arteries. If Dr. Torres was not careful, the procedure could put pressure on the coronary arteries and squeeze them shut, depriving the heart of oxygen and, potentially, killing me. So he wanted to be careful.

Once that first catheter was in place, Torres's team began to work on the right side of my groin. They cut an incision there, into the femoral vein, and slid a wire up all the way into the pulmonary vein, and up my torso and into my heart, so the far end of this catheter's wire rested against the wall of my right ventricle. This wire would act as a pacemaker during the procedure to make sure that my heart kept beating.

A second wire was slid into the femoral vein alongside the first. This was the guidewire for the Edwards Commander—the brand-new valve delivery system that Dr. Torres believed was right for my heart. Before sliding the Edwards Commander into my thigh, Torres retracted the leading edge, just above the balloon, and a technician, a representative from Edwards Pharmaceuticals, placed the Sapien III valve on the catheter's tip.

It was a tiny thing at the top of the catheter, all its magic powers compacted to a diameter slim enough to slide through my veins without touching the flesh. The cobalt-chromium mesh that contained the valve was coiled tight into a stubby little tube. Not until the balloon inside the catheter expanded would the Sapien III reveal itself. The balloon would push the cobalt-chromium mesh wide, and inside would be the valve removed from a cow's jugular vein.

Torres slid the Commander up and down into my heart and into the pulmonary position. He had to wrestle with the catheter to get the valve into place. I can only guess at his struggles by the marks they left on my body. The wound on the left side of my groin, where the monitoring catheter had entered my heart, was tiny, just a dot, a speck a couple of days after the procedure, and then invisible two weeks later—that's typical of a catheterization. The wound on the right side was bloody, with a tough wad of sutures under the skin and big, black threads hanging out of the scab. He must have been tugging and twisting the catheter, pulling it in and out, pulling it left and right.

My heart objected to Torres's work. It flew into wild arrhythmias, like it was trying to spit the metal and plastic right out of itself. But Torres got the tip of the catheter into place. The Sapien III sat right between the calcifying flaps of the old pig valve that had been implanted in 1999. When it was in place, Torres called out to the nurse operating the pacemaker: "On!"

A flick of a switch, and the current jolted my heart, pulsing fast, making it beat more than 180 times per minute, a rate so fast the heart was rendered incompetent. It could not generate movement of the blood. My heart was, for practical purposes, standing still.

He inflated the balloon inside the Sapien III. The balloon pushed open the cobalt-chromium cover of the valve, which transformed as it expanded into a honeycombed structure of miniature wires and prickles that gripped tight to the ring of my old implanted valve. In the center, some twenty-seven millimeters wide, was the valve itself, two slips of mammal flesh, flapping like a jellyfish.

Valve in place, Torres released the pressure from the catheter and the balloon deflated. He pulled back the Commander system. The new valve was in. The catheter and fluoroscope images showed it there on the screen: it held in place.

"Off," called Torres to the nurse with the pacemaker.

The electrical stimulation stopped. My heart eased into its normal rhythm. My ventricles squeezed. Blood shot upward from my heart through the new valve toward my lungs. When the ventricle expanded, the twin leaflets of the valve shut. They held steady, and blood stopped pouring backward from my lungs toward my heart. Then the heart squeezed, and the blood flew through the valve. The heart expanded, and the valve held firm. The catheter in the left side of my heart measured the new pressures. The function had changed immediately. My heart was healthier than it had been in a decade.

The team removed all the equipment out of my heart and down through my groin. They pulled the breathing tube from my throat. They woke me, and a beaming Dr. Torres reached his hand across the operating table toward me.

"IT WORKED!!!"

The moment comes to me through a drugged-out haze. Time seems to have been recorded fast and played back slow. In my memory, Torres's face is big, his hand enormous. He laughs.

The next morning I was on the cardiac ward, walking the halls. I was discharged by the afternoon and home in time for dinner. Then I woke up in my own bed, a little stiff, a little sore, but otherwise quite fine, thank you.

I ate breakfast. I dressed in a T-shirt and shorts. After I read the paper, I took a walk. A couple blocks from home, I bumped into a friend, a rock-and-roll dad, something of a celebrity in the alternative music scene. We shook hands, smiling.

"Whassup?" he asked. He was walking his dog.

I blurted it out, that the day before I'd had a new valve put in my heart.

"No shit," he said, looking me up and down. He shook his head.

Then I went to the park. I took a selfie, and I sent it to my mom.

ACKNOWLEDGMENTS

I N THE WRITING of this book, I've had a lot of help. Thank you to Belen Altuve Blanton, Chris Halverson, Alan Sabal, Danny Spandau, Bridgette Ratliff, Meg Balke, Jenny, Amanda, and all the patients who shared their stories with me. Thank you to Michael Freed, Welton M. Gersony, Sylvia P. Griffiths, James R. Malm, Davendra Mehta, Marlon Rosenbaum, Abraham Rudolph, Alejandro Torres, and Ali Zaidi. Thanks to the Adult Congenital Heart Association, members and staff.

Thanks to my family for putting up with this: my mother, Rachel Brownstein (a constant, boundless source of support), my brothers, Daniel and Ezra, and my daughters, Eliza and Lucy. None of these people asked to be in this book. None of them complained about it. All of them encouraged me in my work.

Thanks to my dad, too, who died between the writing and publication of the book and who would have been so proud to hold it in his hands. (He once bought twenty copies of *Glimmer Train Stories* when I had a story in that magazine.) My brother Daniel was particularly helpful in the writing about early modern anatomy. Thanks also to Dr. Lucas Dreamer for his careful reading of the book.

The New York Public Library gave me space to work, and St. John's University gave me research support.

Friends kept me afloat: Anne Trubek read the proposal, Sam Greenhoe and Amy King read lumpy early drafts, Rafael ("Thank You, Masked Man") Heller and J. P. Olsen heard me out as I talked (and talked) through it.

I've been lucky to collaborate with talented people. Ben Adams, my patient and thoughtful editor, has been a joy to work with, and his insights have helped me clarify my writing both in general and in particular. David McCormick, my literary agent, is a rock-solid ally and brilliant reader and has stood by me for years, and in this book he helped me at every stage, from conception to book jacket. A shout-out to Alia Hanna Habib at McCormick Literary for her help with the proposal.

Most of all, I want to thank my wife, Marcia Lerner, who was there for every draft, every crisis in confidence, every imagined title and subtitle, every trip to the ER, the OR, the cath lab, and every time I was up with an arrhythmia late at night—who is also my first, last, and best reader and critic.

Thanks.

NOTES

THIS IS A book about my good fortune, and it began with two purposes: to thank my doctors and to figure out how they saved my life. All the doctors who treated me were still alive at the time I was writing, so I've been able to interview many of them and thank them in person. They helped me write this book, and they have been the sources for this book's most intimate information about congenital heart disease and adult congenital cardiology, so though they're in the acknowledgments and in the book, their names appear again here as sources: Michael Freed, Welton M. Gersony, Sylvia P. Griffiths, Davendra Mehta, Marlon Rosenbaum, Alejandro Torres, and Lucy Swift. I also want to thank their colleagues, doctors who didn't treat me but helped me with this book: Jamil Aboulhosn, Eugenia Doyle, David Hoganson, Douglas Moodie, Abraham Rudolph, Roberta Williams, and Ali Zaidi. Nada Farhat, Stephen Fishberger, Deborah Gersony, John Mayer, and the doctor I call Danforth Zhee all discussed my health with me in their offices at the time I saw them, so they are sources too.

Whenever I mentioned I was writing a book about congenital heart disease to anyone outside the community of doctors and patients, eyebrows raised. People seemed to think it was an odd subject. I kept wondering, if I were to say that I was writing a book about any other medical condition—tuberculosis, anxiety, Tay-Sachs disease, backaches, acne, or the flu—would anyone find it odd? Heart defects are the most common serious birth defect, and there's a kid with a surgically repaired heart in most every school, but still the phrase "congenital heart disease" remains almost unmentionable, a turnoff. Even Mark Roeder, the president of the Adult Congenital Heart Association (ACHA), agreed it was not a good idea to put the phrase in the title or subtitle of a book. So as this project came toward its conclusion, I came to a third purpose in writing: to make the condition more recognizable as a part of ordinary social conversation, so that patients like me could tell the stories of their lives and be understood.

The patients (and their parents) who shared their stories with me became the second chief reference source for my book, and though many of these names appear in the book (and the acknowledgments), they deserve to be repeated here: Bob Avery, Meg Balke, Belen Altuve Blanton, Darcie Farella, Chris Halverson, Melissa Hartman, Pauline Loh, Aliza Marlin, Paula Miller, Michael Pernick, Rick Puder, Bridgette Ratliff, Alan Sabal, Josh Sarantis, Danny Spandau, Ian Steele-Avery, Judy Vincent, Corey Joy Williams, Ken Woodhouse, and the patients I call Jenny and Amanda. There were others I spoke to, in recorded interviews and informally, in gatherings of adult congenital heart defect patients. Some of them preferred not to have their names printed; some of them spoke off the record; some of their names have been lost to me. They all deserve acknowledgment. If I talked to you at a lunch or a convention or other ACHA gathering, but you don't find your name here and are disappointed, sincere apologies. No matter how short our conversation, you helped me. I'd also like to thank Mark Roeder and the ACHA—Danielle Hile deserves particular mention, as she acted sometimes like a volunteer research assistant for me.

I have browsed scientific papers, conference reports, oral histories, and other testimonials, but for a significant part of my research I've depended on secondary sources, chiefly on other writers' histories of medicine. Three deserve to be named at the outset, as they were the first I read, and they formed the spine of my understanding of my subject: Roy Porter's *The Greatest Benefit to Mankind: A Medical History of Humanity* (Norton, 1999), Paul Starr's *The Social Transformation of American Medicine: The Rise of a Sovereign Profession and the Making of a Vast Industry* (Basic, 1982), and Dr. James S. Forrester's *The Heart Healers: The Misfits, Mavericks, and Rebels Who Created the Greatest Medical Breakthrough of Our Lives* (St. Martin's, 2015).

This is my first attempt at a long, serious work of nonfiction. I've tried to tell a true story here, but up to now I've mostly written fiction, and I have discovered (as so many other writers have told me) that the phrase "true story" is almost an oxymoron. All the business of putting together a comprehensible narrative—the selecting, omitting, ordering, and condensing of events, the sustaining a particular point of view, just the attempt to take the noisy mess of experience and history and squeeze it into words—all of that skews the truth. This book is primarily a record of my memory, which I know is faulty. When people corrected me (my parents, my wife, my brothers, and my doctors), I accepted their changes. But there was a lot that could not be corroborated or contradicted. I did my best. With other patients, the guiding principle for me was reporting their narratives accurately—I didn't check that they were getting every detail right, because I cared mostly about how they felt about their lives. I tried to present their stories faithfully, as they were related to me.

In interviews of living physicians, I checked one story against another and came up with the most authoritative account I could manage. When I encountered differing accounts—in my interviews or in my reading—I tried to resolve them by offering what seemed to me most plausible, given the context and what I had learned. (Here and there, in the notes below, you'll find a few places where I felt my resolution wasn't reasonably authoritative, and I have been forced to admit it.) When I encountered strikingly similar accounts—when every writer or interview subject told me the same exact story—that's when I knew for sure that the truth had been lost, and (dutifully) I printed the legend. Occasionally I've allowed myself a fiction writer's prerogative and imagined events more dramatically than a scrupulous historian might. In the notes below I've tried to point out the places where my imagination ran away with me.

A couple of points on language: I've used the phrases "congenital heart disease" and "congenital heart defects" almost interchangeably. There are physicians who feel one usage is correct and the other misleading. I don't come down on either side. Another name that I've been slippery with: the hospital where I have been treated for most of my life has changed its name many times over the years and is now called New York–Presbyterian/Columbia University Medical Center. Babies Hospital, where Dr. James Malm operated on me, is part of this complex institution and is now Children's Hospital of New York. I think of the whole as a unit: Columbia Presbyterian. That's the name I've used most often, in several abbreviated forms.

My life was both the impetus and the limiting factor in my storytelling. What you learn in these pages is the history of cardiology and heart surgery as they relate to me. This means that I've left out many of the most famous heart doctors in history. Christiaan Barnard, the South African physician who was the first doctor to successfully transplant a human heart, is not in my book. Neither is Andreas Gruetzig, the German doctor who was the first to perform a coronary balloon angioplasty. Nor is Francis Fontan, the French surgeon who invented the repair of single-ventricle defects that bears his name. Nor are any of the doctors who have been working over decades to build an artificial heart. This is because I've not (yet) needed a heart transplant or a balloon angioplasty, and I will never need a Fontan procedure. Many subjects of urgent current medical interest—in particular, heart defects' relation to genetic disorders and medicine related to genetic research—get thin treatment here. Because this history is told through an autobiographical lens, the book is perhaps overly focused on North America, but it's where I've lived. It's also where heart surgery developed, between 1935 and 1975.

In many ways, this is a story about medicine in the United States, how US medicine flourished and changed the world and provided us with miracles and how more recently its successes have been dimmed by an increasingly chaotic and inequitable system.

PART ONE

Chapter 1

pp. 3–6: The account of the Spandaus' lives comes from interviews with Danny Spandau, on the phone and in person, and in subsequent email exchanges. It was Dr. James R. Malm who gave me Danny Spandau's name. I spent a great deal of time with Danny at the Adult Congenital Heart Association conference in Orlando, Florida, in May 2017 and spoke and corresponded with him before and after. Dr. Sylvia P. Griffiths, who was working as a pediatric cardiologist in the late 1950s, corroborated the likely medical details around Danny's Blalock procedure. For detailed sources on the Johns Hopkins blue baby surgery, see notes to Chapters 21, 23, and 25.

Chapter 2

p. 8: The seven out of eleven number comes from J. R. Malm et al., "An Evaluation of Total Correction of Tetralogy of Fallot," *Circulation* 27 (April 1963): 805–811.

p. 8: The "top ten causes of death" is from B. M. Patten, "Retrospect and Prospect," in *Congenital Heart Disease: A Symposium Presented at the Washington Meeting of the American Association for the Advancement of Science, December 29–30, 1958*, edited by Allan D. Bass and Gordon K. Moe (Washington, DC: American Association for the Advancement of Science, 1960).

p. 8: *Time* magazine issue is March 25, 1957.

p. 12: The description of Danny Spandau's surgery, here and in the following chapter, comes from Malm et al., "An Evaluation of Total Correction," as well as from interviews with Spandau, Malm, and Griffiths.

Chapter 3

p. 13: For statistics on congenital heart defects, I've relied on the Adult Congenital Heart Association, with a big shout out to Danielle Hile, who answered everything warmly, promptly, and accurately; Douglas Moodie's "Adult Congenital Heart Disease: Past, Present, and Future," *Texas Heart Institute Journal* 38, no. 6 (2011), says that the population of adult congenital heart disease (ACHD) patients is growing at about 5 percent a year and that over 85 percent of all infants with congenital heart disease are now expected to reach adulthood; Moodie approximates that 5 percent of ACHD patients who needed follow-up were getting appropriate care in 2011.

p. 14: A number of books recount Taussig's resistance to open-heart surgery, and I heard about it firsthand from Dr. Michael Freed, Dr. Welton Gersony, Dr. Eugenia Doyle, and others.

p. 14: My interviews with Dr. Malm were all over the telephone; when we met in person, he was very gracious, very funny, and very intimidating and dispensed with me quickly.

p. 15: "Median" and "vertical" are from Malm et al., "An Evaluation of Total Correction," 86.

p. 15: I'm grateful to Dr. David Hoganson, a heart surgeon at Boston Children's, one of the few pediatric heart surgeons in the world who is also a congenital heart defect patient; he described to me the trabeculated interior of the heart.

Chapter 4

p. 18: For the phrase "Knights of Taussig," see Joyce Baldwin, *To Heal the Heart of a Child: Helen Taussig, M.D.* (New York: Walker & Co., 1992).

p. 21: William Safire, "Holmes' Horse's Dogs," *New York Times*, February 7, 2002; Thomas Morris, in *The Matter of the Heart* (New York: Thomas Dunne, 2017), points out that the word "tetralogy" is used to refer almost always to works of art and almost never to physiological conditions and that "tetrad" would be more appropriate.

p. 23: The phrase "well balanced" comes from an interview with Welton Gersony.

p. 24: Susan Sontag, *Illness as Metaphor* (New York: Farrar, Straus, and Giroux, 1977), 6; Menninger quoted in Sontag, *Illness as Metaphor*, 6.

p. 25: Lorrie Moore, "People Like That Are the Only People Here," in *Birds of America* (New York: Knopf, 1998), 220.

Chapter 6

p. 34: I have not found the phrase "The Open Heart Club" in any printed materials, but I remember it and the confusion with the title of the Beatles album; the phrase could not have originated in my family, and someone must have said it at the assembly.

p. 36: As early as Maude Abbott's 1936 *Atlas of Congenital Cardiac Disease* (the first book to describe the varieties of congenital heart disease), tetralogy was described as the most common complex congenital defect (see **p. 141** of this book); a good general guide is "Facts About Tetralogy of Fallot," Centers for Disease Control and Prevention, https://www.cdc.gov/ncbddd/heartdefects/tetralogyoffallot.html. I'm grateful to physicians who have described the condition to me again and again over my life, but I'm particularly grateful to Welton Gersony, who is the cardiologist quoted on **p. 37**; one of the best sources for descriptions of congenital heart defects is the Mayo Clinic's website: https://www.mayoclinic.org/diseases-conditions/congenital-heart-defects-children/symptoms-causes/syc-20350074.

p. 38: The "sew together two farts" quote comes from an elderly cardiologist, sitting slightly off-screen, in a video of a Boston Children's Hospital interview between Dr. Michael Freed and Dr. Abraham Rudolph; I'm grateful to Dr. Wayne Tworetsky for providing me with the video.

p. 38: There's a good description of Mustard's organic heart-lung machine in James S. Forrester, *The Heart Healers: The Misfits, Mavericks, and Rebels Who Created the Greatest Medical Breakthrough of Our Lives* (New York: St. Martin's, 2015), 57.

p. 39: I'm grateful to Dr. Gersony for the "100 percent mortality rate" line; for a biography of Mustard, see Oktay Tutarel, "Profiles in Cardiology: William Thornton Mustard," *Clinical Cardiology* 29 (2006): 424–425; also see Canadian Medical Association, "Mustard's Operation," *Canadian Medical Association Journal* 93 (1965): 372; Forrester, *The Heart Healers*, also covers Mustard's career.

Chapter 7

p. 42: For "done in lieu of the Blalock," see this book, **p. 245**.

p. 42: On the percentages: as noted, Himmelstein had an over 50 percent mortality rate. For Kirklin, the rates progressed from an initial 50 percent on open-heart surgery to correct atrial septal defects, a rate that lowered rapidly as the 1950s ended and the 1960s began (see interview with Kirklin in Alan B. Weisse, *Heart to Heart: An Oral History* (New Brunswick, NJ: Rutgers, 2002]). For complex conditions like tetralogy, however, mortality rates remained higher; according to Malm et al., "An Evaluation of Total Correction," the mortality rates among tetralogy correction in 1963 ranged from 16 to 35 percent.

p. 42: Gersony's description of Gross's early failures were confirmed by Abraham Rudolph.

p. 43: Sylvia Griffiths told me she only went to Cotuit once.

p. 44: On Lillehei's drunkenness, see Denton Cooley's *100,000 Hearts: A Surgeon's Memoir* (Austin: University of Texas, 2012), 244.

Chapter 8

p. 47: See "Dr. Dorothy Hansine Andersen," in *Changing the Face of Medicine*, US National Library of Medicine, National Institutes of Health, https://cfmedicine .nlm.nih.gov/physicians/biography_8.html.

p. 48: Additional notes on Malm are from Leora B. Balsam and Abe DeAnda, "Historical Perspectives of the American Association for Thoracic Surgery: James R. Malm," *Journal of Thoracic and Cardiovascular Surgery* 146, no. 3 (September 2013): 501–503.

p. 50: John Norman, "Histrionics, Vignettes, and Quartets: A Syndrome of Stress in Heart Surgeons," *Cardiovascular Diseases, Bulletin of the Texas Heart Institute* 7, no. 4 (December 1980): 339–343.

Chapter 9

p. 53: The thumbnail history of the classical and early modern study of the heart in Chapters 9 and 11 covers so much history so quickly that it is inevitably full of distortions. The compacted history focuses on single well-known transfiguring men, like Galen, Vesalius, and Harvey, and tells the story as if it were one of straightforward progress; a closer view of the subject would reveal almost infinite complexities of progress and regress. Thanks to Daniel Brownstein.

p. 53: Egyptians, from Roy Porter, *The Greatest Benefit to Mankind: A Medical History of Humanity* (New York: Norton, 1999), 50; Crusaders, from Porter, *The Greatest Benefit*, 132; Al Nafis, from Porter, *The Greatest Benefit*, 102.

p. 54: Shakespeare, *Henry VI, Part 3*, II:i, 82–88.

p. 54: For competition in Galen's dissections, see Maud Gleason, "Shock and Awe: The Performance Dimension of Galen's Anatomic Demonstrations," Princeton/Stanford Working Papers in Classics Paper No. 010702, Stanford University, January 2007, doi:10.2139/ssrn.141427007.

pp. 54–56: My discussion of anatomy from Galen to Leonardo da Vinci is largely drawn from Porter, *The Greatest Benefit*, 73–77, as well as from Charles Singer's classic *Short History of Anatomy and Physiology from the Greeks to Harvey* (New York: Dover, 1957), and Thomas Wright's excellent *William Harvey: A Life in Circulation* (Oxford: Oxford University Press, 2012), 30–31.

pp. 55–56: For Servetus, see Porter, *The Greatest Benefit*, 184, which connects his burning at the stake to his hypotheses about anatomy. The extremely complex relation between Servetus's ideas about the circulation of the blood and his heretical ideas (in both the Catholic Church and Calvin's eyes) about the Holy Trinity is, again, one of those subjects well beyond the scope of this book.

Chapter 10

p. 58: Menninger quoted in Sontag, *Illness as Metaphor*, 46–47; Schopenhauer in Sontag, *Illness as Metaphor*, 43.

p. 58: Kafka in Sontag, *Illness as Metaphor*, footnote 44.

p. 60: Frigyes Karinthy, *Journey Around My Skull* (New York: New York Review of Books Classics, 2008), 85.

p. 61: Average tetralogy at 75 percent, from Dr. Rush Waller at 2017 ACHA conference in Orlando.

p. 63: My thumbnail history of adult congenital cardiology comes from conversations with Dr. Ali Zaidi, Dr. Michael Freed, and Dr. Marlon Rosenbaum, all dates and numbers confirmed by ACHA.

p. 64: William James, *The Varieties of Religious Experience* (New York: Modern Library, 2002), 101, 88.

Chapter 11

p. 68: On Eustachi and Fallopia, see Porter, *The Greatest Benefit*, 182–183. For a longer description of Colombo and the clitoris, see David Stringer and Inés Becker, "Colombo and the Clitoris," *European Journal of Obstetrics & Gynecology and Reproductive Biology* 151, no. 2 (August 2010): 130–133. On anatomy before Vesalius, see Wright, *William Harvey*, 36. On Vesalius, including the sentence quoted, see Porter, *The Greatest Benefit*, 177–180.

p. 69: C. D. O'Malley, *Andreas Vesalius of Brussels, 1514–1564* (Berkeley: University of California Press, 1964): medical students, 40; plague dead, 59; "observing the body," 64 (originally *Fabrica* [1543]).

p. 69: "There is no truth," in O'Malley, *Andreas Vesalius of Brussels*, 99.

p. 70: "Greatly driven to wonder," in Porter, *The Greatest Benefit*, 180; "In considering the structure of the heart," in Wright, *William Harvey*, 39.

p. 70: "between the ventricles of the heart," in Wright, *William Harvey*, 110.

pp. 70–71: "display the glory" and "teachers, tailors," in Wright, *William Harvey*, 61; description of Fabricus's dissections from Wright, *William Harvey*, 65–68.

pp. 71–72: My discussion of Harvey is drawn largely from Wright, *William Harvey*, and Porter, *The Greatest Benefit*.

p. 73: "I do not believe," in Wright, *William Harvey*, 151; "Daily experience," in Wright, *William Harvey*, 152. For more on Harvey and Aristotelian thoughts, see Thomas Fuchs, *The Mechanization of the Heart: Harvey and Descartes* (Rochester, NY: University of Rochester Press, 2001).

p. 73: Jefferson quoted in Porter, *The Greatest Benefit*, 303; Dr. Howard Markel, "Dec. 14, 1799: The Excruciating Final Hours of President George Washington," *PBS/Newshour*, December 14, 2014, https://www.pbs.org/newshour/health/dec -14-1799-excruciating-final-hours-president-george-washington. Again, centuries of history are compressed here. More sophisticated contemporary historians would argue that Vesalius did not "invent" autopsy, as Porter says, and the complex relations between Vesalius, Colombo, Fabricus, and Harvey have all been simplified.

Chapter 12

p. 75: Dr. Sylvia P. Griffiths invited me to see Dr. Jamil Aboulhosn and Dr. Marlon Rosenbaum present cases at Columbia Presbyterian. It was exciting for a patient to see how vigorously two top physicians could disagree over the specifics of a complex case. Aboulhosn's remarks of April 20, 2017, are quoted from my notes, and he confirmed them.

pp. 75–76: I interviewed Mark Roeder and Danielle Hile in the Philadelphia offices of the Adult Congenital Heart Association on September 11, 2018.

p. 76: I met Dr. Ali Zaidi and Bridgette Ratliff at the ACHA regional conference at Montefiore Hospital in the Bronx on October 21, 2017. When Bridgette appeared after the procession of cardiologists, she wore a leather jacket, she danced, and she laughed. I spoke to her afterward and met her daughter Rachel.

pp. 76–82: I interviewed Bridgette on the phone and in person, and I visited her at work on February 7, 2018; we also had several email exchanges. I interviewed Dr. Zaidi in his office in Montefiore on February 9, 2018, and the story I tell combines what was told to me by doctor and patient.

Chapter 13

pp. 85–86: Marlon Rosenbaum and I have been discussing these issues for years now, over several visits to his office and in conversations about this book, and I have done my best to tell the story both as it appeared to me twenty years ago and as it appears to me now, through my best understanding of his perspective.

Chapter 14

pp. 89–96: Broadly, the Steno material depends on four books: (1) Troels Kardel and Paul Maquet, eds., *Nicolaus Steno: Biography and Original Papers of a Seventeenth Century Scientist* (New York: Springer, 2013) (this is a translation of Gustav Scherz's German biography, *Neils Stensen*, and a compilation of Steno's thirty-four known scientific papers); (2) Alan Cutler, *The Seashell on the Mountaintop* (New York: Dutton, 2003); (3) Raffaello Cioni, *Neils Stensen, Scientist Bishop* (New York: P. J. Kennedy and Sons, 1962); and (4) Matthew Cobb, *Generation* (London: Bloomsbury, 2006).

p. 91: "When I was very small," in Cioni, *Neils Stensen,* 21.

p. 91: Entry into Copenhagen University, in Kardel and Maquet, *Nicolaus Steno,* 41; "I fear that," in Kardel and Maquet, *Nicolaus Steno,* 56.

p. 92: Quotes from *Chaos* in Kardel and Maquet, *Nicolaus Steno,* 55–57.

p. 93: Description of Amsterdam owes a lot to Cobb, *Generation;* "I felt the point of my knife," in Kardel and Maquet, *Nicolaus Steno,* 65.

p. 94: "I seem to have discovered," in Cioni, *Neils Stensen,* 33; Cutler, *The Seashell,* 37.

p. 95: "penis of a whale," in Simon Schama, *The Embarrassment of Riches: Dutch Culture in the Golden Age* (New York: Vintage, 1997); dates of anatomy performances in Kardel and Maquet, *Nicolaus Steno,* 70; description of Dutch bars in Cobb, *Generation,* 41–42.

p. 96: "He was of fine appearance," in Cioni, *Neils Stensen,* 26; Dutch anti-sodomy laws, from Schama, *The Embarrassment of Riches;* see also Brian Fone, *Homophobia: A History* (New York: Picador, 2001). I believe that my hypothesis about Steno's sexuality is original; that is, no one I read stated it outright.

Chapter 16

pp. 100–102: "Imagine Steno": as the word "imagine" implies, I've taken some liberties here, mostly in condensing facts. In 1663, Steno did perform a dissection-cum-lecture of a human brain, and Baruch Spinoza did come to see him. Sylvius, Thévenot, Swammerdam, and de Graaf all attended Steno's performances, but it's not clear that they were all present on the same day. The lecture I quote from here, *The Discourse on the Anatomy of the Brain,* was given in Paris two years later; see Kardel and Maquet, *Nicolaus Steno,* 508–523. In condensing it I have altered the translator's syntax.

p. 103: The dialogue with Spinoza is invented, but it's true that Spinoza invited Steno to his home in Rijksberg, that Steno went, and that Steno walked most everywhere he traveled. It seems likely that Steno and Spinoza conversed about Descartes. I didn't feel I could fake the conversation between two geniuses, and there is no record of exactly how Steno felt upon leaving Spinoza; however, he did go home and begin to investigate the heart of a deer, and in doing so felt he was in his empiricism destroying the godless rationalism of Descartes and Spinoza. My imagined image of Spinoza himself is largely derived from Rebecca Newberger Goldstein's gorgeous *Betraying Spinoza: The Renegade Jew Who Gave Us Modernity* (New York: Nextbook, 2008).

p. 104: "the first fibers," in Kardel and Maquet, *Nicolaus Steno,* 94; "*not* that seat," in Kardel and Maquet, *Nicolaus Steno,* 110; "I knocked down," in Kardel and Maquet, *Nicolaus Steno,* 99.

p. 104: Tuileries, in Kardel and Maquet, *Nicolaus Steno,* 119; "To say it straight," in Kardel and Maquet, *Nicolaus Steno,* 132.

p. 105: Steno, *Dissection of an Embryo Monster for Parisians,* in Kardel and Maquet, *Nicolaus Steno,* 537–539.

p. 106: "After all is finished," in Edward Dolnick, *The Seeds of Life* (New York: Basic Books, 2017).

p. 106: Again, my entry into Steno's dreams is entirely hypothetical; "the thought came into my mind," in Cioni, *Neils Stensen,* 70.

pp. 107: I do not know if Steno was in fact shown Galileo's instruments, but the Medicis did keep them; see Eric Cochrane, *Florence in the Forgotten Centuries* (Chicago: University of Chicago Press, 1973).

pp. 107–108:: "How the present state," in Cutler, *The Seashell,* 115.

p. 108: Cobb, *Generation,* 97–99.

p. 109: Liebniz, in Kardel and Maquet, *Nicolaus Steno,* 226.

p. 109: Cutler, *The Seashell,* 164–165.

p. 110: Lacan, quoted in Zadie Smith, "Man vs. Corpse," *New York Review of Books,* December 5, 2013.

Chapter 17

pp. 112–113: Letter from Dr. Michael Freed, August 17, 1995.

Chapter 18

p. 116: I met Alan Sabal at a bar in a gathering of adult congenital heart patients in New York in May 2017, and I interviewed him in person near his home soon thereafter; we've spoken at several ACHA events and gatherings.

p. 119: Don DeLillo, *White Noise* (New York: Viking, 1984), 289.

p. 120: On Magendie, see W. Bruce Frye, "A History of Cardiac Arrhythmias," in John A. Kastor, MD, *Arrhythmias* (London: W.B. Saunders, 1994); for transplants and nerves, see Charles Siebert, *A Man After His Own Heart* (New York: Crown, 2004), 185.

pp. 121–122: I had the pleasure of talking to Dr. Abraham Rudolph over the phone in June 2018; we had several long subsequent email exchanges. I am grateful to Dr. Wayne Tworetsky for providing me with access to videos of several interviews and speeches Dr. Rudolph gave at Boston Children's Hospital.

p. 122: Moore, "People Like That Are the Only People Here," 227.

p. 123: The Henry James quote comes from the story "The Middle Years."

PART TWO

Chapter 19

pp. 127–145: Maude Abbott material derives largely from two biographies: H. E. MacDermot, *Maude Abbott: A Memoir* (New York: Macmillan, 1941), and Douglas Waugh, MD, *Maudie of McGill: Dr. Maude Abbott and the Foundation of Heart Surgery* (Toronto: Hannah, 1992).

pp. 127–128: The train ride is obviously another one of my flights of the imagination, but everything about Maude Abbott's body—the dress with food stains, the mass of work, the absentmindedness, the way she walked—is based on descriptions of Abbott, largely in MacDermot, *Maude Abbott*, and Waugh, *Maudie of McGill*.

p. 129: Her father's murder trial is detailed closely in Waugh, *Maudie of McGill*; MacDermot skirts the story entirely.

p. 129: The journal entries are from MacDermot, *Maude Abbott*, 10; Waugh seems to have been unable to locate these papers.

pp. 129–130: "very enthusiastic," in Waugh, *Maudie of McGill*, 28.

p. 130: "People say," in David Oshinsky, *Bellevue: Three Centuries of Medicine and Mayhem at America's Most Storied Hospital* (New York: Doubleday, 2016), 150; information on Hopkins is from Paul Starr, *The Social Transformation of American Medicine: The Rise of a Sovereign Profession and the Making of a Vast Industry* (New York: Basic, 1982), 117; Osler quotes are from Porter, *The Greatest Benefit*, 526, 347.

p. 131: "Can you think," in MacDermot, *Maude Abbott*, 42.

p. 131: "If you do for me," in MacDermot, *Maude Abbott*, 67.

p. 132: Waugh, *Maudie of McGill*, 56.

p. 133: Robert Willis, trans., *The Works of William Harvey* (Philadelphia: University of Pennsylvania 1989), 47.

p. 133: "A surgeon who tries," in Forrester, *The Heart Healers*, 30. Thomas Morris, in *The Matter of the Heart*, doubts that Billroth actually said it.

pp. 133–134: "Surgery of the heart," in Forrester, *The Heart Healers*, 30; Osler quote in Porter, *The Greatest Benefit*, 580; Romero information from Alejandro Aris, MD, PhD, "Francisco Romero, the First Heart Surgeon," *Annals of Thoracic Surgery* 64, no. 3 (September 1997): 870–871.

pp. 134–135: For the description of Daniel Hale Williams, I am indebted to Rob Dunn, *The Man Who Touched His Own Heart* (Boston: Little Brown, 2015), 10–14.

p. 135: For Rehn, I am indebted chiefly to Forrester, *The Heart Healers*.

p. 136: For the material on Eintoven, I'm indebted to John Burnett, "The Origins of the Electrocardiograph as Clinical Instrument," in *The Emergence of Modern Cardiology*, ed. W. F. Bynum, Christopher Lawrence, and Vivian Nutton (London: Welcome, 1985).

p. 136: "the doctors focused," in Christopher Lawrence, "Moderns and Ancients: The 'New Cardiology' in Britain, 1880–1930," in Bynum, Lawrence, and Nutton, *The Emergence of Modern Cardiology*.

p. 136: Porter, *The Greatest Benefit*, 582.

p. 137: Sir William Osler, *The Principals and Practice of Medicine* (New York: Appleton, 1920), 824; "I shall never forget him," in Waugh, *Maudie of McGill*, 59;

"I knew you would," in MacDermot, *Maude Abbott*, 78; "the mood at McGill," in Waugh, *Maudie of McGill*, 84.

p. 138: Jill Lepore, *The Secret History of Wonder Woman* (New York: Vintage, 2015), 18. Abbott's "Women in Medicine" lecture is available online through the Arthur and Elizabeth Schlesinger Library on the History of Women in Medicine, Harvard University.

p. 138: Data on women in medicine is from Starr, *The Social Transformation*, 117; Abbott's letter and Adami's response are from MacDermot, *Maude Abbott*, 127.

pp. 140–141: *Atlas of Congenital Cardiac Disease* (Toronto: McGill University Press, 2006), facsimile of 1936 edition.

Chapter 21

p. 146: Oddly, most books about Helen Taussig are geared toward younger readers. I'm particularly indebted to Baldwin, *To Heal the Heart of a Child*.

pp. 146–147: Again I have indulged my tendency toward dramatization, but all facts and figures come from Helen B. Taussig and Faith L. Meserve, "Rhythmic Contractions in Isolated Strips of Mammalian Ventricle," *American Journal of Physiology* 72, no. 1 (1925): 89–98, and Baldwin, *To Heal the Heart of a Child*, 26–27.

p. 147: "Who is going," in Baldwin, *To Heal the Heart of a Child*, 23.

pp. 148–149: Information on William Taussig is from Baldwin, *To Heal the Heart of a Child*, and from William Hyde and Howard L. Conrad, eds., *Encyclopedia of the History of St. Louis: A Compendium of History and Biography for Ready Reference* (New York: The Southern History Company, 1899).

pp. 149–150: Information on Frank Taussig is from Baldwin, *To Heal the Heart of a Child*, and Joseph Schumpeter, *Ten Great Economists from Marx to Keynes* (Oxford: Oxford University Press, 1965), 191–221.

p. 150: "a sound lesson," in Baldwin, *To Heal the Heart of a Child*, 14.

p. 150: There's some discrepancy among the sources about whether Taussig lost her spot because of her GPA or because of an exam, but so few exams are graded to tenths of a point that I've assumed it's GPA, and Geri Lynn Goodman, in her 1983 Yale dissertation on Taussig, *A Gentle Heart*, reports that it was the GPA.

pp. 150–152: The correspondence between Park and Taussig is from William N. Evans, "Helen Brooke Taussig and Edwards Albert Park: The Early Years (1927–1930)," *Cardiology in the Young* 20, no. 4 (2010): 387–395.

p. 150: For Thomas Lewis and the history of British cardiology in the early twentieth century, see Lawrence, "Moderns and Ancients."

pp. 150–151: "Cardiac Causes and the Care of Cardiac Children," Board of Education, City of New York, Harold W. McCormick director, committee appointed 1936, quoting from pp. 21 and 31: "Rheumatic fever and rheumatic heart disease represent a public health problem of the greatest magnitude which must be attacked from many different angles. . . . The problem of heart disease in children is primarily that of rheumatic fever and rheumatic heart disease. 95% of all heart diseases in children are the result of rheumatic fever."

p. 153: I'm grateful to the New York Academy of Medicine for providing me the program of the 1931 fortnight.

pp. 153–154: I'm grateful to Drs. Freed, Gersony, and Griffiths for help with understanding Taussig's progress; for more on the relationship between Abbott and Taussig, see William N. Evans, "The Relationship Between Maude Abbott and Helen Taussig: Connecting the Historical Dots," in *Cardiology in the Young* 18, no. 6 (December 2008): 557–564.

p. 154: For statistics about PDA, see "Patent Foramen Ovale (PFO)," American Heart Association, http://www.heart.org/en/health-topics/congenital-heart-defects /about-congenital-heart-defects/patent-foramen-ovale-pfo.

p. 155: I interviewed Dr. Eugenia Doyle in her home on June 30, 2018.

Chapter 22

pp. 157–164: I met Chris Halverson first at the Adult Congenital Heart Association convention in Orlando on June 1, 2017, then conducted several phone interviews thereafter and visited his church on January 14, 2018. He was kind enough to share with me some of his autobiographical writing, which I quote.

p. 160: "I feel the pressure" and "I tried to move my hands," from Halverson's story "Thinking and Feeling."

p. 162: "Cocooned," from "Thinking and Feeling."

p. 165: James, *The Varieties of Religious Experience*, 234.

Chapter 23

pp. 166–173: The material on Lorraine Sweeney and Robert Gross comes largely from Lindsay Murray, "'A Thrill of Extreme Magnety': Robert E. Gross and the Beginnings of Cardiac Surgery" (PhD diss. Harvard Medical School, 2015); Francis D. Moore and Judah Folkman, *Robert Edward Gross, 1905–1988: A Biographical Memoir* (Washington, DC: National Academy of Sciences, 1995); and Forrester, *The Heart Healers*.

p. 166: "Music came on," in Murray, "A Thrill of Extreme Magnety," 18.

p. 167: "At the time of admission," in Robert E. Gross and John P. Hubbard, "Surgical Ligation of a Patient with Ductus Arteriosus," *Journal of American Medical Association* 112, no. 8 (February 25, 1939): 730.

p. 168: "If God wants her," in Murray, "A Thrill of Extreme Magnety," 19.

p. 169: For a biography of Carrel, read W. Sterling Edwards, *Alexis Carrel: Visionary Surgeon* (Springfield, IL: Thomas, 1974).

p. 170: Alexis Carrel, *Man the Unknown* (New York: Harper, 1939) (page numbers here from online reprint by archive.org): "The democratic principle," 141; "the extinction," 2; "never have the European races," 2; "number of misfits," 2.

p. 171: Bing quoted in Allen B. Weisse, *Heart to Heart: The Twentieth Century Battle Against Cardiac Disease, An Oral History* (New Brunswick, NJ: Rutgers, 2002), 60.

pp. 171–172: Harold Foss, "The Surgeon and His Nurse Anesthetist," *Bulletin of the National Association of Nurse Anesthetists* 5, no. 3 (August 1937): 351.

p. 172: From Murray, "A Thrill of Extreme Magnety."

p. 172: All quotes are from Gross and Hubbard, "Surgical Ligation of a Patient."

pp. 173–174: Baldwin, *To Heal the Heart of a Child*, 52, except "Madame, I close ductuses," which is quoted in Weisse, *Heart to Heart*, 43, in Weisse's interview with Taussig's protégée Mary Allen Engle.

p. 175: Vivien Thomas, *Partners of the Heart* (Philadelphia: University of Pennsylvania, 1985). The question of exactly who deserves credit for the idea of the shunt is blurred—some sources will say it is Blalock and others Thomas. My sense is that Taussig outlined a specific plan to Gross and was rejected out of hand. Her language with Blalock was much more open, and it seems to me likely that she altered her approach to allow more intellectual space for the surgeon and his technician to invent the particulars of the operation. For a scholarly description of the Blalock-Taussig-Thomas collaboration, see William N. Evans, "The Blalock-Taussig Shunt: The Social History of an Eponym," *Cardiology in the Young* 19 (2009): 119–128.

Chapter 24

p. 177: I met Dr. Michael Freed at Zaftig's Diner in Brookline, Massachusetts, for lunch on May 16, 2018. Subsequently, we had discussions over the phone and a correspondence through email. He was extraordinarily generous with his time, and the historical information in this chapter, both about my case and about the development of cardiology, emerges from those conversations.

Chapter 25

p. 181: The Blalock-Taussig-Thomas history is probably the most chronicled of all the twentieth-century stories I recount in this book. Katie McCabe's 2007 article in the *Washingtonian*, "Like Something the Lord Made," is the first important work to retell what had been called the story of the Blalock shunt so that Thomas was given due credit for his role in the invention; the 2004 film of the same title was based on McCabe's work. For my retelling, I've relied on the books about Taussig and Thomas's article cited above, as well as the oral histories and interviews cited below.

p. 181: Technically speaking, Dr. Koko Eaton is a cousin of Vivien Thomas, but he grew up around Thomas and always called him Uncle Vivien; I interviewed Dr. Eaton on March 27, 2018.

p. 182: "Stop-gap," in Thomas, *Partners of the Heart*, 11.

p. 183: "I soon overcame," in Thomas, *Partners of the Heart*, 14; "a reputation," in Thomas, *Partners of the Heart*, 17.

p. 183: "The profanity," in Thomas, *Partners of the Heart*, 16; Woods quoted in Thomas, *Partners of the Heart*, 77; "She was tall . . . tetralogy of Fallot," in Thomas, *Partners of the Heart*, 80.

p. 183: Jim Murphy's book for young readers, *Breakthrough! How Three People Saved Blue Babies and Changed Medicine Forever* (Boston: Clarion, 2015), does a lovely job describing these events; see also C. D. Kensinger, W. H. Merrill, and S. K. Geevarghese, "Surgical Mentorship from Mentee to Mentor: Lessons from the Life of Alfred Blalock," *JAMA Surgery* 150, no. 2 (February 2015): 98–99.

p. 185: "After eating," in Alfred Blalock and Helen Taussig, "The Surgical Treatment of Malformations of the Heart in Which There Is Pulmonary Stenosis or

Pulmonary Atresia," *JAMA* 128 (1945):189–202; see also Anne Murphy, MD, and Duke E. Cameron, MD, "The Blalock-Taussig Thomas Collaboration: A Model for Medical Progress," *JAMA* 200, no. 3 (July 16, 2009): 328–330; "During her recurrent spells," in Baldwin, *To Heal the Heart of a Child*, 57.

p. 186: On Blalock's being anxious, see Murphy, *Breakthrough!*, 66; "Suture materials," in Thomas, *Partners of the Heart*, 92.

p. 186: "I guess you better call," in Murphy, *Breakthrough!*, 67; "Many of us," in Murphy, *Breakthrough!*, 64.

pp. 186–188: The description of surgery prep depends largely on Cooley's *100,000 Hearts* and Thomas's *Partners of the Heart*, as well as the original publication by Blalock and Taussig, "The Surgical Treatment of Malformations of the Heart."

p. 187: "no bigger," in Baldwin, *To Heal the Heart of a Child*, 63; "The patient's vessels," in Thomas, *Partners of the Heart*, 93; Longmire quoted by Mike Field in "Hopkins Pioneered Blue Baby Procedure 50 Years Ago," *Johns Hopkins Gazette*, May 30, 1995.

p. 188: Cooley quoted in Murphy, *Breakthrough!*, 70.

p. 188: "Well you watch," in Thomas, *Partners of the Heart*, 95; Harmel quoted in Murphy, *Breakthrough!*, 71; "You've never seen something so dramatic," Thomas quoted in McCabe, "Like Something the Lord Made." Though Thomas, Cooley, and the original Blalock/Taussig article (as I understand it) assert that Eileen Saxon became pink immediately after surgery, and though all my interview subjects tell me that this sudden color change was typical of a successful procedure, Thomas Morris, whose research in *The Matter of the Heart* is likely more thorough than mine, suggests that the color change was achieved in subsequent Blalock-Taussig-Thomas blue baby surgeries but not in the first.

p. 189: Whittemore quoted in Evans, "The Blalock-Taussig Shunt," 124; Thomas quoted in Murphy, *Breakthrough!*, 77; description of influx of patients is from Thomas, *Partners of the Heart*,.

p. 189: Description of operating conditions is from Thomas, *Partners of the Heart*, 100.

p. 190: On Blalock's disparagement of Taussig and women, see Cooley, *100,000 Hearts*, 55; for Taussig biographies, see also Mary Allen Engle's reminiscence, "Helen Brooke Taussig: The Mother of Pediatric Cardiology," in the Biographies of Great Pediatricians series in *Pediatric Annals* 11, no. 7 (July 1982): 629.

pp. 191–193: I had several conversations with Belen Altuve Blanton over the course of the ACHA convention in 2017, and I spoke with her over the phone and corresponded via email thereafter.

Chapter 26

p. 194: The history of MRI diagnosis of cardiac function is from a conversation with Dr. Freed.

p. 196: Dr. Freed's letter, June 1999.

PART THREE

Chapter 28

p. 206: Cooley, *100,000 Hearts*, 101–102.

p. 207: W. H. Auden, *The Dyer's Hand* (New York: Vintage, 1968), 13.

pp. 207–208: Here and in much of my writing on Lillehei, I've relied on two sources: Forrester, *The Heart Healers*, and G. Wayne Miller's biography of Lillehei, *King of Hearts* (New York: Crown, 2000); "I didn't necessarily," in Miller, *King of Hearts*, 22.

p. 209: "I've certainly seen," in Miller, *King of Hearts*, 28.

p. 209: For figures on the federal budget, see Starr, *The Social Transformation*, 343; on penicillin, see Starr, *The Social Transformation*, 341.

pp. 210–211: My history of Harken depends largely on Forrester, *The Heart Healers*, and Morris, *The Matter of the Heart*.

p. 211: "suddenly, with a pop," in Forrester, *The Heart Healers*, 32–33.

pp. 211–215: This section on Forssmann comes from his autobiography, *Experiments on Myself* (New York: St. Martin's Press, 1974), and also from David Monagan, *Journey into the Heart* (New York: Gotham, 2007).

p. 211: "cheerful, colorful," in Forssmann, *Experiments on Myself*, 22; "golden twenties," in Forssmann, *Experiments on Myself*, 42; "I'm afraid," in Forssmann, *Experiments on Myself*, 55.

p. 212: "I cannot," in Forssmann, *Experiments on Myself*, 83; "I made a point," in Forssmann, *Experiments on Myself*, 84.

p. 213: "I knew," in Forssmann, *Experiments on Myself*, 84.

p. 213: "You idiot," in Forssmann, *Experiments on Myself*, 85.

pp. 213–214: "I had a mirror," in Forssmann, *Experiments on Myself*, 85.

p. 214: On Forssmann and the Nazis, see David Siegel, letter to the editor, *American Journal of Cardiology* 80 (1997): 1643–1644.

p. 214: "I put a call through to Goebbels," in Forssmann, *Experiments on Myself*, 239; "wanted to tell Himmler," in Forssmann, *Experiments on Myself*, 241.

pp. 215–216: For material on Cournand and Richards, I've relied on Oshinsky, *Bellevue*, and also Weisse's oral history with Cournand in *Heart to Heart*; "had been received very critically by the cardiologists of the time," in Weisse, *Heart to Heart*, 33; "You have your grant," in Weisse, *Heart to Heart*, 34; Dr. Freed helped me understand Joyce Baldwin's relation to Cournand and her work, as well as Richard Bing's and Abraham Rudolph's work catheterizing children.

p. 216: National Institute of Health figures are from Starr, *The Social Transformation*, 342.

p. 216: On NIH grants to build catheter centers, see Kirk Jeffrey, *Machines in Our Hearts* (Baltimore: Johns Hopkins, 2003), 48.

p. 216: Lillehei and Wagensteen dialogue, in Miller, *King of Hearts*, 29.

Chapter 30

p. 221: The section on Bailey depends largely on Forrester, *The Heart Healers*, and Weisse, *Heart to Heart*; also Lorenzo Gonzalez-Levin, "Charles P. Bailey and Dwight E. Harken—the Dawn of the Modern Era of Mitral Valve Surgery," *Annals of Thoracic Surgery* 53 (1992): 916–919.

pp. 221–222: "There are no more egotistical," in Weisse, *Heart to Heart*, 79; "There is an old saying," in Weisse, *Heart to Heart*, 80; "He died," in Weisse, *Heart to Heart*, 81; "My mother," in Weisse, *Heart to Heart*, 81; "I didn't come from," in Weisse, *Heart to Heart*, 92; "Early on," in Weisse, *Heart to Heart*, 76.

p. 223: "Severe bleeding," in Forrester, *The Heart Healers*, 42.

p. 223: "ended up telling me," in Weisse, *Heart to Heart*, 78.

p. 225: "Obviously," in Weisse, *Heart to Heart*, 77.

p. 226: "Surgical procedures," in Miller, *King of Hearts*, 150.

pp. 226–227: For material on Ishii, see Porter, *The Greatest Benefit*, 650.

p. 227: For Father Miechalowski's testimony, see "Testimony: Father Leo Miechalowski," United States Holocaust Memorial Museum, https://www.ushmm.org/information/exhibitions/online-exhibitions/special-focus/doctors-trial/testimony-father-miechalowski.

pp. 227–228: For Bigelow and Gibbon, see Forrester, *The Heart Healers*, and Miller, *King of Hearts*.

p. 229: "Now that you've done that," in Miller, *King of Hearts*, 41.

Chapter 32

pp. 233–235: Forrester, *The Heart Healers*, and Miller, *King of Hearts*.

p. 235: "The others were taking risks," in Forrester, *The Heart Healers*, 85.

Chapter 34

p. 240: On eighteen attempts, see William S. Stony, "Evolution of Cardiopulmonary Bypass," *Circulation* 119, no. 21 (June 2009): 2844–2853; "A two-hundred percent," in Forrester, *The Heart Healers*, 65.

pp. 241–242: The description of surgery is largely from Miller, *King of Hearts*.

pp. 242–245: For the Pamela Schmidt and Mike Shaw surgeries, see Forrester, *The Heart Healers*, and Miller, *King of Hearts*.

p. 246: "Admit you have a vegetable," in Forrester, *The Heart Healers*, 73; "Too bad," in Forrester, *The Heart Healers*, 74.

pp. 246–247: On Calvin Richmond, see Miller, *King of Hearts*, 162–164; "I wonder," Miller, *King of Hearts*, 163.

p. 247: "I think the medical world," in Weisse, *Heart to Heart*, 98; "Dewey Dodrill's machine," in Weisse, *Heart to Heart*, 97.

pp. 247–248: On early heart-lung machines, see Forrester, *The Heart Healers*, Miller, *King of Hearts*, Cooley, *100,000 Hearts*, and Weisse, *Heart to Heart*.

Chapter 36

pp. 255–256: For Zoll, Lillehei, and Bakken again, see Forrester, *The Heart Healers*, and Jeffrey, *Machines in Our Hearts*.

p. 255: "How easily excitable," in Jeffrey, *Machines in Our Hearts*, 50; "poor background," in Jeffrey, *Machines in Our Hearts*, 51.

p. 256: "The problem with the external," in Weisse, *Heart to Heart*, 168; "Even my cardiac fellow," in Weisse, *Heart to Heart*, 164; "We had a patient," in Jeffrey, *Machines in Our Hearts*, 53.

p. 257: "Getting a shock," in Jeffrey, *Machines in Our Hearts*, 61–62; "drove the heart," in Jeffrey, *Machines in Our Hearts*, 63.

p. 257: "Many of these," in Jeffrey, *Machines in Our Hearts*, 64.

p. 259: Medtronic statistics, in Jeffrey, *Machines in Our Hearts*, 139, 151.

Chapter 37

pp. 262–264: I have given Dr. Davendra Mehta all the exposition here; the truth is that we did meet that day, and he did describe my arrhythmia and my defibrillator, and I took notes—but I took notes as a patient and not as a writer, and those notes are lost. Much of this information has been gleaned over the years from other doctors, including Dr. Fishberger, Dr. Rosenbaum, and also Nada Farhat, RN, who works with Dr. Rosenbaum. For information on conduction, arrhythmias, and defibrillators, I have relied on Forrester, *The Heart Healers*, Jeffrey, *Machines in Our Hearts*, and Kastor, *Arrhythmias*; for a good description, see "Conduction Disorders," American Heart Association (AHA), http://www.heart.org/en/health -topics/arrhythmia/about-arrhythmia/conduction-disorders. The AHA website also has a good description of the function of an implanted pacemaker-defibrillator: "Implantable Cardioverter Defibrillator (ICD)," AHA, http://www.heart.org/en /health-topics/arrhythmia/prevention—treatment-of-arrhythmia/implantable -cardioverter-defibrillator-icd. The AHA's website is searchable, friendly, and a good, reliable place for patient information on cardiac disorders. For a description of ATP, see Elia de Maria et al., "Antitachycardia Pacing Programming in Implanted Cardio-verter Defibrillator: A Systematic Review," *World Journal of Cardiology* 9, no. 5 (May 16, 2017): 429–436. I was able to review all this material with Dr. Mehta after I'd written it, and I'm grateful to him for that conversation.

Chapter 38

p. 266: For Mirowski's story, see Forrester, *The Heart Healers*, Jeffrey, *Machines in Our Hearts*, and John Kastor, "Michel Mirowski and the Implantable Defibrillator," *American Journal of Cardiology* (April 15 and May 1, 1989): 977–982 and 1121–1126.

p. 267: "An imperfect solution in search of": these words come from Dr. Bernard Lown, and they're quoted in Kastor, "Michel Mirowski," 1123; "I had a liberal view," in Kastor, "Michel Mirowski," 978; "Even the police," in Kastor, "Michel Mirowski," 977; "The schools were closed," in Kastor, "Michel Mirowski," 978.

pp. 268–269: "I saw the camp," in Kastor, "Michel Mirowski," 979; "I knew I wouldn't be staying," in Kastor, "Michel Mirowski," 980; "A typical German professor," in Kastor, "Michel Mirowski," 980; "My wife," in Kastor, "Michel Mirowski," 981.

Chapter 39

p. 271: Everything about Damon Weber comes from Doron Weber's book, *Immortal Bird* (New York: Simon & Schuster, 2012), and the breakfast interview with Weber in March 2018.

p. 272: Weber, *Immortal Bird*, 63.

p. 273: Weber, *Immortal Bird*, 121.

p. 273: "My son bends," in Weber, *Immortal Bird*, 169; "I think you're overreacting," in Weber, *Immortal Bird*, 87.

p. 273: "D-man, listen to me," in Weber, *Immortal Bird*, 335.

Chapter 40

p. 275: "He felt porous," and so forth, in Vladimir Nabokov, *Pnin* (New York: Doubleday, 1957), 20–21.

pp. 276–277: Interview with Meg Balke at the ACHA conference in Orlando and subsequently in email and phone conversations; Jenny interviewed at the ACHA conference in Orlando.

pp. 279–280: The information here is from decades of conversations with Dr. Marlon Rosenbaum, including interviews specifically for this book, but mostly in his office when he was examining my heart.

p. 281: Forrester, *The Heart Healers*, 20.

Chapter 41

p. 282: "Everyone who is born," in Sontag, *Illness as Metaphor*, 1.

P 282: Laurie Edwards, *In the Kingdom of the Sick* (New York: Bloomsbury, 2014), 11.

p. 293: Elaine Scarry, *The Body in Pain* (Oxford: Oxford University Press, 1985), 5, 7; "It is the intense pain," in Scarry, *The Body in Pain*, 35.

p. 294: "I do not know," in Nabokov, *Pnin*, 20.

Chapter 42

p. 297: Norman Mailer, *Miami and the Siege of Chicago* (New York: Random House, 2016), 3.

Chapter 43

p. 308: Interview with Mark Roeder and Danielle Hile at the Philadelphia headquarters of ACHA on September 11, 2018.

Chapter 44

p. 312: "the single most," in Forrester, *The Heart Healers*, 325.

p. 312: Quotes from Dr. Lin and Dr. Aboulhosn are from the ACHA Orlando conference.

pp. 313–319: Description of valve replacement surgery comes from discussions with Dr. Torres, in particular the interview in his office in August 2017.

INDEX

in 1950s, 20, 42–44, 240–241, 244,
247–248
two-patient, 10, 122
Byrne, David, 276

Calvin, John, 56
Campbell, F. W., 131
Canis carchariae dissectum caput (Steno),
108
cardiac arrhythmias, 61, 191–192,
250–254
cardiac catheterization
Cournand's and Richards's work on,
215–216
fear of, 115, 179, 194
Forssmann and, 211–215
historical development of, 209,
211–216, 226
measurements taken with, 22–23
risks of, 86–87
Rudolph's use of, 121
scheduling, 85–86
Spandau, D., and, 11
valve replacement surgery via, 312
cardiac cirrhosis, 192
Cardiac Surgery (Kirklin), 248
cardiology, 74. *See also* pediatric
cardiology
founding of, 216
historical development of, 151
hypothermia and, 226–228
Carrel, Alexis, 169–171, 228
Carter, Richard, 307
catheterization. *See* cardiac
catheterization
certification, of adult congenital heart
centers, 299–300
Chaveau, Jean-Baptiste Auguste, 211,
213
chest surgery, Malm's training in,
49–50
children, open-heart surgery
preparation for, 116–117
Christianity, 159–161
chromosome 18p deletion, 298
chronic illness, future rates of, 282–283
Cioni, Raffaelo, 95

circulation. *See also* cross-circulation
discovery of, 73
Steno demonstrating, 105
Circulation, 52
Clinton, Bill, 46
Cobb, Matthew, 108
Colombo, Realdo, 68, 70
Columbia Presbyterian Hospital
Babies Hospital at, 8, 19, 42
Mayo Clinic compared to, 45
operating rooms in, 14
returning to, 32–33
"complete repair," "total correction"
compared to, 39
conal septum, 37
congenital heart disease, 128–129.
See also tetralogy of Fallot
Abbott on, 133, 139–141
adult, 62–63, 75, 86, 279–281,
299–300, 305
common types of, 36–38
complexity of, 36
environmental factors of, 38
frequency of, 13, 38
genetic factors of, 38
Halverson's childhood with,
158–159
religion, faith and, 164
as secret, 23–26
survival rates of, 13
Taussig, H., studying, 152–156
triumph over, 30
Congenital Malformations of the Heart
(Taussig, H.), 190
Cooley, Denton, 119, 186–188, 191,
206–207, 248, 299
Cooley's Coffee Pot, 248
Copenhagen University, 91–92
Cornish, James, 134–135
costs, of valve replacement surgery, 314
Cournand, Andre, 215–216
cross-circulation
complications of, 241
Lillehei's experiments with,
240–241
Lillehei's first operations using,
241–243

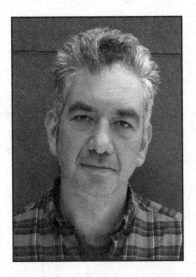

Gabriel Brownstein has published a novel, *The Man from Beyond,* and a book of stories, *The Curious Case of Benjamin Button, Apt. 3W.* For his short stories, he's won a PEN/Hemingway Award and a Pushcart Prize. He teaches at St. John's University in Queens, New York, and lives in Brooklyn with his wife and two daughters.

PublicAffairs is a publishing house founded in 1997. It is a tribute to the standards, values, and flair of three persons who have served as mentors to countless reporters, writers, editors, and book people of all kinds, including me.

I. F. STONE, proprietor of *I. F. Stone's Weekly*, combined a commitment to the First Amendment with entrepreneurial zeal and reporting skill and became one of the great independent journalists in American history. At the age of eighty, Izzy published *The Trial of Socrates*, which was a national bestseller. He wrote the book after he taught himself ancient Greek.

BENJAMIN C. BRADLEE was for nearly thirty years the charismatic editorial leader of *The Washington Post*. It was Ben who gave the *Post* the range and courage to pursue such historic issues as Watergate. He supported his reporters with a tenacity that made them fearless and it is no accident that so many became authors of influential, best-selling books.

ROBERT L. BERNSTEIN, the chief executive of Random House for more than a quarter century, guided one of the nation's premier publishing houses. Bob was personally responsible for many books of political dissent and argument that challenged tyranny around the globe. He is also the founder and longtime chair of Human Rights Watch, one of the most respected human rights organizations in the world.

. . .

For fifty years, the banner of Public Affairs Press was carried by its owner Morris B. Schnapper, who published Gandhi, Nasser, Toynbee, Truman, and about 1,500 other authors. In 1983, Schnapper was described by *The Washington Post* as "a redoubtable gadfly." His legacy will endure in the books to come.

Peter Osnos, *Founder*